HANDBOOK OF
PSYCHIATRIC
EDUCATION

HANDBOOK OF
PSYCHIATRIC
EDUCATION

Edited by

Jerald Kay, M.D.
Edward K. Silberman, M.D.
Linda F. Pessar, M.D.

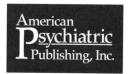

American
Psychiatric
Publishing, Inc.

Washington, DC
London, England

Copyright © 2005 American Psychiatric Publishing, Inc.
ALL RIGHTS RESERVED

Manufactured in the United States of America on acid-free paper
09 08 07 06 05   5 4 3 2 1
First Edition

Typeset in Adobe's Janson Text and Univers.

American Psychiatric Publishing, Inc.
1000 Wilson Boulevard
Arlington, VA 22209-3901
www.appi.org

WM
18
H2362
2005

Library of Congress Cataloging-in-Publication Data
Handbook of psychiatric education / edited by Jerald Kay, Edward K. Silberman, Linda Pessar.—1st ed.
    p. ; cm.
    Includes bibliographical references and index.
    ISBN 1-58562-189-7 (pbk.: alk. paper)
    1. Psychiatry—Study and teaching—United States—Handbooks, manuals, etc. 2. Psychiatry—Study and teaching (Residency)—United States—Handbooks, manu-als, etc.
    [DNLM: 1. Psychiatry—education. WM 18 H2362 2005] I. Kay, Jerald. II. Silberman, Edward K., 1944–. III. Pessar, Linda, 1944–.
    RC459.5.U6H36 2005
    616.89'0071'173—dc22

2005014182

British Library Cataloguing in Publication Data
A CIP record is available from the British Library.

CONTENTS

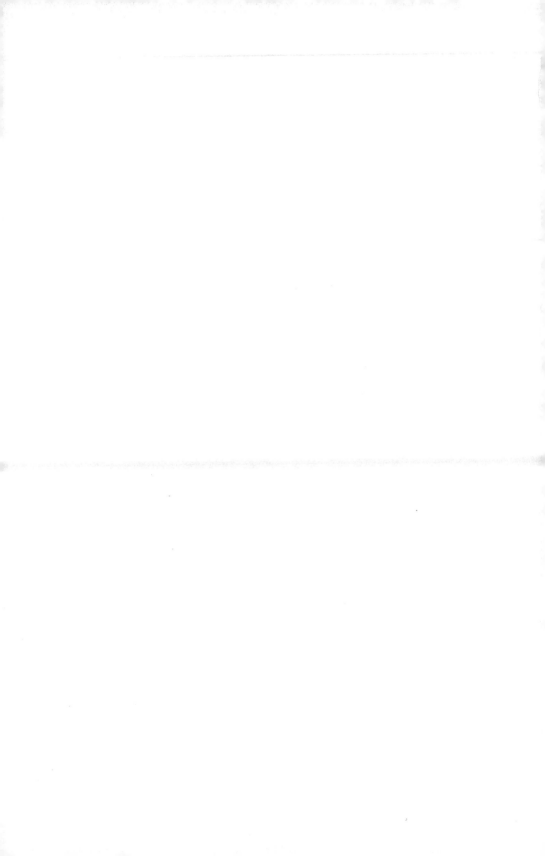

CONTRIBUTORS

Carol A. Bernstein, M.D.
Associate Professor of Psychiatry, Designated Institutional Official and Senior Assistant Dean for Graduate Medical Education, Vice Chair for Graduate Medical Education, and Director of Residency Training in Psychiatry, New York University School of Medicine, New York, New York

David Bienenfeld, M.D.
Professor, Vice Chair, and Director of Residency Training, Department of Psychiatry, Wright State University, Dayton, Ohio

Greg Briscoe, M.D.
Associate Professor of Psychiatry, Clerkship Director, Eastern Virginia Medical School, Norfolk, Virginia

Amy C. Brodkey, M.D.
Clinical Associate Professor of Psychiatry, University of Pennsylvania School of Medicine, Philadelphia, Pennsylvania

Carlyle H. Chan, M.D.
Professor of Psychiatry, Vice Chair for Education and Informatics, Director of Residency Education, Department of Psychiatry and Behavioral Medicine, Medical College of Wisconsin, Milwaukee, Wisconsin

Theodore B. Feldmann, M.D.
Associate Professor of Psychiatry, Department of Psychiatry and Behavioral Sciences, University of Louisville School of Medicine, Louisville, Kentucky

Carl Greiner, M.D.
Professor of Psychiatry, Assistant Dean for Clinical Affairs, University of Nebraska Medical Center, Omaha, Nebraska

Jerald Kay, M.D.
Professor and Chair, Department of Psychiatry, Wright State University School of Medicine, Dayton, Ohio

Ze'ev Levin, M.D.
Clinical Associate Professor of Psychiatry, Associate Director, Residency Training in Psychiatry, New York University School of Medicine, New York, New York

Myrl R.S. Manley, M.D.
Associate Professor, Director of Medical Student Education in Psychiatry, New York University School of Medicine, New York, New York

Lisa A. Mellman, M.D.
Clinical Professor of Psychiatry, Department of Psychiatry, College of Physicians and Surgeons, Columbia University; Associate Director of Residency Training, New York State Psychiatric Institute; and Director, New York State Psychiatric Institute Psychotherapy Clinic for Research and Training, New York, New York

Paul C. Mohl, M.D.
Professor, Vice Chair of Education, Residency Training Director, Department of Psychiatry, University of Texas Southwestern Medical Center, Dallas, Texas

Brock P. Nolan, M.D.
Staff Psychiatrist, Luke AFB, Phoenix, Arizona

Linda F. Pessar, M.D.
Professor of Clinical Psychiatry, University at Buffalo, State University of New York, School of Medicine and Biomedical Sciences, Buffalo, New York

Nyapati Rao, M.D.
Professor of Clinical Psychiatry, Director of Psychiatric Residency Training, State University of New York Downstate Medical Center, Brooklyn, New York

Ronald O. Rieder, M.D.
Professor of Clinical Psychiatry and Vice Chairman for Education, Department of Psychiatry, College of Physicians and Surgeons, Columbia University; Director of Residency Training, New York State Psychiatric Institute, New York, New York

Brenda Roman, M.D.
Associate Professor, Director of Medical Student Education, Department of Psychiatry, Wright State University School of Medicine

Frederick S. Sierles, M.D.
Professor and Director of Medical Student Education in Psychiatry and Behavioral Sciences, Rosalind Franklin University of Medicine and Science, North Chicago, Illinois

Edward K. Silberman, M.D.
Clinical Professor of Psychiatry and Director of Residency Education, Jefferson Medical College, Philadelphia, Pennsylvania

Bryce Templeton, M.D., M.Ed.
Professor of Psychiatry; Associate Director, Medical Student Education in Psychiatry, Drexel University College of Medicine, Friends Hospital, Philadelphia, Pennsylvania

David Trachtenberg, M.D.
Clinical Instructor of Psychiatry, New York University School of Medicine, New York, New York

Sidney H. Weissman, M.D.
Professor of Psychiatry and Director of Residency Training, Department of Psychiatry and Behavioral Sciences, Feinberg School of Medicine, Northwestern University, Chicago, Illinois

Joel Yager, M.D.
Professor and Vice Chair for Education and Academic Affairs, Department of Psychiatry, University of New Mexico School of Medicine, Albuquerque, New Mexico; Professor Emeritus, Department of Psychiatry and Biobehavioral Sciences, David Geffen School of Medicine, University of California at Los Angeles

PREFACE

We are pleased to respond to the request from American Psychiatric Publishing, Inc. (APPI), for a brief paperback version of the *Handbook of Psychiatric Education and Faculty Development*, published in 1999. Bob Hales, editor-in-chief of APPI, and John McDuffie, its editorial director, believed that a book focusing on undergraduate and graduate medical education issues would be helpful to directors of medical student education and general psychiatry residency programs. Although we hope that this book will be of assistance to program directors, we also intend to provide a resource for the many faculty members who are active in teaching students and residents. This new book will undoubtedly also be helpful to program administrators and assistants because it addresses issues such as evaluation of students and residents, curriculum development, administrative challenges, and accreditation issues on the graduate medical education level.

Since the publication of the *Handbook of Psychiatric Education and Faculty Development*, there have been a number of changes and advances in the education field. A greater interest in research training, a reassuring residency recruitment trend, the renewed quest for assessing competency, and the introduction of technology into pedagogical approaches are but a few of these advances. We have included both new and updated chapters addressing these topics. The reviews of the *Handbook* were exceptionally positive, but we have also incorporated reviewers' suggestions about how to improve our treatment of a number of topics. Readers should still refer to the larger *Handbook* for more broad-based discussion of careers in academic psychiatry, psychiatric research, psychiatric administration, psychiatric fellowships, certification, and continuing medical education.

As we noted in the introduction to our previous volume, we are indebted to the chapter authors for their willingness to share their wisdom about how to develop and assess increasingly sophisticated and responsive educational programs. This new book is especially timely in light of the rapid turnover of residency training directors and directors of medical student education. Providing continuity to the educational mission in psychiatry is therefore of great importance to us. We welcome comments from our colleagues about the usefulness of these chapters, as well as their ideas about what might be included in future publications.

Jerald Kay, M.D.
Edward K. Silberman, M.D.
Linda F. Pessar, M.D.

CHAPTER 1

PRECLINICAL UNDERGRADUATE CURRICULA

Myrl R.S. Manley, M.D.

David Trachtenberg, M.D.

COURSE CONTENT

Courses in psychiatry for preclinical medical students have conventionally included a survey of psychopathology and something called behavioral science. Behavioral science was traditionally taught in the first year and psychopathology in the second year. This pattern has been substantially altered over the last decade because many schools have undertaken extensive curriculum reorganization. To cite one example among many, the revised medical curriculum at the University of California, San Francisco, is now divided into three stages over 4 years of training: the Essential Core (lasting 16 months), the Clinical Core, and Advanced Studies (Satterfield et al. 2004).

BEHAVIORAL SCIENCE

Describing a behavioral science curriculum is like shooting at a moving target. The scope and content of this area are in flux, with considerable variation between schools and over time within schools. Some programs have abandoned teaching behavioral science altogether, and many have replaced courses taught exclusively by departments of psychiatry with multidisciplinary courses.

Behavioral science courses became widespread in the late 1960s when the National Institute of Mental Health made grants available to academic departments of psychiatry to expand their preclinical teaching. The courses became universal and fixed in medical school curricula when the National Board of Medical Examiners (NBME) added behavioral science questions to its Part I examination in 1971 and 1972 and then began reporting a behavioral science subsection the following year (Brownstein et al. 1976).

From the beginning there was widespread disagreement on what should be taught in behavioral science courses. The NBME proved to be of limited help in defining course content when it designated as "behavioral science" an impossibly comprehensive list of topics ranging from sociology to medical anthropology to medical economics, including subjects such as epidemiology and biostatistics that were already taught by nonpsychiatry departments.

A 1983 survey of North American medical schools by Arnett and Hogan (1983) revealed that only a single topic was taught in more than 50% of behavioral science courses and that only five topics were included in at least a quarter of all programs. A decade later (two decades after the courses were first required), another study found an emerging consensus in the content of behavioral science courses. However, the consensus topics appeared to be heavily centered on psychoanalytic theories of development and relatively neglectful of the extraordinary advances that were being made in the neurosciences and molecular biology (Manley 1994). A follow-up study in 2004 by D. Signorelli, F.S. Sierles, and M.J. Schrift ("A National Survey and Catalogue Review of the Teaching of Behavioral Science–Related Topics in the Pre-Clinical Years at U.S. Medical Schools," unpublished data, Keck School of Medicine, University of Southern California, Los Angeles, May 2004) revealed continuing changes in the topics taught in behavioral science courses. Presented in Table 1–1 is a comparison of the findings from the 1994 and 2004 surveys. These data cannot be regarded as definitive, because of the diversity of course offerings, the likelihood of some content duplication from one course to another, and the possibility that some topics are taught in nonpsychiatry courses. Nevertheless, they suggest a trend away from psychodynamic concepts and increasing emphasis on the neurobiology of behavior.

The 2004 survey by Signorelli and colleagues also documents the variety of ways in which preclinical psychiatry topics are packaged. Although a slim majority of schools (55%) still offer behavioral science topics in the first year, and two-thirds of schools teach psychopathology in the second year, the extraordinary variability in the amounts of time devoted to these areas suggests that schools are teaching quite different things in different

TABLE 1–1. Teaching of selected topics in medical schools, 1990 and 2004

Topic	Percentage of schools teaching	
	1990	2004
Child development	94	73
Psychodynamic theory	88	67
Adult development	83	70
Human sexuality	83	70
Doctor–patient relationship	82	80
Behavioral learning theory	75	64
Coping and adaptation	68	66
Behavioral neuroscience	57	72
Sleep physiology	52	57
Behavioral genetics	31	52

Source. Manley 1994; Signorelli D, Sierles FS, Schrift MJ: "A National Survey and Catalogue Review of the Teaching of Behavioral Science–Related Topics in the Pre-Clinical Years at U.S. Medical Schools," unpublished data, Keck School of Medicine, University of Southern California, Los Angeles, May 2004.

ways. The number of hours devoted to teaching behavioral science ranged from 8 to 174, and for psychopathology the range was 6–170 hours.

We would like to pose three key questions as the necessary first steps in designing a course in behavioral science:

1. *What should be taught?* Considerable time, attention, and thought should be given to defining the core topics of behavioral science. It is a mistake to cobble together a course out of existing resources. Such a pastiche is likely to be perceived by students and deans as makeshift. Whether the core is defined by the individual course director or by a committee of basic scientists and clinicians, the process of definition is important.

   We are including three different approaches to the content of behavioral science courses. The outline contained in Table 1–2 was prepared by the American Psychiatric Association Committee on Medical Student Education (1994). Table 1–3 is based on the content outline of the 2004 United States Medical Licensing Examination (USMLE; Federation of State Medical Boards of the United States 2004).

   Our proposal is presented in Table 1–4. It is divided into primary subject areas (those of likely importance to a broad spectrum of schools) and secondary subject areas (those more likely to be of interest to indi-

TABLE 1–2.   Behavioral science topics proposed by the Committee on Medical Student Education of the American Psychiatric Association, 1994

A. Medical interviewing and physical diagnosis
   1. Cultural influences on health and health-related behaviors
   2. Health and illness in relation to social identity, role, and social context
   3. Family interactions and how they contribute to developing and maintaining illness and facilitating recovery
   4. The explicit and implicit "contract" between doctor and patient
   5. The use of various forms of psychotherapies in medical treatment
B. Behavior and neuroscience
   1. Human development throughout the life cycle
   2. Neuroanatomical, biochemical, genetic, physiologic, and immunologic correlates in normal behavior and in psychiatric and medical illnesses
   3. The doctor–patient relationship
   4. The application of psychodynamic understanding to patient, physician, and family behavior
   5. Learning theory
   6. Health behavior
   7. Psychological issues related to gender
   8. Human sexuality
   9. Chronobiology
  10. Domestic violence
  11. Suicidal and homicidal behavior
  12. Alcoholism and other forms of substance abuse
  13. Psychosocial responses to acute chronic illness and disability

Source.   American Psychiatric Association Committee on Medical Student Education 1994.

vidual programs based on available teaching hours and faculty re-sources). It is intended to be minimal rather than comprehensive, a foundation on which given departments and medical schools may build according to their particular strengths and orientations.

2. *What is already taught elsewhere?* Having defined a core, the course director needs to ascertain whether individual topics are being taught in other courses and if they are, whether they should remain there, be duplicated in behavioral science, or be shifted to behavioral science.

3. *Who should teach?* The course director must decide which areas will be better taught in collaboration with another department. A variety of solutions are being implemented across the country; although it is not possible to describe them all, we can give some representative examples.

TABLE 1–3. Behavioral science topics listed in the content description of Step 1 of the USMLE, 2004

A. General principles: gender, ethnic, and behavioral considerations affecting disease treatment and prevention, including psychosocial, cultural, occupational, and environmental

1. Progression through the life cycle, including birth through senescence
   a. Cognitive, language, motor skills, and social and interpersonal development
   b. Sexual development (e.g., puberty, menopause)
   c. Influence of developmental stage on physician/patient interview
2. Psychological and social factors influencing patient behavior (includes psychodynamic and learning theory, doctor–patient relationship)
   a. Personality traits or coping style, including coping mechanisms
   b. Psychodynamic and behavioral factors, related past experience
   c. Family and cultural factors, including socioeconomic status, ethnicity, and gender
   d. Adaptive and maladaptive behavioral responses to stress and illness (e.g., drug-seeking behavior, sleep deprivation)
   e. Interactions between the patient and the physician or the health care system (e.g., transference)
   f. Patient adherence, including general and adolescent
3. Patient interviewing, consultation, and interactions with the family
   a. Establishing and maintaining rapport
   b. Data gathering
   c. Approaches to patient education
   d. Enticing patients to make lifestyle changes
   e. Communicating bad news
   f. "Difficult" interviews (e.g., anxious or angry patients)
   g. Multicultural ethnic characteristics
4. Medical ethics, jurisprudence, and professional behavior
   a. Consent and informed consent to treatment
   b. Physician–patient relationships (e.g., ethical conduct, confidentiality)
   c. Death and dying
   d. Birth-related issues
   e. Issues related to patient participation in research
   f. Interactions with other health professionals (e.g., referral)
   g. Sexuality and the profession; other "boundary" issues
   h. Ethics of managed care
   i. Organization and cost of health care delivery

TABLE 1–3.   Behavioral science topics listed in the content description of Step 1 of the USMLE, 2004 *(continued)*

B. Central and peripheral nervous system: normal processes

1. Brain, including gross anatomy and blood supply; cognition, language, memory; hypothalamic function; limbic system and emotional behavior; circadian rhythms and sleep; and control of eye movement

C. Central and peripheral nervous system: abnormal processes

1. Psychopathological disorders, processes, and their evaluation
    a. Early-onset disorders (e.g., learning disorders)
    b. Disorders related to substance use
    c. Schizophrenia and other psychotic disorders
    d. Mood disorders
    e. Anxiety disorders
    f. Somatoform disorders
    g. Personality disorders
    h. Physical and sexual abuse of children, adults, and elders
    i. Other disorders (e.g., dissociative, impulse control, posttraumatic stress disorder)
2. Principles of therapeutics: psychopharmacological agents (e.g., anxiolytics, antidepressants, antipsychotic agents, mood-stabilizing agents)
3. Gender, ethnic, and behavioral considerations affecting disease treatment and prevention, including psychosocial, cultural, occupational, and environmental
    a. Emotional and behavioral factors (e.g., drug abuse, dementia, sleep deprivation, accident prevention, pets)
    b. Influence on person, family, and society (e.g., developmental disabilities, dementia, generational reversal, nutrition, seizures, sleep disorders)
    c. Occupational and other environmental risk factors (e.g., boxing, carbon monoxide exposure)
    d. Gender and ethnic factors

Source.   Federation of State Medical Boards of the United States 2004.

Many schools now offer a first-year course called "Introduction to Clinical Medicine," "The Doctor and Patient," or something similar. It is often interdisciplinary, is sometimes run from the department of medicine, and typically includes active involvement by the department of psychiatry. It provides supervised, small-group clinical exposure during the first year of medical school. Common to many such courses are medical interviewing, physical diagnosis, and a range of issues con-

TABLE 1–4. A core curriculum in behavioral science

I. Primary topics

  A. Human growth and development

  From infancy through old age and senescence, a survey of the interplay between physical maturation and cognitive, emotional, and social growth; in childhood and adolescence (more emphasis on brain plasticity and environmental triggers, and milestones of development than on purely theoretical models of staged development)

  B. Human sexuality

  Female and male sexuality, anatomy, and physiology; sexual response cycles; full range of normal sexual behaviors across the life span

  C. Behavioral medicine

  The doctor–patient relationship; compliance; acute stress syndromes; adaptation to chronic illness

  D. Neurobiology of behavior

  Memory; mood and anxiety regulation; chronobiology; psychoneuroimmunology; behavioral genetics; sleep physiology

II. Secondary topics

  A. Culture and medicine

  B. Death, dying, and bereavement

  C. Drug- and alcohol-related topics

  Neurobiology of addictions, epidemiology, and sociology of drug/alcohol use; specific disorders may be included in psychopathology

cerned with the doctor–patient relationship (e.g., medical ethics) and behavioral medicine (e.g., compliance). Where they exist, "Introduction to Clinical Medicine" courses have largely supplanted the clinical component of conventional behavioral science courses.

Some medical schools include a separate course on reproductive medicine. Nearly always multidisciplinary, it may include obstetrics–gynecology, urology, endocrinology, and physiology. The psychiatry department may take responsibility for topics in normal and abnormal sexual behavior (including sexual response cycles in men and women) and a discussion of sexual dysfunctions.

A course in neurosciences may be expanded to include, in addition to the usual neuroanatomy and neurophysiology, behavioral neurobiology. This attractive solution firmly grounds psychiatry in the medical model and establishes that normal and abnormal behavior derive from biological brain processes.

PSYCHOPATHOLOGY

Compared with behavioral science, developing courses in psychopathology is a breeze. The subject matter is clearly defined, the clinical focus catches students' interest, and the topics are thoroughly familiar to the faculty. Nevertheless, it is helpful to think of some key questions while planning a course in psychopathology:

1. *Which psychiatry?* Most psychiatry residency programs are now described as being eclectic. It is understandable that over the course of 4 years of intensive, full-time training and exposure to multiple schools and clinical approaches, residents would be expected to forge their own synthesis. This is unrealistic for medical students, whose time with psychiatry is much briefer. Unless students are presented with a single, clear theoretical focus, the field will seem anarchic. We believe that the appropriate model of psychiatry for medical students is medical: phenomenological–descriptive psychiatry, strongly grounded in biology.

2. *Which disorders?* It is unlikely that any psychopathology course will be able to present all known psychiatric disorders, and some will be very restricted indeed. Judgments will have to be made about what to include and what to omit. The following principles will help in deciding:

   a. Choose common disorders over uncommon ones: schizophrenia instead of erotomanic delusional disorder, and human immunodeficiency virus (HIV) encephalitis instead of neurosyphilis.

   b. Emphasize diagnostic categories. It may be sufficient to give a few representative examples of the broader category—for example, to teach a few personality disorders to illustrate the general concept of a personality disorder.

   c. Play to your strengths. If your department includes a world expert on multiple personality disorder, that would be a good topic to include in the course.

   d. Consider including disorders that illustrate important principles. Alzheimer's disease, in addition to being common, is useful for making correlations between brain pathology and clinical symptoms (degeneration of amygdala and hippocampus associated with memory loss). HIV encephalitis helps to illustrate the difference between cortical and subcortical dementias. Narcolepsy—identified by sleep-onset rapid eye movement—is the exception that helps clarify the broader generalization that there are not yet biological markers for psychiatric disorders.

e. Make sure students understand that the list of disorders is incomplete. It may be useful to suggest additional topics for self-study or USMLE preparation.

3. *What to do with the DSM?* DSM-IV-TR (American Psychiatric Association 2000) is great for getting psychiatrists to think in the same conceptual categories and speak the same language. It is pretty good for increasing diagnostic reliability. It is not meant to be a textbook of psychopathology for beginners. Trying to understand schizophrenia by reading diagnostic criteria is a bit like trying to visualize a truck by reading a parts manifest listing gear ratios and axle lengths. Although DSM-IV-TR is useful in providing the organization for diagnostic categories and common agreement about what the diagnoses mean, students should not be made to memorize diagnostic criteria. The criteria do not appear as questions on the board examinations and will change in a few years anyway.

As medical schools across the country continue to reshape preclinical curricula, psychopathology courses have also been affected. One common model promotes "vertical integration," in which traditional, department-based basic science topics are organized around organ systems and are taught as a block. For example, a unit on the cardiovascular system will include study of the physiology and pathophysiology of the heart, cardiac histology and pathology, and cardiac medications.

Psychiatry of course is a clinical rather than a basic science preclinical discipline, and it fits uncomfortably into vertically integrated organ system blocks. For the great majority of psychiatric disorders, the pathophysiology remains unknown and there is no consistently identifiable pathology. The obvious organ system under which psychiatry could be subsumed is the brain, but to present all psychiatric disorders as brain disorders conveys a subtle falsehood.

The understanding of the neurobiology of psychiatric symptoms and disorders is important and growing. It would be a mistake to omit this material from medical student courses in psychiatry, and colleagues from the neurosciences can be a great help in teaching it. Nevertheless, the methodology of clinical psychiatry—establishing precisely defined descriptive phenomena to enhance diagnostic reliability—is different from both clinical neurology and bench neurosciences. Moreover, common psychiatric disorders such as depression may more helpfully be conceptualized as medical disorders than as brain dysfunctions. Overwhelmingly, psychiatrists do not attempt to repair brain lesions but to control (or soften the impact of) abnormalities of thinking, feeling, and behavior. Grouping psychiatry with the neurosciences may anticipate a future reality but does not represent the field as it exists today.

How common is the pairing of psychopathology and neurosciences in preclinical medical education? The curriculum directory on the Web site of the Association of American Medical Colleges (AAMC) lists the titles of required first- and second-year courses of medical schools in the United States, Canada, and Puerto Rico (http://services.aamc.org/currdir/section2/courses.cfm). A review of courses currently required for first- and second-year classes graduating in 2006 and 2007 reveals that of the 70 schools providing information, more than half (53%) listed freestanding psychiatry courses, typically called "Psychopathology," "Clinical Psychiatry," or "Introduction to Psychiatry." Twenty-three percent listed an integrated neuroscience–psychiatry course such as "Brain and Behavior" or "Mind and Brain." (The remaining 24% listed either ambiguous course titles or courses that were part of a curriculum that is broadly multidisciplinary, such as problem-based learning.)

These data need considerable qualification. Slightly more than half of the schools listed provided no information on required preclinical courses. In addition, there is no certainty that listed courses accurately describe how students are actually taught. However, a similar review conducted by D. Signorelli, F.S. Sierles, and M.J. Schrift ("A National Survey and Catalogue Review of the Teaching of Behavioral Science–Related Topics in the Pre-Clinical Years at U.S. Medical Schools," unpublished data, Keck School of Medicine, University of Southern California, Los Angeles, May 2004) had virtually identical results. Taken together, the two reviews do not provide evidence for widespread or growing integration of psychiatry and neurosciences. The positioning of psychiatry in preclinical curricula remains a work in progress.

However it is organized, a successful psychopathology course (or psychopathology topics in a broader course) will emphasize the clinical. Lecturers will illustrate key phenomena with video demonstrations, readings will include case descriptions, and students will be given the chance to talk with psychiatric patients. They can meet in small groups once a week on the psychiatry services to interview patients, perform mental status examinations, take psychiatric histories, and see in person the clinical reality of what they are hearing in lecture. Above all, psychopathology courses can help to demystify psychiatric illnesses. The majority of students will enter fields other than psychiatry. They should take with them the knowledge that these disorders can be medically understood, rationally diagnosed, and in most cases treated or controlled.

ROLE OF THE COURSE DIRECTOR

Course directors are like Hollywood producers. They assemble the component parts of the course—topics, reading assignments, lecturers, small-group preceptors, examinations—and oversee the production through its completion. Successful course directors also remain highly visible and personally identified with a course. They should attend all lectures, sit in on small-group discussions, personally proctor examinations, and be easily accessible to students. Course directors represent the course at departmental meetings and schoolwide curriculum meetings and stand accountable for a course's failures as well as its triumphs.

For a lecture-based course, it is desirable for the course director to personally give, if not all the lectures, a great proportion of them. A single lecturer over several weeks is able to give a course unity, cohesiveness, and direction. He or she can make the course tell a story, drawing from earlier topics and expanding on them. By personally lecturing over several weeks, course directors develop a rapport with their class, recognize faces, call on students by name, understand more quickly when a topic is clear or mysterious, and perfect their timing so the jokes don't fall flat.

Some lucky course directors face the dilemma of departmental superstars—widely published faculty members with national or international reputations who travel extensively, conducting grand rounds and lecturing at meetings of professional associations. The course director may be tempted (or pressured) to use superstars in preclinical courses. They are, after all, part of the unique richness of an institution, and they advertise the strength of the individual department.

There is no question that students should be engaged with the most talented, productive, and creative people within a department, but required preclinical courses may not be the best forum for this contact. Superstars tend to be extraordinarily busy. Their lectures are likely to be prepackaged and delivered from a series of slide projections that may not hit the appropriate level of training and knowledge. The very depth of their knowledge may make it harder for them to appreciate which topics are conceptually difficult for beginners and which vocabulary is foreign. It is often wiser to introduce students to superstars outside the confines of a specific course: at local grand rounds or special lectures, psychiatry club meetings, or discussions in informal settings.

Course directors have two constituencies: their students and their teaching faculty. Attention to the former should not result in neglect of the latter. Much of a course director's time and energy is spent in faculty development. Course directors need to continually recruit new lecturers and group leaders, often from among the junior faculty who are eager to begin building an academic career. Becoming coach, mentor, and senior adviser to beginning teachers can be among the most rewarding parts of a course director's work. Like students, faculty members are eager for feedback. They need encouragement and supportive criticism. Course orientations, teaching workshops, and instructional packets are part of the standard armamentarium of faculty development. It has been our experience, however, that none of these devices are as helpful in the long run as frequent, informal, personal, one-to-one conversations, which serve to sustain the vision of a particular course while solidifying personal relationships.

COLLABORATION WITH OTHER DEPARTMENTS

In 1984 the AAMC issued a report, titled "Physicians for the Twenty-First Century," calling for fewer classroom hours and more interdisciplinary teaching (Physicians for the Twenty-First Century 1984). The trend was strengthened in 1992 when Parts I and II of the NBME examination were reorganized as Steps 1 and 2 of the USMLE. Topics on the old examinations were organized and reported as categories that corresponded to preclinical courses: anatomy, biochemistry, physiology, and so on. The new examinations have a section on general principles and another on organ systems, each of which includes normal and abnormal processes. Among the normal and abnormal processes are psychosocial, cultural, and environmental considerations. A given question may require knowledge from several disciplines. Many schools have responded to these changes by attempting to weaken departmental boundaries to decompartmentalize preclinical courses (and perhaps to strengthen central control over the curriculum).

Problem-based learning (PBL), pioneered at McMaster University and Michigan State University in the early 1970s, became widely popular in the mid-1980s as a way not only to increase interdisciplinary teaching but also to radically revamp preclinical medical student education and strengthen self-directed learning (Neufeld et al. 1989; Schmidt 1983; Tosteson 1990). In PBL, students meet in small groups to discuss written cases. As students work through the cases, they must first identify what they need to know, then seek out the information on their own and report back to the group. The cases are constructed to draw on information from all disciplines. For example, the case of a patient with renal failure may raise questions about acid–base balance, renal anatomy and physiology, adaptation to chronic illness, patient–doctor communication, and medical economics. The groups are led by a "facilitator"—by design not an expert in a given field—whose task is more to monitor and guide discussion than to impart factual information or answer questions of content. The PBL group discussions may be supplemented by lectures and laboratories, but in their purest form these are optional resources from which students may draw to work through the written cases.

Proponents such as Kaufman et al. (1989) have argued that PBL would teach problem solving, increase motivation, promote self-directed learning skills, and impart knowledge better than traditional teaching. Above all, it would be more fun. Advocates and converts have at times displayed an almost messianic zeal. Unfortunately, their enthusiasm has not been supported by research data. By all available measures, the graduates of PBL and traditional schools are indistinguishable (Berkson 1993). Moreover, there are serious difficulties with PBL. Because all learning is confined to cases and only one or two cases are prepared each week, there are limits on the number of topics that can be taught. It is not uncommon for all of psychopathology to be limited to discussions of schizophrenia, mood disorders, and anxiety disorders. The demands on faculty teaching time are heavy and sustained. Because most group leaders are nonexperts, students miss out on the valuable experience of thinking *along with* a senior colleague, to observe how a seasoned clinician reasons from the information at hand. There may be great differences in students' abilities to use a self-directed curriculum. (It should also be remembered that the clinical years in traditional schools have always employed problem-based teaching techniques.)

Less radical approaches to multidisciplinary teaching are also being implemented by many medical schools. Course boundaries and departmental identification with a given course may be preserved while the course director recruits lecturers, discussants, and group leaders from other departments. A pharmacology course might include lectures by clinical psychiatrists on psychopharmacology; an anatomy course might include lectures and prosections by surgeons. In addition, the sequence of topics in conventional, department-based courses may be coordinated so that all courses deal with a particular organ system simultaneously (sometimes called vertical integration).

In the past few years, considerable controversy has been generated over the issue of psychiatry collaborating with primary care or family practice. The debates have been impassioned, fueled by uncertainty over the future direction of psychiatry as a medical specialty and changing patterns of reimbursement. Because there is a trend among health maintenance organizations to establish primary care physicians as gatekeepers to specialist services, and because of concern that the gatekeepers will refer services traditionally supplied by psychiatrists to lower-cost nonphysician providers, some have argued that psychiatry must establish itself as a primary care specialty (Shore 1996). Others have argued for increasing specialization, citing the advances in criterion-based diagnosis, growing knowledge of the neurobiology of psychiatric disorders, and absence of empirical evidence that psychiatrists are better psychotherapists than trained psychologists, social workers, and nurses (Lieberman and Rush 1996). Although we hope preclinical course directors will remain involved with these issues, we also urge them to recognize that their responsibilities to their students and their responsibilities to their field are not coterminous. Medical students in the first 2 years are not being taught psychotherapy. If their introduction to the doctor–patient relationship, medical interviewing, and medical ethics can be strengthened through collaboration with primary care and family practice, we strongly support such cooperation. It will help keep those topics from becoming marginalized, and it further serves to establish psychiatry as a medical discipline, fully integrated in the work and culture of the medical center. The areas in which psychiatrists do hold unique expertise—the assessment and treatment of psychiatric disorders—will be presented in the psychopathology course and more thoroughly in the psychiatry clerkship.

One word of caution: When curriculum hours or course ownership are relinquished, they are seldom regained. It is not realistic to think that psychiatry teaching time can be given over to interdisciplinary courses on an experimental basis. Once it is gone, it is likely gone forever.

TEACHING FORMATS

LECTURES

Lecture courses have long been the mainstay of preclinical medical school education. Although recent efforts have been undertaken to limit the number of hours students spend attending them, lectures remain the predominant form of teaching at most medical schools. Lectures have been criticized by just about everyone. Students tend to see them as dull, irrelevant to clinical work, and inefficient ways to learn material for examinations. Faculty members often feel frustrated trying to teach complicated, rapidly evolving topics in such a short period of time. Deans and course directors worry about adding to the biotechnology information overload that risks leaving students confused, overwhelmed, and focused on memorization and examination preparation. In its 1984 report, the American Association of Medical Colleges published the following conclusion:

> Medical faculties should examine critically the number of lecture hours they now schedule and consider major reductions in this passive form of learn-

ing. In many schools, lectures could be reduced by one third to one half. The time that is made available by reducing lectures should not necessarily be replaced by other scheduled activities. (Physicians for the Twenty-First Century 1984, p. 12)

The idea that lectures are a "passive form of learning" has been repeated so frequently that it has become a truism. Too often, bad lectures obscure the potential for lectures as a teaching modality. We believe that lectures can be an exciting, dynamic, active process with strengths not shared by other teaching formats.

At its best, when it is not simply a recitation of facts for students to copy and memorize, a lecture is a place where students are asked to think and reason along with a senior colleague. Thinking is active and should be cherished as one of a physician's most important activities. Good lecturers provide the conceptual scaffolding around which knowledge is constructed. They identify what is core and what is subsidiary. They draw from their own clinical experiences and critical analysis of current issues.

Good teachers also help students develop their own capacities for self-learning and critical thinking by identifying key principles and by demonstrating how to formulate and solve problems. For example, rather than asking students to memorize twin concordance data, a lecturer on the genetics of schizophrenia may stress the interpretation of that data and ask students to identify and critique some of the underlying assumptions of twin studies. Similarly, a lecturer on personality disorders may present the problem of categorical versus dimensional diagnosis instead of outlining DSM-IV-TR diagnostic criteria. Lectures are for ideas, not lists.

When lecturers pose problems, ideas are generated, new questions get formulated, and creative thinking is most likely to take place in students' minds. Students who attend a lecture (unlike those reading a transcript) can see the teacher thinking, outlining main ideas, clarifying points, and giving examples. The student can ask questions and challenge assumptions.

Videos, movies, slides, and other audiovisual aids can help a lecture. Used promiscuously, however, they can sink it. The development of computer software for generating slide projections such as Microsoft's Power-Point has proved to be a mixed blessing. It has certainly enabled lecturers to quickly and easily develop interesting, attention-grabbing, uniquely individual visuals to accompany a spoken idea. The process is in fact so easy that such presentations have become standard whether in the corporate boardroom or the medical classroom. Junior faculty sometimes think that a PowerPoint presentation is required of lecturers. On the contrary, there is increasing recognition that when this technical medium is overused, the results can be numbing. Edward Tufte—a professor emeritus of political science, computer science and statistics, and graphic design at Yale University—has achieved national recognition for his argument that PowerPoint's emphasis on format over substance trivializes subjects. Vint Cerf, one of the inventors of the Internet and chair of its chief oversight body, stated that avoiding PowerPoint "actually improves communication because people have to listen rather than being distracted by fancy PowerPoint charts" (Konrad 2003).

In an editorial in the *New York Times* titled "The Level of Discourse Continues to Slide," John Schwartz (2003) called attention to "Power-Point's tendency to turn any information into a dull recitation of lookalike factoids," and he criticized "the lazy use of the program as a replacement for real discourse." Schwartz's essay prompted a remarkable letter from David Weingarten (2003), a medical student in Louisiana. We believe the sentiments he expressed are widespread and are on target, and so we include the letter here in its entirety:

> To the Editor:
> I am in my first year of medical school, where we are being taught almost exclusively by PowerPoint presentation. Gone are the days when a professor had to pause to write something on the blackboard. Lecturers can now read directly from their PowerPoint presentations, flipping through slides so quickly that it is impossible to take notes fast enough. Medical education lectures by PowerPoint are often so unhelpful (or even counterproductive) that our school's student survival guide recommends that we not go to class, a recommendation that many of my fellow students now follow. I firmly believe that PowerPoint presentation is deleterious to the education of future doctors. (Weingarten 2003)

The power of a lecture is the personal connection between teacher and student. When the personal is repeatedly disrupted by the technological, the power is weakened. We do not favor the practice of lecturing from a series of slide projections. The practice is widely used by faculty members who are too busy to adequately prepare a lecture. The technique focuses students' attention on the projection screen rather than on the person of the lecturer. Dimming the houselights breaks the immediacy of the connection between speaker and students. Here are some tips for better lecturing:

1. Don't read the lecture. Nothing is deadlier. Use notes sparingly or not at all. Don't hide behind a lectern. Get out in front and look at your audience. Make them look at you.

2. Use the blackboard. Write while you are talking and thinking. Students will keep better pace with you as they write their own notes.
3. Use slides only for what cannot be easily written on the blackboard, such as complicated diagrams or photographs of brain pathology. Students should receive printed copies of all projected diagrams.
4. If your lecture is built around a series of slides with list after list of facts, take them out and burn them. Once again: lectures are for ideas, not lists.
5. Video clips should be short (i.e., no more than 3 minutes) and should be shown for a clearly defined purpose. The lecturer should introduce the taped segments by telling students what to look for and at the conclusion should summarize what they have seen. It will engage students' interest to pose a problem for them to solve; for example, "The manic patient on this tape uses a clang association. See if you can identify it."

SMALL GROUPS

Small-group learning has become an increasingly popular alternative to lecture-based courses. Small teaching groups are presumed to require more active participation by students in the form of preparation and in-group discussion. They facilitate faculty–student interaction and encourage student self-education. Small-group preceptors get to know their students as individuals, appreciate their strengths and areas of need, and observe firsthand their skills and attitudes. Some modalities of small-group teaching are outlined in Table 1–5.

Careful attention to patient selection will increase the success of clinical small groups. A common difficulty among beginning students is overidentification with patients and minimization of pathology ("Of course he's depressed; I would be too if I were in his situation"). On the other hand, the life circumstances of some patients may be so alien to students that they find it difficult to summon up any compassion, empathy, or even curiosity. The ideal patient will be willing and sufficiently verbal to be interviewed, with obvious pathology but with whom empathic resonance is still possible. If a given site is relentlessly homogeneous, having, for example, only deteriorated patients with chronic schizophrenia, efforts should be made to rotate students among different sites.

Small-group teaching inevitably means the recruitment of a large teaching faculty. Residents can be quite helpful, especially in clinical groups. Voluntary faculty may be needed as well, and department chairs can be extremely useful in reminding voluntary faculty of the teaching obligation

TABLE 1–5.   A sampling of small-group formats

Clinical small group—Live patient interview with a preceptor; case is then discussion. *Example:* Medical students and preceptor meet with a psychiatric inpatient, take a history, and perform a mental status examination.

Case conference—Similar to clinical small group; faculty member typically conducts the interview. Focus is often on the case findings rather than the patient. *Example:* Demonstrating memory impairment or neurological signs in a patient with dementia.

Seminar discussions—Readings and/or topics are assigned (there is no "live" patient); discussion is usually guided by a faculty member. May involve formal preparation and questions. *Example:* Reviewing and critiquing a paper describing structural brain abnormalities in schizophrenia.

Problem-based learning—Groups are assigned a facilitator, often a nonexpert, who encourages group discussion and team interaction around investigating a written clinical case presented in several parts. *Example:* The case of a woman with heart disease raises questions of cardiac physiology, adaptation to chronic illness, complications of tricyclics, possible panic disorder, and medical economics.

Case-based learning—Discussion proceeds from a printed case history and is usually led by a person with some clinical expertise. The conference intermixes discussion of the case with didactic material. The printed case provides the starting point for elucidating previously defined objectives. *Example:* The case of a woman with major depressive disorder and hypertension who makes a suicide attempt is used as a forum for discussing the major classes of antidepressant medications.

Small-group tutorial—A group focuses on a specific topic, paper, or patient or meets for exam preparation. Usually involves only a few students together with a preceptor. Allows for more student-preceptor interaction, individualization of learning. *Example:* Students who do poorly on the midterm receive tutoring in preparation for the final.

that comes with university appointment. Wherever they are recruited, faculty members will need guidance. An orientation allows the course director to personally welcome faculty members, distribute course materials, and discuss the mechanics of the course. In our experience, the most valuable part of any orientation is providing teachers with clearly defined goals and objectives.

GRADING, PROMOTION, AND REMEDIATION

Grading practices vary. Some schools give only pass/fail grades; some give pass/fail with honors. Some use letter grades in preclinical courses and pass/

fail in clinical courses; others do just the opposite. Some schools have expanded pass/fail grades (e.g., Honors, High Pass, Pass, Low Pass, Unsatisfactory) to the point that they are functionally equivalent to letter grades. Whatever the grading policy of an individual school, three principles should guide the course director in this area:

1. The basis for evaluation should be made explicit at the start of a course, preferably in writing, including requirements for passing, the relative weights of examinations, small-group and clinical exercises, and what remediation will be required in the case of unsatisfactory work.
2. Timely midcourse evaluations should be given so that students with deficiencies are given the chance to bring their work up to passing standards. (This is not possible, of course, when a grade is determined by a single final examination—one reason why grading by a single examination is undesirable.)
3. Evaluations should be meaningful; it must be possible for a student to fail. It is unfair to students who work hard, and a terrible disincentive to all students, to routinely pass everyone without regard to the quality of his or her work or whether the standards of the course have been met.

During the past 10 years, "grade inflation" has received increasing recognition at all levels of education throughout the United States, not excluding medical schools. As ever greater proportions of a class receive the highest possible grade, the significance of that grade is diluted and the ability to discriminate different levels of achievement among students is weakened.

Grade inflation is less an issue for preclinical courses than it is for clinical courses. The dean's letter, which serves as a school's official summary of evaluations for a student's residency application, routinely de-emphasizes both between-course and within-course differences in achievement. Commonly, a summary statement is made, such as "The student successfully completed all required courses of the first 2 years." Evaluations for clinical courses, on the other hand, are more likely to include both a specific grade and a narrative summary of the student's strengths and weaknesses. There are no data to indicate that any one grading scale—whether 3 points or 7 points, letters, numbers, or adjectives—is more effective than others in curbing grade inflation.

We favor a pass/fail grading system in the preclinical years. Preclinical basic science grades are unreliable predictors of future work with patients. Moreover, preclinical courses—even those with small-group components—typically include only modest amounts of direct faculty–student interactions; final course grades are often determined by performance on one or two multiple-choice examinations. It is possible to design a pass/fail system in which the threshold for passing is rigorous enough to guarantee adequate preparation for all students progressing to clinical training.

Preclinical psychiatry courses are in the advantageous position of routinely including small-group discussions and clinical sessions. It may be more possible in these than in other basic science courses to evaluate professional behavior and personal social interactions. These are important aspects of professional education, and students should be evaluated on their behavior as well as on exam scores. It should be possible for a student to fail a course because of unprofessional conduct despite receiving passing grades on examinations. Behavioral evaluations must be purely descriptive and nondiagnostic. "John was 20 minutes late for each small-group session" is an acceptable descriptive evaluation. "John was passive-aggressive (or hostile, entitled, narcissistic, depressed, etc.)" is inappropriate.

Medical schools and individual departments also vary in the work required to remediate a failing grade. Makeup examinations are often given for students who score below passing on the initial examination. Students who do poorly in small groups or clinical exercises may be required to undertake a series of tutorials or to submit a paper. In extreme cases, students may be required to repeat the course. (Course directors and lecturers usually dread having someone in class who has already heard all the jokes.) For a fuller discussion of evaluations, see Chapter 4, "Evaluation of Students," in this book.

STANDARDIZED PATIENTS

"Standardized patients" are actors (sometimes trained laypeople) who play the part of patients to help in teaching and evaluating medical students. Clinical evaluations using actors are sometimes called objective structured clinical examinations (OSCEs; pronounced "oskies"). The actors are given a rough script, including presenting symptoms and medical history, from which to prepare. They usually work with a clinical specialist who explains nuances and answers questions, and they are commonly instructed not to reveal a critical piece of information unless a specific question has been asked by the student. Because all students taking an examination with standardized patients deal with identical clinical material, the examinations are more reliable than those using real but highly variable patients.

A clinical skills examination using standardized patients was added to the USMLE in 2004. The clinical skills examination became a requirement of Step 2 beginning with the graduating class of 2005. As a result, the use of standardized patients is becoming even more widespread throughout American medical schools in the preclinical as well as the clinical years. Standardized patients are being used not only as an instrument for assessing students' clinical skills, in which the standardization has a rationale, but also for clinical instruction.

This development is a particular problem for psychiatry. Because external validating criteria (such as laboratory markers) for establishing a diagnosis do not yet exist, psychiatrists depend on the careful elucidation of cognitive, behavioral, and emotional signs and symptoms. The accuracy of this information depends on the physician's ability to establish rapport and engender trust and on the patient's willingness and capacity to report current and past subjective states of mind. Whether this can be meaningfully simulated with an actor-patient is open to debate.

Lois Krahn and colleagues (2002) at the Mayo Medical School reported the results of a fascinating study in which second-year medical students in a psychopathology course were randomly assigned to interview standardized patients and real patients in a small-group outpatient setting. Students and faculty preceptors were both blind to which patients were real and which were actors. At the end of the course, students and faculty members completed questionnaires about their reactions to the different patients they had seen. Ninety-one percent of students reported difficulty feeling empathy with patients who were subsequently revealed to have been standardized patients. Faculty members and students alike had little difficulty in guessing which patients were standardized, and both groups expressed a strong preference for working with real patients.

The findings of Krahn and colleagues are consistent with our own observations. One sensitive and insightful clerkship student commented that the only feeling she could summon up in an interview with a virtual patient was virtual empathy. The problem, of course, is that students feel pressure to demonstrate empathy in test situations using standardized patients. Students know that their ability to appear compassionate and understanding will be one of the dimensions on which their performance is evaluated. As a result, we run the risk of debasing empathy with our students by letting external signifiers such as facial expressions, gestures, and stock phrases displace the powerful internal response to a patient's suffering that a physician experiences.

Nevertheless, the use of standardized patients is likely to increase, and psychiatric educators must be mindful of its limitations. Above all, it is important that work with standardized patients and preparation for clinical skills assessments not be allowed to crowd out work with real patients in all their bewildering complexity. Presented in Table 1–6 is a summary of some of the pros and cons of using standardized patients.

TABLE 1–6. Pros and cons of standardized patients

Advantages	Disadvantages
1. **Standardization**—Because the clinical experience is identical from student to student, the use of standardized patients in clinical examinations enhances the reliability of the exam.	1. **Empathy**—It is difficult for students to feel real empathy for a patient who is only pretending to be sick.
2. **Feedback**—Standardized patients can be trained to give helpful critiques from the patient's perspective about the student's performance.	2. **No psychological depth**—Standardized patients do not bring to the examination the memories and experiences of a lifetime. Questions that stray beyond the script may elicit answers that are psychologically inconsistent, confusing, and nonsensical.
3. **Variety**—Standardized patients can be scripted for any clinical presentation, thereby ensuring that students have some exposure to an essential core, even if real patients are not available.	3. **Clinical oversimplification**—To provide material on which students can be tested, standardized patients tend to present with unambiguous signs and symptoms and clearly delineated diagnoses. This is inconsistent with the clinical reality of psychiatry.

COURSE EVALUATIONS

Centrally administered course evaluations are mandated by the AAMC for accreditation and are now fixtures of all medical schools. Students are asked to anonymously rate a range of items such as quality of lectures, course organization, and accessibility of faculty and to indicate a global rating of satisfaction. Rating questionnaires are commonly distributed at the time of major examinations to maximize student participation. (It is worth pausing to consider the implicit assumption in this decision, that students will not be in full attendance at lectures, laboratories, or small-group activities.) A summary of the data is returned to each course director and usually to the respective department chair. Comparisons over time within and between departments are compiled and often widely circulated.

These evaluations are almost certain to remain a fact of course directors' lives for the foreseeable future, and it is wise to consider their strengths and weaknesses, uses and misuses. They have the advantage of providing regular, detailed feedback about student satisfaction. They offer a way to monitor the impact of innovations and changing curriculum, and they provide a means for the formal recognition of superior teaching.

There are a number of potential problems, however, in overreliance on evaluations of this sort. Because the ratings are collected at examinations, they are vulnerable to the distorting effect of an unusually difficult or unpopular exam. Obviously invalid ratings on one item (e.g., a course receives midrange ratings on its computer instruction when it offers none at all) may call into question the validity of the whole.

There is also the risk when course evaluations are given strong emphasis that course directors will begin to play to the numbers, subordinating their own judgment to the annual ratings, embracing the safe and familiar and becoming reluctant to innovate. For example, if a potentially exciting clinical exercise receives bad ratings its first year out, there may be the temptation to drop it rather than to work on improving it over the next several years. Moreover, evaluations are of little use to a course in progress. They cannot identify the profoundly disaffected students who will go on to give the lowest possible rating for every item. They are of no help with midcourse corrections.

Students can indicate their level of satisfaction with a course, but there is much information they cannot provide. They cannot tell if courses are teaching what they should or if the content is widely accepted, accurate, and up to date. This is critical for a field as rapidly changing as psychiatry. (It is sometimes argued that scores on Steps 1 and 2 of the USMLE provide a check on course content, but of course they may be more of an indication of students' ability to supplement the formal curriculum with self-study.) Some schools are now addressing this problem by supplementing student course evaluations with external reviews. Members of other departments, representatives from other medical schools, or other outside experts are invited to meet with the director and faculty of a course to review the curriculum, interview students, read examinations, and in some cases to serve as external examiners at students' oral exams. The outside reviewers then prepare individual reports offering comments and suggestions.

Above all, it is critical that course directors not rely on central evaluations to the exclusion of their own judgment. They must monitor lectures, sit in on small-group discussions, and attend clinical exercises. They must arrange to meet regularly and frequently with students to attend to early dissatisfactions, and they must be willing to respond quickly to students' comments. If a particular lecture was incomprehensible, the material may be summarized in a handout, additional reading may be recommended, or a clarifying makeup lecture may be offered. If there are complaints about a group preceptor, the course director must be willing to work with that person and, in extreme circumstances, find a replacement. Boring lecturers may be (tactfully) interrupted with intriguing and provocative questions.

Course directors who take this active role and who remain at the center of a course are positioned to intelligently use the information from central evaluations within the context of their own experience. They will be able to accept and make use of criticisms that they agree with but also to reject those with which they disagree.

Some departments supplement central course evaluations with internal departmental evaluations. Although they may put students at some risk of evaluation overload (resulting in more superficial, thoughtless responses), internal evaluations can be tailored to the specific needs of a course, identifying unique areas of strength and weakness. They may also be a source of information that can be used to identify teaching excellence for departmental recognition and promotion.

SPECIAL PROBLEMS

ANTIPSYCHIATRY BIAS

Beginning course directors are sometimes jarred to find not only skepticism among their students, but outright hostility. Numerous surveys have found that medical students consider psychiatry to be soft and unscientific and psychiatrists fuzzy thinkers (Eagle and Marcos 1980; Nielson and Eaton 1981). In preclinical courses this bias may reveal itself in nonattendance, sarcasm, and cheekiness. When combined with the heavy academic demands of gross anatomy, biochemistry, pathology, and physiology, a milieu may be established in which dismissive disregard for psychiatry courses is tolerated.

The origins of antipsychiatry bias are multiple and are often beyond the reach of an individual course director: the culture and traditions of the medical school, school admission policies, societal stereotypes. Although they are widespread, the negative attitudes are neither intractable nor inevitable. In many schools, psychiatry courses are highly rated and their faculty win best-teaching awards. Although course directors may not be able to completely eradicate preexisting bias, they can create a climate of scientific curiosity in which the course material is taken seriously. Some suggestions include the following:

- *Be unapologetic.* Course directors themselves must believe in the value of their material. Saying "I know most of you aren't interested in psychiatry" is instantly self-fulfilling. Skepticism is healthy and scientific. Uninformed antagonism is not and should not be accepted.

- *Don't try to buy respect with kindness.* A kindly, indulgent, forgiving attitude reinforces stereotypes and fosters dismissive contempt. The greatest kindness a course director can show students is giving them their money's worth with a solid, well-organized, high-level academic course—a course that challenges the intellect and stimulates creativity. It must be possible to fail the course; otherwise, passing has no meaning.
- *Be visible.* Course directors and psychiatry faculty should take active, visible roles in the medical school community, chairing committees, serving as academic advisers, participating in campuswide clinical pathology conferences, interviewing applicants, performing at talent nights, and taking part in student–faculty athletic events. Psychiatry will not be seen as an integrated medical discipline if its representatives maintain disdainful isolation.
- *Be honest.* Students have extraordinarily well-tuned radar for intellectual dishonesty. If you don't know something, say so. Discuss how you can find the answer. Look it up and bring it back to class.
- *Be respectful.* Disparaging remarks about surgeons or other medical specialists are totally out of place. Many of your students are thinking of becoming surgeons, and such comments will sound defensive and insulting.
- *Don't analyze students.* Your position with students is as educator, not therapist. It is desirable that the teaching functions and student counseling functions of the department be kept as separate as possible. It is a conflict of interest for faculty members to treat students and also judge their academic performance. Students need the reassurance that in the classroom your concern is with their learning and not with their hidden emotional conflicts or private behavior. Students who do bring personal problems to the course director can be listened to sympathetically and, if necessary, guided to independent evaluation and treatment.

RECRUITMENT

During the late 1980s and early 1990s, the number of American medical students matching psychiatry residencies declined to all-time lows. There was considerable concern that the number of new psychiatrists entering the field would not be sufficient to sustain even a minimally adequate supply. Since 1998, the number of students matching into psychiatry residencies has steadily increased. Unsurprisingly, high rates of student career interest in psychiatry are correlated with a department's commitment to medical student education and faculty development (Sierles et al. 2003). Despite the ever-increasing numbers, recruitment into psychiatry remains a concern.

Psychiatry course directors need to recognize dual obligations. They should be able to identify, nurture, and mentor the small number of students who express an intense interest in psychiatry. At the same time, they must not forget or neglect their responsibilities to the entire class, the great majority of whom will be going into other fields.

If a program has no graduates choosing psychiatry, it is worth asking whether the teaching is turning off potential interest, but the success of a program should not be measured by the number of students entering the field. It should be possible, however, to make students comfortable with choosing psychiatry. High-quality, demanding, and well-organized courses will help the most. Psychiatry clubs may establish a cohort of self-support. Strong, happy, productive faculty members provide good role models. When psychiatry teaching is well respected and thoroughly integrated among the medical disciplines, a career choice in psychiatry appears less culturally deviant. In Chapter 3, "Undergraduate Electives," Theodore Feldmann discusses positive ways to encourage psychiatry education.

COMPUTER INSTRUCTION AND THE INTERNET

The use of computers and online learning in medical education is at an all-time high. Most students now enter medical school with some degree of computer literacy; some students have highly sophisticated expertise. Some schools require all students to own personal computers; many students own portable laptops, use wireless networks, or carry handheld computers, also known as personal digital assistants (PDAs). All schools make computers available. The consequence of these trends is unknown but is a fertile area for speculation. Some observers, such as Chodorow (1996), predict an utter transformation in teaching:

> The development of new multimedia teaching materials will break apart the old molds we have used for centuries to organize teaching and learning. Our effective contact with students will not be bound by time and place; our distinction between elementary and advanced will be virtually impossible to maintain; our traditional pacing of teaching and learning will lose some of its usefulness and justification. (p. 224)

Others have urged that we not be caught in a stampede of enthusiasm and that we consider the meta-effects of supplanting the personal with the electronic:

> Perhaps our networked world isn't a universal doorway to freedom. Might it be a distraction from reality? An ostrich hole to divert our attention and

resources from social problems? A misuse of technology that encourages passive rather than active participation? What's most important in school? Working with good teachers who can convey method as well as content. Except to the extent that students are involved with a caring teacher, schooling is limited to teaching facts and techniques. In this sense, network access is irrelevant to schooling—it can only prevent this type of interaction. The computer is a barrier to close teaching relationships. (Stoll 1995, p. 118)

What seems certain is that preclinical course directors will not have the option to ignore these powerful tools. They will need to educate themselves or have ready access to good computer consultants to ensure that the tools are used wisely. For those of us made uneasy by the fact that we have less experience and facility with these modalities than do our students, it is useful to review what interactive computer programs and the Internet do well and what they do rather more poorly. Among their greatest strengths are the following:

1. *Information storage and retrieval:* Information that would fill a library shelf can be efficiently sorted through and accessed. Literature searches, once requiring laborious review of volume after volume of *Index Medicus* or *Psychological Abstracts*, can now be done in a few minutes with the point and click of a mouse over high-speed Internet connections. Information on drug interactions and the newest available antidepressants, glossaries of terms, textbooks, reference guides, and abstracts of current journal articles are all immediately at hand.

2. *Visual information:* The extraordinary sophistication of computer graphics offers imagery unequaled by any other medium. It is possible, for example, for a student studying Alzheimer's disease not only to move back and forth through serial sections of a head computed tomographic (CT) scan but also to move back and forth through time to study the disease progression on sequential CT scans. It is possible to call up a three-dimensional model of the basal ganglia and rotate it so that it can be viewed from different perspectives.

3. *Rote review:* Several software programs and Internet sites such as those of the American Association of Directors of Psychiatric Residency Training (AADPRT; http://www.aadprt.org) and Student Net (http://www.student.net) provide series of questions on selected topics, including immediate feedback and suggested references and reading lists for follow-up study. These resources offer great flexibility in permitting students to practice in their own time and at their own pace.

4. *Computer-based quizzes and assessment tools:* Traditional methods of testing can now be administered and graded online, creating potential time

savings. The development of improved educational software has made it possible for students to work through basic science problems or try their hand at medical decision making. Such software is available through Web sites such as those of Medical & Science Media (http://www. msmedia.com.au) or Immersion Corporation (http://www.immersion. com).

5. *Curriculum sharing:* The "For Educators" page on the AADPRT Web site (http://www.aadprt.org/public/educators.html) provides resources for neurosciences curriculum development. It is possible to sign up for specialized forums and mailing lists to exchange materials and ideas with other medical professionals.

A list of some useful Internet sites is provided in Table 1–7.

We believe that computers are less effective for presenting new concepts and for clinical training. The most brilliant interactive program cannot approach the interactive quality of a person-to-person encounter—the teacher's ability to detect the faint shadow of doubt or uncertainty on a student's face, or the ability to grasp the misperception embedded in a poorly worded question and to rephrase the question before answering. No computer training can be a substitute for working with living patients, for touching their bodies and hearing their words, for fine-tuning our powers of perception and learning to deal with the near infinity of unexpected and idiosyncratic responses of patients.

The best education is personal. Our minds have evolved an extraordinary capacity to learn from one another, and the relationship between teacher and student can be one of the strongest motivating forces available. When our students begin to know us, when we become important people in their educational lives, when we are seen to embody the knowledge and discipline to which they aspire, our personal knowledge and judgment of their progress become extremely important. The experience of sitting face to face with a respected and admired teacher and hearing the teacher say, "I'm disappointed in your work; I know you can do much better" is more powerful than receiving an examination grade or reviewing a transcript. When education is personal, our students will gradually internalize the judgments and expectations of valued teachers. They will learn to set and meet their own demands and will be started on the difficult road of self-education.

TABLE 1–7. Useful Internet sites

Educational resources

1. The Association of American Medical Colleges Web site (http://www.aamc.org/meded/start.htm) has a Listserv and a national curriculum database.

2. The e-journal *Medical Education* (http://www.mededuc.com/thisissue/thisissue.asp) features articles such as "Small Group Teaching: What Students Really Think."

3. Another electronic journal specifically for educating health professionals is *Medical Education Online* (http://www.med-ed-online.org). This site hosts forums for discussion as well.

4. One of the best all-around Web sites for psychiatric educators is the "For Educators" page (www.aadprt.org/public/educators.html) on the American Association of Directors of Psychiatric Residency Training (AADPRT) Web site. The AADPRT site has many links for online learning and also features a good reading list for students interested in psychiatry.

5. There is even a Web site just for medical students, called The Student Doctor Network (http://www.studentdoctor.net), that features tips on study skills, learning tactics, and medical mnemonics.

6. For those interested in neurosciences, Neuroguide.com (http://www.neuroguide.com) has tutorials on a wide range of clinical and basic science topics such as spinal cord disorders and multiple sclerosis.

7. Neuroanatomy models and full-body skeletal radiographs are available from the University of Washington Diagnostic Radiology Residency Programs (http://www.rad.washington.edu/anatomy).

8. The Student Source at the University of Virginia School of Medicine (http://www.med-ed.virginia.edu/menu/otherMedEd.cfm) provides links to tutorials and sample questions for students to practice.

Retail sites for software and materials

1. A leading provider of handheld and Web-based clinical reference tools such as drug databases is ePocrates (http://www.epocrates.com).

2. Immersion Corporation (http://www.immersion.com/medical) features software that permits students to practice physical examination skills on virtual patients.

3. Studica (http://www.studica.com) offers software programs on genetics, anatomy, and fluids and electrolytes.

4. Medical & Science Media (http://www.msmedia.com/au) retails software, slides, and videotapes on a variety of clinical and basic science topics.

REFERENCES

American Psychiatric Association: Diagnostic and Statistical Manual of Mental Disorders, 4th Edition, Text Revision. Washington, DC, American Psychiatric Association, 2000

American Psychiatric Association Committee on Medical Student Education: Guideline for a Medical Student Curriculum in Psychiatry and Behavioral Science. Washington, DC, American Psychiatric Association, 1994

Arnett JL, Hogan TP: The role of behavioral sciences in North American medical schools: an overview. J Med Educ 58:201–203, 1983

Berkson L: Problem-based learning: have the expectations been met? Acad Med 68 (10 suppl):S79–S88, 1993

Brownstein EJ, Singer P, Dornbush R, et al: Teaching behavioral science in the preclinical curriculum. J Med Educ 51:59–62, 1976

Chodorow S: Educators must take the electronic revolution seriously. Acad Med 71:221–226, 1996

Eagle PF, Marcos LF: Factors in medical students' choice of psychiatry. Am J Psychiatry 137:423–427, 1980

Federation of State Medical Boards of the United States and National Board of Medical Examiners: United States Medical Licensing Examination: USMLE, 2004. Step 1: General Instructions, Content Description, and Sample Items. Philadelphia, PA, Federation of State Medical Boards of the United States and National Board of Medical Examiners, 2004

Kaufman A, Mennin S, Waterman R, et al: The New Mexico experiment: educational innovation and institutional change. Acad Med 64:285–294, 1989

Konrad R: Does PowerPoint make us stupid? New York, Associated Press, 2003. Available at: http://www.cnn.com/2003/TECH/ptech/12/30/byrne.powerpoint.ap/index.html. Accessed June 7, 2004.

Krahn L, Bostwick JM, Sutor B, et al: The challenge of empathy: a pilot study of the use of standardized patients to teach introductory psychopathology to medical students. Acad Psychiatry 26:26–30, 2002

Lieberman JA, Rush AJ: Redefining the role of psychiatry in medicine. Am J Psychiatry 153:1388–1397, 1996

Manley MRS: An emerging consensus in behavioral science course content. Acad Psychiatry 18:30–37, 1994

Neufeld VA, Woodward CA, MacLeod SM: The McMaster M.D. program: a case study of renewal in medical education. Acad Med 64:423–432, 1989

Nielson AC, Eaton JS: Medical students' attitudes about psychiatry: implications for psychiatric recruitment. Arch Gen Psychiatry 38:1144–1154, 1981

Physicians for the twenty-first century. Report of the Project Panel on the General Professional Education of the Physician and College Preparation for Medicine. J Med Educ 59(11 Pt 2):1–208, 1984

Satterfield JM, Mitteness LS, Tervalon M, et al: Integrating the social and behavioral sciences in an undergraduate medical curriculum: the UCSF Essential Core. Acad Med 79:6–15, 2004

Schmidt HG: Problem-based learning: rationale and description. J Med Educ 17:11–16, 1983

Schwartz J: The level of discourse continues to slide. New York Times, September 28, 2003, sec 4, p 12

Shore JH: Psychiatry at a crossroads: our role in primary care. Am J Psychiatry 153:1398–1403, 1996

Sierles FS, Dinwiddie SH, Patroi D, et al: Factors affecting medical student career choice from 1999 to 2001. Acad Psychiatry 27:260–268, 2003

Stoll C: Silicon Snake Oil. New York, Anchor Books, 1995

Tosteson DC: New pathways in medical education. N Engl J Med 322:234–237, 1990

Weingarten D: The art of persuasion, by PowerPoint (letter). New York Times, October 3, 2003, p A23

CHAPTER 2

PSYCHIATRY CLERKSHIPS

Frederick S. Sierles, M.D.

Linda F. Pessar, M.D.

Amy C. Brodkey, M.D.

To be accredited, every medical school must have a psychiatry clerkship (Liaison Committee on Medical Education 2003). For the vast majority of future physicians, the psychiatry clerkship is the only time they will be taught intensively about the diagnosis and management of psychiatric disorders, despite the fact that more psychiatrically ill persons are treated by nonpsychiatrist physicians—particularly generalists—than by psychiatrists (Regier et al. 1993).

To further illustrate this point, approximately 45% of persons who commit suicide visit primary care professionals during the month before the suicide, and approximately 77% of persons who commit suicide visit primary care clinicians during the prior year. In contrast, 19% of persons who committed suicide visited mental health professionals in the previous month, and 32% did so in the prior year (Luoma et al. 2002).

The characteristics of a good psychiatry clerkship—the student's taking considerable responsibility for patient care under the close supervision of enthusiastic and accessible teachers, supplemented by a good formal didactic program and a fair grading system—have remained the same since the

The authors thank Terrie Stengel for her suggestions about the manuscript.

early 1970s, when psychiatry clerkships became required nationally (Pessar 2000; Sierles and Taylor 1995). However, changes in the health care system during the past decade, particularly the expansion of managed care, have resulted in increased requirements for documentation of educational planning, supervision, and educational outcomes in all medical specialties (Halpern et al. 2001; Kassebaum 1997; Leach 2004; Long 2000) and reductions in the time available for clinicians to teach (Brodkey et al. 2002). Simultaneously, more attention has been paid to career development and educational scholarship (Fincher 2000b; Kay et al. 1999) for medical school faculty, including a burgeoning literature about clerkships and clerkship education (Brodkey et al. 1997; Fincher 2000b; Kuhn et al. 2002; Pangaro et al. 2003; Sierles and Magrane 1996). Also, since more psychiatric care is being provided in outpatient settings, more educational focus is directed toward ambulatory care rotations (Gay et al. 2002; Pessar 2000).

GOALS OF THE CLERKSHIP

Psychiatry clerkship directors (PCDs) broadly agree about the goals and objectives of clerkships (Brodkey et al. 1997). Given both the high prevalence of psychiatric disorders in primary care populations (Norquist and Regier 1996; U.S. Department of Health and Human Services 1999) and deficiencies in recognizing and adequately treating these disorders (Luoma et al. 2002; Young et al. 2001), the most important purpose is to impart basic skills, knowledge, and attitudes to future generalists and other nonpsychiatric physicians. These basic abilities include 1) conducting, recording, and presenting an initial psychiatric interview; 2) using the history and mental status examination to identify psychopathology; and 3) being knowledgeable about the differential diagnosis, evaluation, and management or referral of the most common and emergent psychiatric disorders.

In addition, attitudes and skills vital to practitioners of any specialty are reinforced in psychiatry. These include skillful interviewing; developing professionalism, caring, empathy, tolerance, and comfort with a wide variety of patients; communicating effectively; knowing one's limitations and biases; understanding and using biopsychosocial models of causation and treatment; and tolerating ambiguity. Students should appreciate that the absence of pathognomonic laboratory tests for psychiatric disorders means that the history usually takes longer and the mental status examination must be particularly precise, and explains in part why psychiatrists take more time with their patients than other specialists (Sierles et al. 2003b).

Other goals include decreasing prejudice against the field and its patients, emphasizing both the validity of diagnosis (Robins and Guze 1970) and the efficacy of treatments, preparing students for the psychiatry portion (Case et al. 1997) of the United States Medical Licensing Examination (USMLE, Step 2) and the Clinical Skills (CS) examination (Ayers and Boulet 2001), and assisting in the recruitment of students interested in psychiatry (Sierles et al. 2003b). For students who are interested, this goal also includes ensuring that they receive career counseling and advice about obtaining suitable residencies as the third year progresses and the fourth year begins. The clerkship is probably the most important medical school influence on recruitment, and it is likely that high recruitment rates are associated with excellent educational programs in departments that give priority and resources to teaching (Sierles and Taylor 1995).

GOALS AND OBJECTIVES

The Liaison Committee on Medical Education (LCME; 2003), which accredits medical schools, expects that the goals of each medical school and each clerkship in each school will be written as behavioral objectives that address the knowledge, skills, and attitudes that students should demonstrate on completion of the clerkship (Kassebaum et al. 1997). Kassebaum and colleagues (1997, p. 648) wrote that, compared with schools with "robust learning objectives,…those with vapid objectives attracted 40% more accreditation citations for shortcomings in curricular management, course and clerkship quality, and the evaluation of student achievement, especially in the clinical skills domain." In response to the expectation of departments having objectives, every clerkship directors' organization in every core specialty (Fincher 2000a) has published model behavioral objectives.

WRITING GOALS AND OBJECTIVES

Goals and objectives should be written as observable behaviors or outcomes (such as "*Conducts* an interview that facilitates information-gathering and formation of a therapeutic alliance") rather than processes (such as "*Learns* how to interview," "*Knows* about interviewing," or "*Understands* interviewing") (Brodkey et al. 1997; Burkholder et al. 1999; Gronlund 1970).

THE ADMSEP OBJECTIVES

Formulating goals and objectives in psychiatry was facilitated by the introduction of model clerkship objectives by the Association of Directors of Medical Student Education in Psychiatry (ADMSEP) (Brodkey and Sierles 1999; Brodkey et al. 1997). Based on an assessment of what generalists need to know and do to adequately diagnose and treat or refer the psychiatric problems they are likely to encounter, these objectives were developed to facilitate a department's defining its curriculum in light of its priorities and resources.

The ADMSEP objectives can be used verbatim as a clerkship's learning objectives, but it is far preferable that the objectives serve as a starting point for a department's faculty to deliberate about what the students should be able to do at the conclusion of the clerkship. It is crucial to engage key faculty members in curriculum development to generate a sense of ownership and enthusiasm (Brodkey et al. 1997). Too often, "objectives are sent to the faculty and receive a superficial review and stamp of approval" (Sachdeva et al. 2000, p. 217), "…following which they are archived and are not resurrected until it is time for an LCME site visit" (Skochelak and Albanese 2000, p. 47). A thorough departmental review of the teaching program should take place every 4 or 5 years, and it is useful to involve trainees in this process. A departmental educational retreat is one way of achieving this.

The ADMSEP objectives are quite detailed, and not all of them can be mastered during the clerkship. Some can be taught in preclinical courses and other clerkships. In a recent survey of ADMSEP members (A.C. Brodkey, F.S. Sierles, and J.L. Woodard, "Use of Educational Learning Objectives in Psychiatry Clerkships," unpublished data, 2005), approximately half of those surveyed reported that they used the ADMSEP objectives.

NEW LCME REQUIREMENTS

To fulfill the goals and objectives, the LCME requires that the department provide students with a clerkship orientation, supervised patient-care experiences (documented with a logbook), an evaluation and grading system, equivalency among sites, student ratings and other means of assessing the clerkship, and evidence of follow-up of student performance into residency (Alexander et al. 2000; Liaison Committee on Medical Education 2004). In October 2004, the LCME added several requirements regarding student experiences to facilitate development of specified clerkship competencies. Schools must specify the numbers and kinds of patients that students must see in order to achieve the objectives of the learning experience.

It is not sufficient simply to supply the number of patients students will work up in the inpatient and outpatient setting. The school should specify, for courses and clerkships, the major disease states or conditions that students are expected to encounter. They should also specify the extent of student interaction with patients and the venue(s) in which interactions should occur. A corollary requirement is that courses and clerkships will monitor the number and variety of patient encounters in which students will participate, so that adjustments can be made to ensure that all students have the desired clinical experiences (Liaison Committee on Medical Education 2004). Additional new requirements for formal mid-clerkship feedback and timely final grades are also described.

Since the LCME added these requirements, medical schools, departments, and clerkship directors' organizations (including ADMSEP) have deliberated their meaning and strategies for meeting them. The LCME has clarified that the collective judgment of faculty (under leadership of the school and departments) should determine what core expectations are. They should not be left to individual teachers or site directors.

Underlying this is the premise that the school's overall goals and objectives have been determined, and that departmental faculty members have determined clerkship objectives that support those goals. The LCME anticipates that by specifying this as a priority for the clerkship, clerkship directors will receive the time and resources they need to meet the expectations.

The list of core items is the prerogative of the faculty of the individual medical school and should support the objectives of the institution, but it is expected that such a list be defensible and not appear arbitrary to others. Overall, the expected planning starts with the particular school's deciding that a successful graduate looks like, and then determining an overall plan for achieving that success for each student. Once the overall plan is set, resources (patients and reasonable alternatives to patients) should be in place within the clerkships to ensure that the objectives are achieved and the goals are met; in other words, there should be suitable process and outcome measures.

ADMINISTERING THE CLERKSHIP

PSYCHIATRY CLERKSHIP DIRECTOR

The psychiatry clerkship director (PCD) runs the clerkship (Kuhn et al. 2002). The PCD is assisted by a clerkship coordinator and typically an educational site director at each clinical site. The PCD also works closely with other department and school administrators, psychiatry faculty and residents, and, naturally, the students. Phalen and Magrane (2000) wrote, "Managing a clerkship is very much like being the ringmaster for a three-ring circus. The center ring is the medical students and their clinical and academic needs, the right ring includes the faculty and medical school administrators, and the left ring houses your scholarship and research, professional development, and patient care commitments. You (the director) must 'work' each ring variously as a leader and follower, and give due 'applause' frequently."

Characteristics of the Psychiatry Clerkship Director

The most recent survey of PCDs' characteristics (Sierles and Magrane 1996), conducted in 1994, indicated that the average PCD was 46 years old and had been the director for almost 6 years. Over 90% were board-certified psychiatrists. Their distribution in academic ranks of assistant (36%), associate (32%), and full (27%) professor did not differ from that of residency training directors. More than 90% carried one or more additional administrative duties, most often director or co-director of medical student education in psychiatry (66%), course director in psychopathology or behavioral science, or clinical service chief. Half were members of their department's executive committee. It is our impression that these characteristics have remained essentially the same.

In 1994, PCDs worked an average of 51.7 hours per week, including 13.6 hours teaching and another 11.2 on educational administrative duties. Teaching hours were divided among clinical (5.5) and didactic (4.1) instruction of students and of residents (3.9). Other activities included clinical practice (15 hours), which most felt enhanced their teaching, and research (5.9 hours). Some 80.4% of PCDs reported that their jobs were "personally fulfilling," and 65.4% of them wanted to remain as PCDs for the rest of their careers (Sierles and Magrane 1996).

With managed care's expansion, changes have occurred in the hours spent by PCDs in clinical practice and in their attitudes about their work. In a 1997–1998 survey (Brodkey et al. 2002) of clerkship directors in all specialties, 48% of PCDs perceived that their clinical responsibilities had increased because of managed care (46% of clerkship directors in all specialties had the same perception), and 51% of PCDs reported that their morale and the quality of their professional lives as PCDs had decreased because of managed care (vs. 39.6% of clerkship directors overall).

Qualifications of the Psychiatry Clerkship Director

To clarify the duties, roles, competencies, and required resources of the PCD (Table 2–1) in light of changes in the health care system, ADMSEP published "Standards for Psychiatry Clerkship Directors" (Kuhn et al. 2002).

New PCDs may not have all these competencies, and mentoring by the

TABLE 2–1. Duties and competencies of the psychiatry clerkship director

Leadership

— Incorporates departmental views of contemporary clinical psychiatry into curriculum
— Provides overall vision for the clerkship mission in collaboration with chair and key faculty
— Motivates colleagues to teach
— Presents psychiatry as a specialty to nonpsychiatric colleagues
— Demonstrates broad clinical psychiatric skills and familiarity with educational theory and practice
— Encourages peer learning and education along the training hierarchy

Administration

— Provides a full-time clinical experience for every student in the medical school
— Oversees production and distribution of all schedules
— Recruits new teaching affiliates and maintains ongoing affiliations
— Recruits new faculty into teaching roles
— Monitors the effectiveness of all clinical sites, faculty, and the clerkship in achieving their goals
— Ensures that timely formative and summative evaluations are provided to all students
    Serves on relevant medical school education and evaluation committees
— Serves as a link between department, dean's office, other clerkship directors, and all clinical sites
— Delivers narrative evaluations and final grades to dean's office
— Implements changes in clerkship mandated by department, medical school, or Liaison Committee on Medical Education
— Manages support personnel, educational budget, and office space

Education

— Sets core educational goals for the clerkship
— Prepares students to evaluate and treat or refer patients with common psychiatric disorders
— Develops curriculum based on local needs, national standards, and departmental vision
— Establishes mandatory duties and assignments for students (call nights, papers, etc.)
— Delivers strong didactic presentations and clinical teaching
— Establishes and conveys standards for student participation in patient care at clinical sites
— Ensures that myths of psychiatric illness are acknowledged, discussed, and dispelled

TABLE 2–1.   Duties and competencies of the psychiatry clerkship director *(continued)*

— Develops overall assessment strategy for students
— Prepares and implements all examinations
— Develops plan and instruments for evaluation of program's success in meeting clerkship goals

Advising and mentoring

— Fosters personal growth and professional development of students
— Provides career guidance to medical students
— Maintains knowledge of local and national career options
— Counsels students with inadequate knowledge, skills, or attitudes and plans remediation
— Collaborates with and encourages residents and junior faculty interested in teaching
— Models and facilitates lifelong learning and openness to feedback

Scholarship

— Demonstrates educational innovation and research as evidenced by
    — Presentations at national meetings
    — Published abstracts and exhibited posters at academic meetings
    — Peer-reviewed papers, book chapters, monographs, and books
    — Committee service in medical school and in local and national organizations

Source.   Modified from Brodkey AC, Sierles FS: "Psychiatric Clerkships," in *Handbook of Psychiatric Education and Faculty Development.* Edited by Kay J, Silberman EK, Pessar LF. Washington, DC, American Psychiatric Press, 1999, pp. 256–257.

director of medical student education, psychiatry chair, and education dean is necessary for developing these skills.

The PCD's job is made immeasurably more enjoyable and productive by the presence of a supportive, accessible psychiatry chair or vice-chair for education. It is essential for the chair to believe that teaching students is a vital departmental mission and to allot the resources and time necessary for the PCD: 20% full-time equivalent for clerkship administration, 25% for direct teaching, and 10% for educational research or other education-related scholarly work, for a total of 55% of time devoted to clerkship-related activities (Kuhn et al. 2002). This recommendation is consistent with those of other clerkship directors' organizations (Pangaro et al. 2003).

An education budget should cover direct student costs (e.g., printed and audiovisual materials, books, computer programs, National Board of Medical Examiners [NBME] subject examinations), use of the school's educational center for objective structured clinical examinations and stan-

TABLE 2–2. Duties of the administrative assistant (clerkship coordinator)

— Schedules classes, reserves classrooms, and obtains audiovisual and other equipment
— Orders supplies (Scantron answer sheets, markers for board/overhead, slide trays, etc.)
— Makes clinical assignments
— Prepares written materials
— Distributes keys and meal tickets
— Fields questions, relays messages, and handles crises
— Proctors and grades exams
— Tracks evaluations and maintains students' records and databases for research and evaluation
— Communicates with dean's office, office of medical education, and other clerkship administrators
— Provides a sympathetic ear to students and information to the clerkship director
— Assists in preparation of faculty performance evaluations for appointment, promotion, and teaching awards

Source. Modified from Brodkey AC, Sierles FS: "Psychiatric Clerkships," in Handbook of Psychiatric Education and Faculty Development. Edited by Kay J, Silberman EK, Pessar LF. Washington, DC, American Psychiatric Press, 1999, pp. 256–257.

dardized patients, faculty development and the PCD's professional development, and administrative support costs (e.g., computers and software, costs for a psychiatry club, awards). During frequent meetings of the PCD and the chair, the general goals of the clerkship, the teaching program, and outcome measures used to monitor the program's effectiveness should be discussed. The PCD and the chair must keep each other posted about clerkship, medical school, or national trends that might require the other's intervention. The PCD should never surprise the chair in public, and vice versa (Fincher 2000a).

Another indispensable requisite for the clerkship is a competent, organized, pleasant full-time administrative assistant (clerkship coordinator), whose responsibilities are listed in Table 2–2 (Brodkey and Sierles 1999).

CLERKSHIP SITE DIRECTOR

With the possible exception of the medical center in which the PCD treats patients, each teaching site to which students are assigned needs a clerkship site director (CSD), about whom little has been written. The CSD is responsible for the student program at the site and is the students' principal teacher and supervisor there (Sachdeva et al. 2000). An additional responsibility is representing the site at the department's education committee meetings. The CSD should have a practice at the teaching site and should be there at least half-time.

The CSD should have credibility in both the medical school department and the teaching site, delegated or direct authority to implement programs and make changes, some educational expertise, a major commitment to teaching, and adequate protected time for the role (Sachdeva et al. 2000). The CSD is administratively responsible to the teaching site's psychiatry service chief, to the PCD, and (through the PCD) to the medical school's psychiatry chair. The CSD's dual loyalties differ from those of the PCD, whose main loyalty must be to the medical school department. The CSD's capacity to serve both enterprises sincerely is essential. Ideally, both enterprises should contribute to the CSD's salary. Being a CSD is an excellent stepping-stone for eventually becoming a PCD or residency director.

Under some circumstances, particularly when patient care is provided in one building, the service chief could also be the CSD, but only if he or she has a major commitment to and protected time for education. One person could simultaneously be site director for both residents and students, but if so he or she must have even more protected time. In some instances, the dual-role director, or any clinical teacher, can teach clerks and residents simultaneously (e.g., in an interview conference or in caring for patients).

Adequate administrative support for the site's educational program is necessary for preparing teaching schedules; assigning rooms, lockers, and meal tickets; scheduling examinations; conveying messages; and handling other logistics. The CSD's secretary or administrative assistant, if available, is the logical person for this role.

THE DIRECTOR'S OTHER ACADEMIC RELATIONSHIPS

A clerkship committee that sets goals, policies, and standards; informs and advises; monitors performance; and shares responsibility for decisions can keep faculty involved in the medical student program and keep the PCD and CSD from becoming isolated. In programs with associate directors, communication regarding philosophy and expectations must be particularly clear, and the director must delegate some responsibility and authority.

Relationships with the school's other clerkship directors foster exchanges of information, coordination of the curriculum, and moral support. Offices of medical education may provide technical assistance (e.g., automated exam grading and statistical analyses), advice and resources for educational innovation, and research.

Membership in national educators' organizations (e.g., ADMSEP, Association of Academic Psychiatrists) and participation in their annual meetings, e-mail lists, and Web sites give access to like-minded and helpful colleagues and mentors, keep the PCD posted about national developments, and provide a collegial, informative annual meeting at a lovely location. Presenting at these meetings and networking with colleagues help the PCD develop a national reputation and is a source of letters of recommendation.

Also of interest is the PCD's role on student evaluation committees, where two problems may occur. The first is the blurring of the psychiatrist's roles as educator and clinician (e.g., "Please explain this student's problem"). Although the PCD may need to educate committee members on aspects of psychopathology—from learning disabilities to suicide potential—that may affect a student's performance, the roles of educator and clinician must be separated. Second, some faculty members still hold the idea that psychiatry has little content and therefore is less deserving of time, is less rigorous, and certainly cannot be failed. Tactful but firm explanations may help to alter these attitudes.

IMPLEMENTING THE CLERKSHIP

Following a competent preclinical program in behavioral science and psychopathology (see Chapter 1, "Preclinical Undergraduate Curricula"), a good general clerkship orientation and specific site orientation, and some "coaching" for each activity by the CSD or the student's supervisor, the essence of the clerkship is to provide a good balance of supervised patient care and a formal didactic program, with students spending the majority of their time participating in patient care.

PATIENT CARE

The best clerkships are those in which the student has considerable patient care responsibility with good supervision (Skochelak and Albanese 2000). Although some observation of attending and resident psychiatrists' interviewing and diagnostic skills is necessary, when the student spends most of the clerkship as an observer the clerkship will be inadequate. By performing initial and follow-up interviews, observing the patient's mental status, interviewing family members, participating in treatment decisions, making referrals, and meeting with other professionals, the student "tries on the clothing" of a psychiatrist. When the student does this under the watchful eye of an enthusiastic supervisor who prepares the student in advance and provides constructive feedback afterward, most of the goals of the clerkship and of the student will be met. The students should see a reasonable variety of patients, and the formal didactics should supplement the students' clinical experiences.

CLERKSHIP LENGTH

The modal required third-year (rarely, fourth-year) psychiatry clerkship lasts 6 weeks, with a range of 4–9 weeks. Some 49.5% last 6 weeks, about 19% are 8 weeks, and about 20% are 4 weeks (Rosenthal et al. 2005). Most PCDs perceive that 4 weeks is too brief for a meaningful psychiatry clerkship. Educational problems in 4-week clerkships are the limited number of patient care, supervisory, and didactic experiences a student can have and the limited number of goals, objectives, and competencies that the student can fulfill. Administratively, the 4-week clerkship is a problem because it requires a dozen clerkship orientations and formal didactic programs during a 48-week academic year, compared with eight rotations annually for a 6-week clerkship.

Negotiating Clerkship Length

In negotiating with the medical school administration to increase or (if necessary) maintain one's clerkship's length, it may be useful to cite the huge responsibilities of primary care physicians for caring for psychiatric patients; the deficiencies in this care (Luoma et al. 2002; Young et al. 2001); the high population prevalence of psychiatric or addictive disorders, which is approximately 30% per year (Kessler et al. 1996; Luoma et al. 2002; Norquist and Regier 1996; Regier et al. 1993; U.S. Department of Health and Human Services 1999); the large indirect costs of mental illness, which imposes on the economy a loss of $79 billion a year—not counting the additional $99 billion in direct costs of mental health care—resulting from lost productivity due to illness, premature death, and incarceration (U.S. Department of Health and Human Services 1999), yielding a "global burden of disease" exceeding that for cancer and just below that for cardiovascular diseases (Murray and Lopez 1996; U.S. Department of Health and Human Services 1999); and the fact that among persons with general medical disorders, survival is shorter for those who have comorbid psychiatric disorders than for those who do not (Schulz et al. 2002).

In the past 5 years, there has been an increasing frequency of psychiatry clerkships being combined with other clerkships, most often neurology (88%), internal medicine (6%), and family practice (6%). Of these clerkships, 55% were "combined but not merged" and 45% were merged, but only 15% of the latter had a common evaluation (Clegg 2003).

In some cases, the length of the psychiatry clerkship was shortened to make this accommodation. The majority of PCDs perceived that overall, the combined clerkship was not educationally beneficial, having administrative difficulties that impaired the experience. Interestingly, most neurology clerkship directors feel the same way about neurology-psychiatry combinations, in part because of differences in patient populations and administrative problems.

As a result, the American Academy of Neurology and ADMSEP published a memorandum (Olson 2004) raising doubts and urging caution about combining their clerkships, especially if either clerkship must be shortened. To our knowledge, there is no published evidence of or strategy for successfully merging the two clerkships.

Increasing recruitment of medical students into psychiatry should not be used as a justification for increasing clerkship length, because 1) studies have shown that there is no association between clerkship length and proportions of graduates choosing psychiatry (Serby et al. 2002; Sierles 1982; Sierles et al. 2003a), and 2) most medical school administrations do not care about recruiting students into psychiatry.

ASSIGNING STUDENTS WITHIN EACH ROTATION

There are two ways to provide students with clinical variety during the clerkship. One is to divide the rotation into discrete full-time experiences (e.g., 3 weeks of outpatient psychiatry followed by 3 weeks of consultation-liaison psychiatry), and the other is to offer several experiences concurrently throughout the clerkship. The advantage of the former is that it allows students to participate intensively in all the activities of a service. It is particularly successful at sites with rapid patient turnover, such as emergency and consultation-liaison services. With planning, placements can be complementary, such as initial placement on an inpatient unit, followed by assignment to a mobile outreach team that follows chronically ill outpatients. A disadvantage is that split rotations deprive students and their supervisors of the continuity, familiarity, and individualization of teaching that longer experiences provide.

To maximize continuity of supervision while providing a variety of experiences, several services can be utilized concurrently (Brodkey and Sierles 1999). Students are assigned primarily to one site (e.g., consultation-liaison service) throughout the clerkship and have one or two briefer experiences (e.g., interviewing outpatients two afternoons a week, attending a child psychiatry clinic, taking night or day call in an emergency room) each week. This model provides the student an opportunity for mentoring by teachers who come to know his or her clinical work well. A disadvantage is that some students find the multiple assignments distracting and fail to establish roots at any location. Continuity of care and supervision can be maximized in a principal care (firm) model in which physicians care for their patients in all settings (Greenfield 1995; Sierles et al. 1996), but very few medical centers use this model.

CLERKSHIP SETTINGS: INPATIENT, OUTPATIENT, AND OTHERS

We maintain that, on balance, good results are based more on enthusiastic teaching and close attention to students' needs for supervised responsibility than on the place where the teaching occurs. Students' knowledge, as measured by test performance, is greater when they have good teachers (Griffith et al. 1997, 1998; Stern et al. 2000).

Nevertheless, the site itself is important. When the LCME mandated a psychiatry clerkship in the early 1970s, departments established inpatient-based clerkships, which had predominated in medical education since the late nineteenth century (Pessar 2000). Psychiatric inpatient services allowed efficient teaching because patients were always available. It was believed that students needed to see "pathology writ large" before they could benefit from observing milder and subtler conditions. Hospital lengths of stay of several weeks to months allowed students to watch the patients' conditions evolve, assess treatment efficacy, interview families, work with teams of mental health professionals, and participate in discharge planning. The variety of disorders diagnosed was limited, and clerks did not see patients with anxiety disorders, uncomplicated mood disorders, and most personality disorders (Pessar 2000).

With recent changes in health care delivery and reimbursement, the educational milieu in most inpatient units changed dramatically. More patients are treated as outpatients; hospital lengths of stay are shorter and tend to focus on stabilization, not full remission. Most hospital inpatient services are essentially intensive care units. Therefore, students are less likely to obtain the previously described benefits of the inpatient setting.

Progressively more psychiatric care is being provided in ambulatory settings (Pessar 2000), where students are much more likely to participate in the care of patients whose illnesses more closely resemble those that they would see as primary care physicians. Also, it is important for students to learn that many patients with more severe illnesses can work and live independently and that their success often results from family support and mental health resources. The outpatient setting is preferable for teaching about supportive psychotherapy or crisis management. And just as it has been well documented that the majority of patients in primary care clinics are willing to be evaluated by students (Devera-Sales et al. 1999; Purdy et al. 2000), in our experience the vast majority of psychiatric outpatients are similarly willing.

But unlike primary care clerkships, in which progressively more ambulatory teaching occurs, students in most psychiatry clerkships are still assigned most often to inpatient services. Ambulatory teaching has its own limitations. In many programs, "there is not yet a medical student teaching culture in ambulatory settings in psychiatry" (Pessar 2000, p. 65). Faculty, residents, and students typically see large numbers of patients in relatively short periods. Clinic administrators often will not permit the extra time necessary for thorough individualized supervision of students and for teaching that extends beyond each case (e.g., "In some ways, Mr. Jones is very similar to other patients with bipolar disorder"). Most private practitioners and ambulatory care clinics are not paid to teach students.

But some of these problems can be overcome, especially when the clinic has a medical student teaching culture. Some solutions lie in three types of ambulatory settings: 1) clinics in which students interview new or unscheduled (walk-in) patients with supervisors either present (Gay et al. 2002) or immediately available to round out the interview and make recommendations in concert with the student (e.g., intake or walk-in clinics, consultation-liaison clinics in primary care settings); 2) specialty clinics in which the students have been well coached about the common findings and treatments (e.g., mood disorder clinics, behavioral neurology clinics, stress disorder clinics, geriatric clinics) or in which patients are already diagnosed and students can use standardized checklists; and 3) psychotherapy clinics with patients carefully screened in advance by faculty members (Lofchy 2003).

CLERKSHIP SITE SELECTION

It is becoming progressively more common in clerkships to have multiple clinical teaching sites that must be managed effectively. In a recent survey (A.C. Brodkey, F.S. Sierles, and J.L. Woodard, "Use of Educational Learning Objectives in Psychiatry Clerkships," unpublished data, 2005), the median and modal number of psychiatry clerkship sites was 4, and the mean was 4.6.

The clerkship can meet most or all of its goals and objectives in a broad variety of clinical settings, including but not limited to academic medical centers, clinics and emergency departments (Melchiode et al. 1983), com-

TABLE 2–3. Strategies for attaining equivalency between clerkship sites

— Use the same clerkship manual at all sites.
— Orient all students to the clerkship at a central site.
— Have the same goals, objectives, and required clinical experiences.
— Have the formal didactic curriculum at a central site.
— Use the same grading strategies.
— Give the same examinations.
— Document that examination scores and grade distributions are similar across sites.
— Review student logs for equivalency of patient care experiences and diagnoses.

munity mental health centers, affiliate hospitals and clinics, Veterans Affairs medical centers, state hospitals, military hospitals, and even correctional settings (Leamon et al. 2001). The selection of sites should take into account that starting in 2004, the LCME requires that students be assigned only to sites in which there are residents and continuing medical education programs (Liaison Committee on Medical Education 2003). Also, for LCME accreditation, the department must document that the clinical education at each site combined with the formal didactic program enables the students at each site to similarly achieve the clerkship's goals and objectives, which is termed *equivalency between sites*. Listed in Table 2–3 are strategies for attaining this equivalency.

The PCD should regularly visit each clerkship site ("circuit riding"), perhaps every month or two, to show the department's support; to chat with the CSD, service chief, and students about the program; and to conduct a conference or teaching rounds focusing on one or several patients at the site. The residency director and chair should also make similar visits.

DEVELOPING A NEW CLERKSHIP SITE

Most PCDs will eventually help to develop a new clerkship site. To ensure that the prospective site has the resources to fulfill the clerkship's goals and objectives (Sachdeva et al. 2000), the PCD, residency director, and psychiatry chair should, together or independently, conduct a resource audit. After being invited by the site's service chief, they should tour the facilities, guided by the chief, and learn about the patients, the treatment methods, the prospective faculty, the staff and schedules, the site's and clinicians' previous experiences with trainees, and the facilities for students. Each floor where students will work must have offices available for students to see patients; a dedicated conference room; and a dedicated student room where students can relax, read, do paperwork or computer work, make phone calls, leave their coats, and have access to washrooms.

During the same visit, the PCD must simultaneously discuss with the service chief and prospective CSD the timetables, objectives, requisite patient care experiences and supervision, evaluation and grading systems, common problems and suggested solutions, legal considerations (e.g., that the medical school covers each student's malpractice and health insurance), and clerkship documents. The PCD should solicit recommendations from the chief and the prospective CSD about how the school's requests can best be fulfilled at the site. During the same visit or a follow-up visit, these same topics should also be discussed with the prospective site faculty. In turn, the medical school's resources (e.g., libraries, conference rooms) should be made available to the new faculty members.

There should be a mechanism for the prospective faculty members to promptly obtain faculty appointments in the department before the students appear for the first rotation. In turn, the PCD, residency director, and chair should apply for consultant privileges at the site.

Once the affiliation is mutually agreed on, the medical school should generate a written affiliation agreement to be reviewed and signed by appropriate persons from the school and the site. During the first few weeks of the first several rotations, the PCD should call the CSD, and the chairperson should call the service chief, to discuss progress.

IDENTIFYING THE AVAILABLE SLOTS IN EACH CLERKSHIP

Based on regularly obtained feedback about the educational performance of each clerkship site, the PCD should inform the student affairs dean in a timely fashion of how many students can be properly supervised at each site—a number that does not always remain constant. If faculty and staff availability and commitment change, the number of slots may vary as the year progresses. Typically, once the department determines the appropriate number of slots at each site for a given rotation, the students hold a centralized lottery supervised by the student affairs office, to determine which students will be assigned to which site. This arrangement is fair to the students and avoids the hassles associated with a department's determining which students should be assigned to which site. At schools where the department is responsible for student assignment, the lottery should be held as part of the clerkship orientation. The clerkship coordinator can e-mail or fax student names to clerkship sites.

TEACHING AND LEARNING IN THE CLERKSHIP

PSYCHIATRIC INTERVIEWING

Psychiatric interviewing is the core skill of the clerkship. Most of the clerkship objectives center on the student's becoming competent in conducting a psychiatric diagnostic interview of a patient with whom the student is unfamiliar. The need for improving physician interview skills is well documented, and several studies indicate that the performance of medical students may deteriorate from the first to the fourth year (Craig 1992). During the clerkship orientation, there should be presentations on diagnostic interviewing, the mental status examination, and psychiatric diagnosis and treatment.

Then, in addition to students observing faculty members interview patients for role modeling purposes, which should occur during the first week and periodically thereafter, the most crucial clerkship activity occurs when the student interviews an unfamiliar patient under supervision and receives feedback from a faculty member or senior resident. All students *must* be directly observed interviewing and be given immediate feedback (Carroll and Monroe 1980), either on the student's assigned service or in an interviewing conference. The more supervised interviewing with feedback the student does, the better.

Supervised interviews can occur in a broad variety of situations, ranging from the student interviewing a new patient on a service with a faculty member or resident in the same room, to a regularly scheduled interview conference in which a patient is preselected and available, to a scheduled standardized patient interview directly supervised by a faculty member or senior resident. Standardized patient interviews must be supplemented by interviews of real patients.

By the second week of the clerkship, if not sooner, the student should begin seeing some patients alone. After interviewing the patient, the student presents the patient to a supervisor, who completes the interview in the student's presence. At most medical centers, it is legally required for an attending doctor to be present in the clinical area—if not in the same office—while a trainee sees a patient.

For patients for whom this interview determines the patient's diagnosis and treatment, these can be discussed in the patient's presence. If the supervisor perceives that the student is reasonably tactful, the supervisor could ask the patient, "Is it okay if we discuss your diagnosis and treatment now, in your presence?" Then the supervisor could ask the student, "What's your diagnosis for (patient's name)?" and then make the proper adjustments and corrections. In our experience, patients and students handle this situation well, and research suggests that patients prefer this scenario to being asked to wait outside while they are being discussed (Purdy et al. 2000).

Although it is fine to discuss the patient's diagnosis and treatment in the patient's presence, it is best to give feedback to the student about his or her interviewing technique after the patient leaves. Feedback given to students about their clinical skills should be immediate and precise: immediate "because skills that are learned incorrectly are hard to correct later, and precise because just telling a student an action is incorrect does not help him or her to improve" (Brodkey and Sierles 1999; Skochelak and Albanese 2000). Feedback should be both positive and negative. Giving examples of things a student does well in addition to those that require improvement lets students place negative comments in a balanced perspective. Feedback should emphasize specific behaviors. This approach reduces the chance that the student will take feedback as a personal attack and guides students to improve their performance.

In the clinical education literature, it is often asserted that feedback must literally be labeled as feedback:

> When students are asked whether they received feedback on a clinical service, they invariably state that they received little to none. If clinical faculty members on the same service are asked whether they gave feedback, they say that they give students feedback "all the time." Who is right? Probably both. The problem is that what faculty see as feedback, students do not recognize as such....Unless students are told they are being given feedback, they will often not realize they are receiving it. (Skochelak and Albanese 2000)

Students and faculty can utilize one of the many available checklists to specify the skills to be learned, practiced, and evaluated (Appendix 2–A), and ideally the teacher could supplement the verbal feedback by giving the student a completed checklist.

THE CLERKSHIP ORIENTATION

The clerkship orientation typically has two phases, a central presentation by the PCD to all the clerks, followed—on the student's arrival at the assigned site—by a brief site-specific orientation from the CSD or site coordinator and a brief orientation to the day's patient care activities by the student's supervisor. The central orientation includes structuring students' expectations and responsibilities, addressing students' concerns, and nuts-and-bolts items.

Structuring Students' Expectations and Responsibilities

Clear communication of expectations and responsibilities to students, residents, and faculty members is essential for reducing anxiety, achieving the goals of the clerkship, and avoiding the problems that result from failure to meet unclear standards. Written guidelines should be distributed to and verbally reviewed with the entire group of clerks at their central orientation session on the first clerkship day (Brodkey and Sierles 1999).

Third-year students often do not remember much of what they hear about the details of the clerkship organization; therefore, written guidelines are needed. Explicit instructions regarding clinical responsibilities, including the number of assigned patients, hours of attendance, directions for chart documentation, night-call schedules and duties, rounds participation, responsibilities in the assessment of new patients (including the physical examination), what to do in case of absence, and any dress codes should be covered.

A schedule of classes and conferences is distributed and reviewed, along with guidelines on what to do about conflicts between clinical duties and class attendance. Expectations for written assignments (including examples), such as patient assessments and logs, should be distributed. Goals and objectives of the clerkship, textbooks and other learning resources, and evaluation standards and procedures are discussed.

Examinations and evaluations are potent motivators of students, most of whom believe their residency matches depend on their clerkship grades. The grading system must be described explicitly, orally and in writing, and standards must remain the same throughout the academic year.

Students should be told what to expect of faculty, residents, and staff. Guidelines for supervision and teaching, feedback, and general participation by clerks should be reviewed, with directions to report deviations to the CSD and, if they are not resolved immediately, to the PCD.

Student Concerns

Students beginning the clerkship are often anxious about certain issues. Pre-clerkship anxiety is often associated with negative attitudes and is best addressed at this initial meeting. The PCD may begin by eliciting students' ideas of how psychiatric patients may resemble or differ from other patients (Brodkey and Sierles 1999). Concerns about patient assaultiveness should be addressed by discussing the assessment and management of agitated or irritable patients, followed up by a presentation on psychiatric emergencies.

Misperceptions may include the notion that psychiatric patients are more chronically ill or less treatable than other patients, that psychiatrists use only one type of treatment (e.g., psychotherapy or medication) for all problems, or that psychiatrists (and therefore psychiatry clerks) should maintain a blank façade with patients.

Students may need the PCD to address these myths. It is useful to review some of the real differences they can expect with some patients—such as difficulty in communicating, unconventional behavior, stigma and denial associated with psychiatric illness, and involuntary status—and to remind students of the importance of noting and understanding their own reactions.

It is helpful to tell students that they may have distressing emotional reactions to some patients and that they should discuss such reactions with a faculty supervisor or colleague. It is also prudent to discuss maintaining professional boundaries with patients. Clerks should be specifically instructed that they may not date or befriend patients during or after the clerkship. Orientation also provides an opportunity to discuss the high prevalence of psychiatric disorders seen in all specialties (Brodkey and Sierles 1999).

During this first meeting the PCD must convey openness, warmth, respect, a sincere desire for communication, and excitement about this mutual endeavor. Because some students believe that the psychiatry clerkship is a "vacation," expectations that they will be involved in patient care, meet high standards in their learning, and develop important professional skills and attitudes should be apparent.

Often during this orientation, the students do not seem to remember much of what they were taught in their previous behavioral science or psychopathology course. The reason for this apparent lack of retention is probably that in the students' other clerkships, psychiatry and behavior were discussed minimally, so little reinforcement of their previous learning occurred (Case et al. 1997).

Nuts and Bolts

Practical issues such as use of telephones and pagers, storage of personal items, office space, transportation, parking, keys, meal tickets, student credentialing at the affiliate sites, and student memberships in the American Psychiatric Association can be addressed by the coordinator. Other details should be addressed when the students arrive at their assigned sites.

Site-Specific Orientation

On the students' first day at their assigned sites, they should be oriented about site-specific expectations for performance, including daily work schedules, unit conferences, teaching by housestaff, and exact duties. Junior clerks simultaneously crave and fear patient care responsibility; too little or too much direction frustrates them. Some newer or more anxious students may do better "shadowing" a resident or attending physician for a while before seeing patients independently, whereas others thrive on more responsibility (Brodkey and Sierles 1999). Faculty and resident preceptors must identify and respond to these differences.

FORMAL DIDACTIC COMPONENTS OF THE CLERKSHIP

Because patient care experiences and interviewing conferences cannot fulfill all the objectives, clerkships have formal didactic programs. For clerkships with geographically distant sites, the most common strategy is to begin the clerkship with a "didactic day" or two at a central site, typically followed by a weekly didactic day at a central site. If sites are very close geographically, half days or a daily afternoon conference can work well. Although conceivably the teachers at each site could provide a good local formal didactic program without students having to meet at a central site, this arrangement is probably rare.

Broad areas of learning—such as identification of psychopathology, mastery of interpersonal skills, acquisition of knowledge, and attainment of professional attitudes—are often acquired independently of each other and should be taught using the most appropriate methods (Goldney and McFarlane 1986). It helps to map the clerkship objectives onto available teaching opportunities. Didactic formats include lectures, interactive group discussions based on case examples, journal clubs, computer-assisted instruction, self-study, and team learning. In team learning, the teacher divides the class into teams of 4–6 students, each with approximately equal expertise. The students are assigned an advance reading and are given a multiple-choice test on this reading at the beginning of class. Team members each sit together as the teacher re-asks the class the multiple-choice questions one by one. Each team reaches a consensus, displays its answer on a card, and selects a member to justify the answer to the class. Advantages include advance preparation, learning teamwork, and class participation by a large number of students (Levine et al. 2004). Covering important topics with a variety of teaching formats helps to compensate for students' different learning styles and developmental levels. The most useful duplications are between classroom teaching and clinical care. Excellent guides for lecture and small-group teaching are available (Whitman 1982a, 1982b).

It is useful to offer elective enrichment opportunities—created for students with particular interest in psychiatry but available to all clerks—during the clerkship. For example, the chief resident might offer a weekly journal club, or the department might sponsor a once-per-rotation dinner meeting at which a film with a psychological theme is presented and discussed. In our experience, these activities, if well taught, draw about half of the rotation's clerks.

The Interviewing and Diagnostic Conference

Basic principles and functions of interviewing and the mental status examination should be covered during the first few clerkship days. These topics should include 1) developing rapport with the patient through techniques such as open-ended questioning, empathic listening, facilitation, reflection, and recapitulation (see Appendix 2–A); and 2) learning diagnostic scripts for the common disorders.

After these basic themes have been addressed, most clerkships offer a weekly conference or course that covers psychiatric interviewing, clinical reasoning, and diagnosis. The teacher should also use these sessions to identify and discuss attitudes and reactions to patients, help students identify psychopathology, demonstrate clinical reasoning, or discuss other relevant topics (e.g., ethics, psychiatry and medicine, health care financing). Videotapes and role playing can also be used to teach students how to handle emotionally charged or otherwise difficult interviews (Brodkey and Sierles 1999).

Lectures and Case Discussions

Most psychiatry clerkships offer lectures, which typically include psychopharmacology, history and mental status examination, major psychiatric disorders including substance abuse, and suicide; a smaller number of clerkships also cover emergency, child, adolescent, and geriatric psychiatry; sleep disorders; and sexuality (Abrams et al. 1987). These lectures should differ from second-year psychopathology lectures by placing greater emphasis on practical aspects of assessment and management.

The major problem with lectures is audience passivity, which discourages the thoughtful learning necessary to successful understanding, critical thinking, and clinical reasoning (Newble and Entwistle 1986). Most lecturers tire quickly of giving the same speech every 4–8 weeks, even when the lectures are well received.

Alternatives to this repetitiveness include rotating the presentations among several teachers, alternating lectures with vignette- or videotape-based case presentations followed by group discussion, or discussions based on prior preparation by students. For example, students can be assigned vignettes or videotapes designed to elicit learning of specific objectives along with readings prior to a class, using a problem-solving format (Barrows and Tamblyn 1980; Ende et al. 1986; Wilkerson and Feletti 1989). This format stimulates curiosity and resourcefulness, forces students to integrate facts, and increases their feelings of competence. Although this strategy requires advance preparation, one study showed that it results in greater learning and better test scores (Ende et al. 1986).

Other Formats

Other assignments include written patient assessments with case formulations, case conference presentations, and papers on topics of special interest to the student. For any of these assignments, performing a literature search can contribute considerably to the student's learning. Such assignments can be done after hours or during unplanned slack time. Ideally, early in the clerkship, every student should be assessed for personal goals and should be encouraged to pursue these goals. Written assignments must be perceived by students to be useful to their development as clinicians, and not as mere "busy work."

Grand Rounds and Other Presentations Targeted for Faculty or Residents

Students are sometimes expected to attend conferences—typically grand rounds—targeted to faculty or residents. If the PCD anticipates that a given presentation will be too advanced for students but assigning an alternative activity to the students is not feasible, a faculty member or resident could lead a postconference student discussion to supplement the conference, or the speaker could be scheduled—well in advance—to meet the students afterward to supplement and clarify the content of the presentation (Skochelak and Albanese 2000).

RESIDENTS AS TEACHERS

Students receive considerable instruction from residents, who are expected to supervise the students on their services. Because of their closeness in age and professional development, students are often more comfortable with residents than with attending physicians. Housestaff physicians are role models in their attitudes toward patients, staff, and clinical work and must be reminded of their importance in their interactions with students. Each resident group should be oriented to the schedule, objectives, and clinical expectations of the clerkship and to their roles in teaching and evaluating students. The PCD and CSDs should attend residents' meetings periodically to review the residents' roles and performance in the clerkship (Brodkey and Sierles 1999). Residents generally focus on clinical issues of immediate relevance and daily patient management, whereas attending physicians emphasize differential diagnosis and integration of disparate facts, link classroom learning to patient care, and locate the patient and illness in a broad psychosocial context (Brodkey et al. 2002; Skeff and Mutha 1998; Tremonti and Biddle 1982).

Like faculty members, residents vary in their skill and inclination for teaching. They are often anxious about their knowledge and skills, their effectiveness as teachers, and their obligations toward students. They may be unsure how the students' role differs from theirs, and they may feel competitive (Brodkey and Sierles 1999). When access to patients or supervisors is limited, residents sometimes compete with students to perform procedures. These issues are best addressed openly, empathetically, and practically. The value of teaching, both in learning to explain clearly and in stimulating further learning, should be presented to the residents.

The Psychiatry Residency Review Committee (Accreditation Council for Graduate Medical Education 2001) requires that residents be formally trained in teaching. In one exercise, a group of first-year residents are asked to recall attributes of effective and ineffective teachers they experienced in the past, with the instructor writing these attributes on a flip chart. The residents inevitably mention—often passionately and with examples—most of the same attributes that the PCD values. Through Socratic questioning the residents refine these descriptions, and it soon becomes apparent that the characteristics of effective teachers listed by the residents are indeed the most important ones to emulate.

Teaching workshops improve skills but need to be reinforced regularly (Edwards et al. 1988; Katzelnick et al. 1991). Another option is didactic sessions in instructional methods (e.g., how to prepare a presentation using PowerPoint slides). Also, residents should participate in evaluation and grading of students.

Identifying residents who are particularly good teachers is helpful. Such residents can be assigned more students or particular students—such as those interested in psychiatry—whereas more advanced residents may give lectures, supervise students in enrichment experiences, remediate students with deficits, or help new residents learn to teach. These residents should be recognized with teaching awards, and some could be recruited for faculty positions. In some departments, senior residents who have performed well academically and teach considerably well are appointed as instructors, which is a source of pride and a helpful credential for the resident.

At the other end of the spectrum are residents who neglect or abuse students or patients. Reports of such behavior should be investigated, and when warranted, the PCD or residency director should counsel the involved resident. Cases of ethical violations should be presented to the residency director. Examples of abuses include asking a student for personal services (e.g., "Pick up my dry cleaning") or for a date, or making insulting comments about a patient's gender or ethnic group (Brodkey and Sierles 1999).

EVALUATION OF THE CLERKSHIP AND ITS FACULTY

Evaluating how well the clerkship meets its goals is essential. Students' perceptions can be solicited informally during the clerkship, individually and in groups. The PCD and CSDs should maintain frequent contact and encourage feedback. Medical students are often unwilling to rock the boat with criticisms unless they perceive they will be taken seriously and there will be no retribution. An open-door policy for both faculty and students is essential to staying on top of problems (Brodkey and Sierles 1999). An informal weekly meeting with students and the PCD or CSD at which interesting or problem cases of the week are presented allows an opportunity to discuss the successes and failures of the clerkship. Changes made in response to student input should always be announced.

RATINGS BY STUDENTS

Formal evaluation by the students is obtained at the end of the clerkship. This information should be gathered anonymously, and results should not be shared with the faculty until the students' grades are in. The student affairs office usually uses a standard form for all clerkships, and at some schools the form can be completed online. Online systems can analyze the data and collate and print students' narrative comments, saving considerable secretarial time.

A supplemental departmental evaluation can be designed to include questions not asked on the form provided by the student affairs office, and results from a departmental evaluation may be available sooner than results of the generic survey. The PCD should ensure that all students complete these forms by collecting them at the final examination or by withholding grades until they are received.

All aspects of the clerkship—including overall experience, clinical experiences (including night call), attending physicians, residents, texts, other learning resources, and examinations—should be rated on an ordinal scale (e.g., outstanding, good, acceptable, unsatisfactory), and ample room should be provided for narrative comments about each component. Some authors recommend that the checklist for rating each teacher should itself contain multiple components (e.g., "Creates a positive learning climate"; "Stimulates the student to learn more") in addition to space for narrative comments (Litzelman et al. 2000). However, we believe that for each teacher, using a single overall rating and narrative comments is preferable. In the former, students tend to rate all components for a given faculty member identically (e.g., circling the entire "good" column), which produces an unhelpful halo effect.

Other facets of the clerkship—such as students' opinions about its success in preparing them for future practice, clarity of objectives, inclusion of the student on the team, and how often the student was observed interviewing and received feedback—can be incorporated.

Student ratings are the most commonly used method for evaluating teaching performance because of convenience and economy, and because they are reliable and valid (Abrami et al. 1990; Cohen 1981; Costin et al. 1971; Litzelman et al. 2000; Risucci et al. 1992). Collated results can be summarized periodically for review by the psychiatry chair and the clerkship committee. The faculty and department can include these ratings in periodic performance evaluations and as documentation accompanying promotion or tenure applications.

PEER REVIEW

Another valuable evaluation method is the PCD's direct observation of teaching (Beckman 2004). Unfortunately, this is seldom used to assess clinical teaching because it is so time-consuming, awkward for many physicians, and underappreciated. But it has proved effective in enhancing reviewers' insights, affecting curricula positively, and providing a counterweight to trainees' ratings (Beckman 2004). Because of the time commitment required, it could be restricted to new teachers or to those having difficulty with teaching. Feedback to teachers should have the same characteristics as feedback to trainees.

EXAMINATION SCORES

Data about the clerkship are also obtained through assessment of student performance on departmental examinations and on the USMLE Step 2 and the CS exam. Specifying the objectives and ensuring that these are taught and tested can help the PCD to estimate the achievement of clerkship goals. Because broad areas of learning (e.g., assessment of psychopathology, interviewing skills, and knowledge of topics) are acquired separately (Goldney and McFarlane 1986), they should be assessed independently.

Utilizing USMLE scores to measure the effectiveness of the clerkship is less straightforward, because scores are determined by multiple variables, such as characteristics of the student body, quality of teaching, timing in the academic year, and validity (or lack thereof) of content. For a given department, strong upward or downward trends in scores over several years are noteworthy. To control for student body characteristics, scores on the Mental Illness (formerly Psychiatry) section of Step 2 should be compared with the national mean on this section. To control for the quality of the department's teaching, this score should be compared to those obtained on other sections by other departments.

GRADUATING SENIORS QUESTIONNAIRE

Still another source of data is the psychiatry clerkship items in the Association of American Medical Colleges (2004) Graduating Seniors Questionnaire, completed by fourth-year students shortly before graduation. In this questionnaire, students' ratings of the clerkship are compared to ratings of psychiatry clerkships nationally.

LOGBOOKS

The LCME requires that students maintain logbooks, which are submitted to the department and the dean's office, to document that students had a good variety of clinical experiences and have fulfilled objectives (Links et al. 1988; Weissberg 1996). Data from logbooks can be used to improve subsequent clerkships (Ferrell 1991). Information recorded in logbooks may include the level of responsibility the student took (Raghoebar-Krieger et al. 2001) and supervision the student received. The logbook, which must be easy for the student to complete (Withy 2001), is best constructed by the department or dean's office using a checklist with number codes for patient diagnoses and levels of student responsibility. Logbooks can be kept in a notebook or on a personal digital assistant (PDA).

Students receive the logbook during the orientation and are asked to indicate if and when each objective or experience is completed. A study of medicine clerkship logbooks revealed that students underrecord patients' diseases compared with those recorded by attending physicians (Raghoebar-Krieger et al. 2001).

Some schools use computer programs that allow patient encounters—including brief narrative descriptions as well as diagnoses and treatments—

to be logged on personal computers and PDAs. These programs allow the supervisor, PCD, or CSD to review and respond to student cases online and to generate aggregate lists of patients seen by each clerk or site according to diagnoses or treatments, and thus they can enrich student teaching and faculty oversight.

EVALUATION AND GRADING OF STUDENTS

FORMATIVE AND SUMMATIVE EVALUATIONS

While observing students' performance in each activity, the teacher is evaluating the students. In addition to this informal evaluation, the more formal evaluation and grading of students comprises two components, termed *formative* and *summative evaluation* (Pangaro et al. 2000).

Formative evaluation is mid-clerkship feedback about multiple aspects of the student's performance with the goal of improving (forming or shaping) the student's performance well before the end of the clerkship. Formative evaluation is provided by a supervisor or CSD (rarely, by the PCD) during a scheduled meeting with the clerk, or spontaneously if it is mutually convenient. Formative evaluation is primarily for the student's benefit, but documenting its occurrence (e.g., in the student logbook or a departmentally produced form) benefits the school.

The summative evaluation is produced at the end of the clerkship by describing (summing up) the student's performance on the evaluation and grade form. In addition to providing feedback to the student, it fulfills the department's obligation to the school and society by pronouncing the student ready for further training (Pangaro et al. 2000).

THE FINAL CLERKSHIP GRADE

The student's final grade is usually recorded on a standardized evaluation and grading form from the student affairs office. In addition to containing the final grade, it typically includes specific performance ratings (e.g., knowledge, interviewing skill, charting, teamwork) and narrative comments. The PCD is responsible for refining and editing the comments on the form before it is sent to the student affairs office, preferably within a month after the clerkship ends (Stagnaro-Green et al. 1999). Late return of evaluation forms to the student affairs dean is a common problem that can embarrass the department.

The final grade is determined by a formula that includes clinical evaluations by the faculty with grades on one or more exams. Faculty and resident clinical evaluations are employed for grading by 84.6% of psychiatry departments (Rosenthal et al. 2005). In one study, clinical ratings by faculty were significantly associated with students' USMLE scores and residency directors' ratings (i.e., they had predictive validity) for all clerkships except surgery and psychiatry (Callahan et al. 2000). In clinical departments, the student's clinical performance grade most typically counts for about half of the final grade, to convey the importance of patient care. However, in studies of contributions of each component to final grades, the weights of clinical performance ratings range from 0% to 100% (Hemmer 2000).

Before each academic year, the PCD, in conjunction with the clerkship committee and psychiatry chair, determines the formula for calculating final grades during that academic year. The PCD informs the curriculum and student affairs deans of this formula and summarizes it in the clerkship handbook distributed to the students on the first clerkship day. The grading system and the formula must remain the same for the entire class during that academic year. Any variation from this formula is unfair and would make the school legally vulnerable. In rare cases when the grading system is not working out well and must be changed during the academic year, the proposed change must be approved by the education and student affairs deans and must apply retroactively for all the students during that year.

THE CLINICAL PERFORMANCE GRADE

Ideally, the students' final clinical performance grades should be determined in a meeting of the faculty and residents who supervised the students. Ideally, to maximize fairness and equivalency between sites, this meeting should occur at a central site and should include all the clerkship's teachers. The PCD should run this meeting. If, because of geographic and time constraints, a central-site meeting is not feasible, then the teachers at each site should meet, and the CSD should run the meeting.

At this meeting, the students should be discussed one at a time, preferably starting with residents' impressions (to ensure that residents contribute), followed by attending physicians' impressions, followed by a group consensus on the overall grade and suggestions for narrative comments. Everyone's perspective counts, and focusing on different aspects of performance gives a more comprehensive picture of the student (Pangaro et al. 2000). Housestaff tend to place more weight on the students' work ethic and motivation to help the team, whereas attending physicians are likely to place greater value on students' interpersonal skills, knowledge, and reasoning skills (Metheny 1991; Stillman 1984). Residents tend to give higher ratings than faculty to students (Dielman et al. 1980; Hull 1982; Littlefield et al. 1981). However, housestaff evaluations have better internal consistency than faculty evaluations, so that combining resident with faculty evaluations improves the reliability of evaluations (Dielman et al. 1980; Hull 1982; Littlefield et al. 1981). The more raters that comment on the student's performance, the better.

NEGATIVE COMMENTS AND LOW OR FAILING GRADES

Unfortunately, many faculty members in all specialties (and deans) are hesitant or unwilling to record negative comments in descriptive evaluations or checklists (or dean's letters), and to give low or failing grades. This is a serious problem, because it is well documented that even if only one supervisor mentions or records a negative comment, it probably has substantial merit (Pangaro et al. 2000; Papadakis et al. 2004). In a study of their medical school's graduates over 46 years, Papadakis et al. (2004) found that graduates who were eventually disciplined by the state medical board for unprofessional conduct were significantly more likely than control subjects to have had negative comments in their medical school files about their professional or personal attributes. Furthermore, the courts have consistently upheld faculty judgments in cases where students have not met professional or academic standards (Irby and Milam 1989).

Research on faculty members' hesitation to record negative comments and to fail students shows that reasons include fear of legal action, low administrative support for unpopular decisions, hesitation to be involved in following through on difficult cases, "passing the buck" to other evaluators (Hemmer 2000; Tonesk 1986), wanting to be liked, and perceiving that students who work hard automatically deserve a passing or good grade. Despite this hesitancy to *record* negative comments, instructors are often willing to *verbally* discuss their concerns (Hemmer 2000; Tonesk 1983), especially in an evaluation meeting where others have the same impression.

In turn, with group support and good descriptions of problem behaviors, it becomes easier to write negative comments and give low grades. In addition, Magarian (2000) suggested that giving valid grades is facilitated by separating the evaluation and grading functions; by having supervisors present and write detailed descriptions of the student's performance; and by having a small, handpicked group of educationally committed faculty members give the final grade. How often this occurs nationally is not known.

When there is good justification for writing negative comments or giving a low or failing final grade, doing so is much easier if the student's supervisor has given feedback to the student about the weak performance, suggested ways to improve, observed whether the behavior subsequently changed, documented in writing any subsequent failure to improve, and reported the latter to the PCD. This giving of due process is excellently explained in Irby and Milam's 1989 paper. Of course, the teacher has to have adequate time to supervise the student well—which too often is not the case (Albanese 1999)—and the department administration must support the teacher. Faculty should be directed to inform the PCD as soon as a pattern is apparent about any student whose performance places him or her in jeopardy of failing the clerkship. The PCD should meet with the student, outline concerns, and formulate a plan for improvement. The content of the meeting must be carefully documented. Often, performance improves after this meeting. If not, the documentation is important to demonstrate due process.

CLERKSHIP EXAMINATIONS

Almost all psychiatry clerkships give at least one examination that contributes to the clerkship grade. Some 65.5% of departments use the USMLE Psychiatry Subject (Shelf) exam generated by the NBME. Some departments use another type of examination, in addition to or in place of the USMLE Subject examination. The other types include departmentally generated multiple-choice exams (DGMCEs), objective structured clinical examinations (OSCEs), and oral examinations.

The USMLE Subject (Shelf) Examination

In 65.5% of schools (Rosenthal et al. 2005), the psychiatry department uses an NBME subject examination, a 120-item, multiple-choice, end-of-clerkship test. Like the USMLE Step 2, the Subject exam is based on clinical vignettes using one-best-answer and extended matching formats (Case et al. 1997). Most Subject and Step 2 items are interdisciplinary, so the vignette often depicts a primary care setting, and a general medical symptom or condition is a possible correct answer. A sample question is presented below.

> For 7 months, a 65-year-old man was treated with adjunctive chemotherapy with methotrexate after a successful operation for carcinoma of the colon. Over the past several months, he has developed insomnia, fatigue, crying spells, feelings of guilt, and anhedonia. At ages 40 and 55, the patient was treated with an antidepressant and psychotherapy for a depressive illness. Which of the following is the most likely cause of this patient's behavior? Options include reaction to methotrexate, metastatic cancer, normal adjustment, and major depression. (Case et al. 1997)

The advantages of using the subject exam are its well-documented reliability (0.74) and validity (Case et al. 1997), the fact that no department faculty time is needed for item construction, and the opportunity it presents for students to practice with the Step 2 format. Disadvantages are its high cost—$31 per student as of July 2004—and the fact that its content validity tends to be lower than that of well-prepared departmentally generated multiple-choice tests.

Content validity is the correlation between the proportion of test items on a given topic and the extent to which the department taught about the topic. For example, if the clerkship has a strong emphasis on psychopharmacology and the exam tests it minimally, the exam has poor content validity.

Case et al. (1997) studied the results of the psychiatry subject examination and the psychiatry component of Step 2 and found the following: For the subject exams, significantly higher scores were obtained by students who had 8-week rather than 6-week clerkships; that is, the more psychiatry to which they were exposed, the higher they scored. There was minimal difference in scores between students who took the subject exam early in the academic year and those who took it later. This finding contrasts with medicine and surgery subject exams, in which students scored significantly better as the year progressed. Case et al. (1997) hypothesized that the reason for this between-specialty difference is that psychiatry clerks are unlikely to have learned much about psychiatry in prior clerkships, in contrast to medicine or surgery clerks, who are more likely to have learned a lot about medicine or surgery in previous clerkships.

This observation also explains why students taking the psychiatry clerkship later in the academic year—nearer to their Step 2 exams—score significantly higher on the psychiatry component of Step 2 than students who took the clerkship earlier. Case and colleagues (1997) suggested that if clerkship preceptors discuss the causes of presenting complaints such as abdominal pain in a broader context—for example, causes related to medicine, surgery, and obstetrics as well as psychiatry—students will make the necessary connections more easily.

Clerkship length and timing, however, are far less important than student-related factors in determining a given student's grade. Psychiatry clerkship length and timing account for only 2% of the variance in subject test scores (Case et al. 1997), whereas students' Step 1 scores—which reflect their motivation and ability to learn and their test-taking ability—account for 26% of the variance. Similarly, for Step 2, psychiatry clerkship timing and length account for 1% of the variance in Step 2 scores, whereas Step 1 scores explained 62%.

Considering Case and colleagues' (1997) recommendation about preparing clerks for the USMLE subject exam or the psychiatric component of Step 2, the PCD or other teacher could give the clerks a half- or full-day review lecture or problem-based learning session covering psychiatric symptoms, signs, and syndromes in primary care settings. To become familiar with subject and Step 2 exams, the teacher should view actual Step 2 questions during a visit that NBME representatives periodically make to the school to display Step 2 exams. Of course, the teacher may not discuss actual questions from that viewing with the clerks. If the PCD requests, after each administration of the subject exam the NBME will send the department a list of the keywords for each test item, including data about the clerks' performance on each item compared with clerks nationally.

Departmentally Generated Multiple-Choice Examinations

Some 37.3% of psychiatry clerkships (Rosenthal et al. 2005) give a departmentally generated multiple-choice exam (DGMCE). The main advantage of a DGMCE is that if it is well produced by one or several experienced, formally trained test-item writers, its contents will have good content validity and good reliability. On the other hand, if test-item writers are inexperienced, the quality of a DGMCE tends to be poor (Case and Swanson 1998; Jozefowicz et al. 2002). Most medical school educational affairs offices will provide data about a DGMCE's reliability. Giving a DGMCE probably increases the likelihood that the students will study specifically what the department teaches, rather than relying primarily on a generic review book.

If resources permit, giving the DGMCE mid-clerkship and returning the scores promptly to the clerks is a way to provide timely feedback relatively early in the clerkship (Hemmer et al. 1999) that could facilitate the clerks' preparation for subject and step exams. If the DGMCE is the sole exam, it should be given at the end of the clerkship. Case and Swanson (1998) wrote a wonderful primer, with which PCDs should become familiar, about preparing DGMCEs in the USMLE format (see also Chapter 4, "Evaluation of Students").

Most or all DGMCE and USMLE item stems are vignettes. Case et al. (1996) discovered that vignettes do not distinguish between high- and low-performing students any more than nonvignette items. Nevertheless, it may still be preferable to use vignettes (Case et al. 1996), because vignettes place clinical problem solving in center stage, and they may facilitate student preparation for the USMLE subject and Step 2 and 3 exams.

DGMCEs have several disadvantages. In addition to requiring faculty expertise, they also take considerable faculty time: At a typical item-writing rate of 3–4 items per hour, with an additional several hours to further refine the exam, a well-done 60- to 75-item test takes 25–30 hours to prepare. Most clinical faculty members are inexperienced at writing test items and typically do not have free time to write questions, so writing items from scratch or editing poorly written items submitted by others typically falls to the PCD.

One consolation is that if the proctor (typically the clerkship coordinator) collects all test booklets at the end of each exam, the PCD usually has to prepare only one or two exams each academic year. It is better to have two exams than one because this allows for giving a different makeup exam to students who failed their original DGMCE. In our experience, it is relatively rare for students to discuss the exam content with students in subsequent clerkships. In the rare instance that the student grapevine about the content of the clerkship test suddenly becomes active, the exam scores will suddenly jump above those of the previous clerkship, and probably a student will tell the PCD that he or she suspects cheating.

Oral Examinations

Some 24.5% of departments (Rosenthal et al. 2005) give an oral live or videotaped patient exam, typically using a format similar to that used by the American Board of Psychiatry and Neurology (ABPN). If the live patient is representative of the clerkship's patients, the ABPN-style oral (ASO) examination has some face validity, because it tests the clerkship's core skills of interviewing, presenting cases, and diagnostic reasoning. If the videotaped exam is representative, it tests the core skills of presenting and diagnostic reasoning. And since the ABPN examination has a long tradition in psychiatry, a well-organized ASO can be credible to students and faculty.

However, at best, ASOs have only modest reliability and validity, and often they have poor reliability and validity (Hubbard 1978, p. 39; Leichner et al. 1984; Sierles et al. 2001). Even the actual ABPN oral exam—the best live-interview or videotape-based oral exam the specialty can offer (McDermott et al. 1991)—has only modest reliability (weighted $\kappa = 0.56$).

Objective Structured Clinical Examinations

Because multiple-choice exams cannot test interviewing and other clinical skills or traits and behaviors like diligence, caring, and professionalism; because accrediting agencies are becoming more attentive to the documentation of clinical competence; and because ASOs have poor reliability and validity, objective structured clinical examinations (OSCEs) are becoming more popular. First described by Harden and Gleeson in 1979, OSCEs are now used in 16.4% of psychiatry clerkships (Rosenthal et al. 2005). Beginning with the graduates of the class of 2005, fourth-year students will have to pass a primary care–oriented OSCE developed by the NBME—the CS exam—for licensure. To prepare students for the CS exam, progressively more schools will start using OSCEs.

When the tests are developed and administered well, and when students are evaluated in multiple stations over a total testing time of 4–6 hours (whether or not a student has demonstrated a variety of competencies), the major advantages of OSCEs are that they have excellent reliability (Newble and Swanson 1988) and good validity (Ayers and Boulet 2001). An example of a multiple-station, high-reliability (Cronbach $\alpha=0.80$) OSCE is the CS exam, a high-stakes exam whose goal is to determine the candidate's ability to practice under supervision in a residency. The CS exam's validity was demonstrated by its significant correlations with scores on the USMLE Step 1 and 2 and with clerkship grades (Ayers and Boulet 2001). Using an eight-station, 150-minute OSCE in a psychiatry clerkship, Hodges et al. (1997) obtained moderate inter-rater reliability. In contrast, OSCEs lasting 1–2 hours are not sufficiently reliable for high-stakes purposes (Newble and Swanson 1988) such as a requirement for passing the clerkship.

How OSCEs Work.   In OSCEs, each station presents a 5- to 30-minute clinical event such as an initial interview or follow-up visit with a standardized patient (an actor playing a role—e.g., a depressed patient—according to a standardized script), a patient's radiograph, a videotaped vignette, or a typed vignette. Immediately after each clinical situation, in a post-encounter probe (PEP), the candidate answers (on a computer) multiple-choice questions based on the clinical situation (Hodges et al. 2002). Using a checklist, the standardized patient assesses the candidate's interpersonal skills and whether he or she asked the right questions or made the appropriate intervention. The computer scores the candidate's multiple-choice answers.

Several papers describe the use of OSCEs in a psychiatry clerkship or residency (Hodges et al. 2002; Loschen 1993, 2002). The details of developing a psychiatry OSCE—from consulting with OSCE experts, to budgeting the considerable start-up and maintenance costs, to planning out the stations, to training the actors (no small task), to monitoring the exam results—are meticulously described by Hodges and colleagues (2002). Harden and Gleeson's original 1979 description of how an OSCE works is also very helpful. As is the case for OSCEs in any other department, the time and money needed to develop and maintain OSCEs are considerable.

Problems with OSCEs include the following:

1. A large amount of time and expense are needed to develop and maintain them (Hodges et al. 2002).
2. Because most standardized patients are paid by the hour, it may be too costly for students to practice repeatedly on them.
3. An OSCE script may not serve the department's purposes. For example, the OSCE center may provide scripts developed elsewhere, rather than the department developing scripts based on its own objectives.
4. Whereas standardized patients can skillfully grade whether students ask specific questions (e.g., Did the student ask about weight loss?), their ability to grade students' interviewing skills (e.g., Did the student apportion time well? Recapitulate well?) is not established (Hodges et al. 2002, p. 152).

For these reasons, scripts should be developed from scratch and refined in practice before administering the OSCEs to clerks for a grade. In addition, the OSCE should not contribute a substantial amount to the clerkship grade until the department documents its reliability and validity over the academic year. Case ambiguity should be minimized (e.g., "Screen the patient for suicide risk" rather than "Evaluate this patient [i.e., the suicidal patient] whose chief complaint is diarrhea"). Finally, if global interviewing skills are rated, we suggest that psychiatrists should do the rating, in place of or in addition to standardized patients.

In addition to evaluation, standardized patients can also be used for teaching. A hypothetical advantage of this method is that a student can be coached by a faculty member to improve his or her interviewing or other clinical skills without having to repeatedly interview real psychiatric patients. Of course, such a program requires an ample number of available standardized patients. Using standardized patients for teaching purposes is well described by Hall et al. (2004) and by Gay et al. (2002).

COPYEDITING THE EVALUATION AND GRADING FORM

The PCD should read each student's final evaluation and grading form before the completed forms are sent to the student affairs and registrar's offices. To ensure that each student's form is in good order, the PCD should copyedit it to eliminate inconsistencies and insensitive or imprecise comments. The most common problematic inconsistency, which leaves the department vulnerable to successful challenge by the student, is when a student's final grade is lower than the individual performance ratings or narrative comments would suggest. For example, if a student receives a grade of B, C, or F, and the narrative comments or specific performance ratings depict outstanding performance (e.g., "Very good and empathic interviewer, got along excellently with the staff, asked great questions, stayed late"), chances are good that the student will challenge the grade successfully unless the low grade is due to a low exam score.

Another problematic example is a vague, global criticism of a student (e.g., "an unenthusiastic student") in lieu of listing specific behaviors suggesting lack of enthusiasm (e.g., "In my clinic, during discussions, he didn't ask questions, or spontaneously answer my questions. He left early multiple times before all his work was done, despite being told that this was a problem. He didn't do a PubMed search on multiple sclerosis after saying he would do so.").

STUDENT REQUESTS TO CHANGE A GRADE

In several rotations during each academic year, a student or two will ask the PCD to have their grades raised. When this occurs, the PCD should tell the student to write a detailed memo with the reasons for the request. Then the PCD and the student's supervisors will review the memo, after which the PCD will notify the student and the student affairs dean in writing about the decision. This procedure saves faculty time, which is best devoted to teaching students in the current clerkship. Alternatively, the PCD may meet with the student to hear his or her complaints and then proceed as described above. For many students, a respectful hearing settles them down and—with good grace—they accept a decision to let the grade stand.

TROUBLED AND TROUBLESOME STUDENTS

The literature suggests that students who may be particularly vulnerable during the clerkship include those with a family history of psychiatric disorder; those who have suffered abuse; and those whose psychopathology resembles that of their patients. On the other hand, having an ill family member or having previously managed personal problems successfully may enhance empathy and motivation (Brodkey and Sierles 1999).

Troubled students often make themselves known through repeated lateness or absence, failure to complete work, unusually intense affective responses, extreme overidentification with or rejection of patients, or inappropriate interactions with staff members and supervisors. In such instances, the director should investigate promptly and take steps, which may include a conversation, a psychiatric referral, or notification of the student affairs dean.

In addition to troubled students, there are troublesome ones. Some come to the clerkship with skeptical or negative attitudes toward psychiatry. These students are best handled by increasing their understanding and mastery of the field and by asserting requirements for professional behavior. Misunderstandings should be corrected, but it is best not to argue with these students. Students who are disruptive or personally abusive should be counseled and redirected toward their clerkship assignments. They are often well known to the student affairs office and to evaluation committees, and their behaviors should be reported to the student affairs dean (Brodkey and Sierles 1999).

Students whose interpersonal abilities are extremely poor despite adequate examination performance present a particular dilemma. Approaches to this problem may include repetition of all or part of the clerkship, remediation of specific skills, referring the issue to the student affairs office, or psychiatric evaluation if indicated.

ACCESS TO PAST EVALUATIONS OF STUDENTS

There is an unresolved controversy about whether clerkship teachers should be informed about a student's prior performance, particularly if the student had problems. The argument against sharing this information is that it could bias future supervisors' assessments. The case for sharing is that the department could structure an educational program that addresses the student's individual needs and academic development.

In a national survey of student affairs deans, Gold et al. (2002) found that 56% of responding schools had policies that addressed sharing, and of the schools with policies, 53% had policies that supported sharing. Among these, the information was shared with clerkship directors 44% of the time, with faculty mentors 11% of the time, with clinical faculty supervisors 8% of the time, and with resident supervisors 3% of the time. When there were no policies, considerable informal sharing still occurred. Gold et al. (2002) recommended that medical schools share this information, as long as 1) clear written policies describe when and how the information should be shared; 2) the information is shared with clerkship directors only, so that students can be assigned to teachers who are best able to address the student's needs; 3) supervisors who assign grades do not have access to this information; and 4) medical students participate in developing the policies.

THE HIDDEN CURRICULUM

Sometimes overlooked is the hidden curriculum (Hafferty and Franks 1994; Hundert et al. 1996), an important aspect of student socialization related to the culture of medicine, such as attitudes toward patients, organizing work, obtaining good grades, political opinions, dealing with hierarchy, managing affective responses, drug company marketing, and bad-mouthing of other specialists. Aspects of the hidden curriculum are vividly depicted in popular books like *The House of God* (Shem 1978) and *Becoming a Doctor* (Konner 1987). If a hidden curriculum theme presents itself, the PCD should address it explicitly (Brodkey and Sierles 1999).

DRUG COMPANY MARKETING TO MEDICAL STUDENTS

A conspicuous illustration of the hidden curriculum is the extensive exposure of medical students to drug company marketing. Students routinely attend industry-sponsored lunches and grand rounds and frequently receive gifts such as pens, books, and snacks (Bellin et al. 2004; Hodges 1995; Monaghan et al. 2003; F.S. Sierles, A.C. Brodkey, F. A. McCurdy, et al., "A National Survey of Medical Students' Exposure to and Attitudes About Drug Company Marketing," unpublished data, 2005). This marketing has occurred without any prior planning by medical educators nationally, with little or no education of medical students about drug company–physician relationships, and with few if any medical school guidelines about industry–student relationships. This is a serious problem because extensive evidence documents that virtually all information provided by drug companies to doctors and trainees—including scientific articles—is biased in favor of the sponsored products, and because students, like doctors, tend to deny that they can be influenced to prescribe the company's products and tend not to recognize erroneous statements or false advertising (Brodkey 2005).

We think that medical schools should 1) teach students about drug company marketing, 2) have guidelines that restrict contact between medical students and representatives of pharmaceutical companies, and 3) take all steps necessary to eliminate or minimize their own and their faculty members' conflicts of interest in their relationships with drug companies.

DISPARAGING OTHER SPECIALISTS

Disparaging (bad-mouthing) other medical specialties is an unethical but common practice. Doctors in all specialties do it, and it has been demonstrated that for 17% of students, such disparagement contributes to the students' switching their choice of specialty (Hunt et al. 1996). Although we psychiatrists tend to believe that disrespecting psychiatry is more frequent and more likely to affect career choice of psychiatry than any other specialty, recent evidence (Hunt et al. 1996) suggests that students selecting surgery and family medicine were more likely than other students to hear their specialty derided and to change their specialty choice as a result.

Educators should mention other specialties respectfully. Is it ethical to ask a clerk what specialty he or she plans to enter (if the clerk has not mentioned or alluded to the subject spontaneously), since this could raise questions of bias or put the student on the defensive? Clinical teachers should ask students about their specialty preferences only if knowing them could facilitate their teaching with the student's preferred specialty in mind, such as by discussing psychiatric conditions commonly seen in that specialty. If the teacher feels that knowing a student's specialty preference could reduce the teacher's enthusiasm for teaching that student or influence the teacher to lower the student's grade, the topic probably should not be broached.

RECRUITING STUDENTS INTO PSYCHIATRY

PCDs are in positions of ethical compromise when there is a conflict between acting as the students' educator and advisor and acting as a recruiter. This tension may arise when the PCD feels the urge to give a better grade to a student who has expressed interest in the field or make curriculum decisions on the basis of student popularity. Like the boundary between educator and therapist, that between educator and recruiter must be firmly maintained. And although the PCD will inevitably like some students better than others, open favoritism will impair his or her credibility (Brodkey and Sierles 1999).

During the third medical school year, some students will approach the PCD or another senior faculty member to discuss their interest in psychiatry and possibly to ask the PCD to be their senior-year advisor. The PCD can accept this mentorship role enthusiastically and should set aside time for one or two lengthy meetings to discuss the student's interest, plan for fourth-year electives, and review strategies for obtaining the best possible residency. After the initial discussions, the PCD can advise the student responsively by e-mail. If the PCD lacks the time to be the student's mentor, he or she should refer the student to a colleague who would be a caring mentor. Details of this mentorship are beyond the scope of this chapter.

CONCLUSION

Like all roles, that of PCD encompasses difficulties and delights. However skilled PCDs are at middle management, they inevitably come up short in serving all their constituencies (the department chair, the faculty, residents, students, the medical school). Changes in health care financing have resulted in the need to make do with increasingly inadequate time at the very time when major changes in clinical education are occurring.

The good news is that most PCDs view their role as fulfilling, and many want to direct the clerkship for the rest of their careers (Sierles and Magrane 1996). The educational importance of the clerkship is unquestionable. The pitfalls of the position are compensated by the satisfaction of teaching and nurturing the next generation of physicians, the challenge of continued self-education and maintaining a comprehensive perspective, and the gratification of working with colleagues.

REFERENCES

Abrami PC, d'Apollonia S, Cohen PA: Validity of student ratings of instruction: what we know and what we do not. J Educ Psychol 82:219–231, 1990

Abrams HL, Dralle PW, Wallick MM: Psychiatry clerkships at U.S. medical schools. J Med Educ 62:55–57, 1987

Accreditation Council for Graduate Medical Education: Program Requirements for Residency Training in Psychiatry. Chicago, IL, Accreditation Council for Graduate Medical Education, 2001. Available at: http://www.acgme.org. Accessed June 11, 2004.

Albanese M: Rating educational quality: factors in the erosion of professional standards. Acad Med 74:652–658, 1999

Alexander OL, Davis WK, Yan AC, et al: Keep on tracking: following medical school graduates into practice: residency directors' assessments after the first year of residency. Acad Med 75 (suppl):S15–S17, 2000

Association of American Medical Colleges: Medical Student Graduation Questionnaire (GQ). Washington, DC, Association of American Medical Colleges, 2004. Available at: http://www.aamc.org/gg/start. Accessed June 11, 2004.

Ayers WR, Boulet JR: Establishing the validity of test score inferences: performance of 4th-year U.S. medical students on the ECFMG Clinical Skills Assessment. Teach Learn Med 13:214–220, 2001

Barrows HS, Tamblyn RM: Problem-Based Learning: An Approach to Medical Education. New York, Springer, 1980

Beckman TJ: Lessons learned from a peer review of bedside teaching. Acad Med 79:343–346, 2004

Bellin M, McCarthy S, Drevlow L, et al: Medical students' exposure to pharmaceutical industry marketing: a survey at one U.S. medical school. Acad Med 79:1041–1045, 2004

Brodkey AC: The role of the pharmaceutical industry in teaching psychopharmacology: there is no middle ground. Acad Psychiatry 29:222–229, 2005

Brodkey AC, Sierles FS: Psychiatric clerkships, in Handbook of Psychiatric Education and Faculty Development. Edited by Kay J, Silberman EK, Pessar LF. Washington, DC, American Psychiatric Press, 1999, pp 255–304

Brodkey AC, Van Zant K, Sierles FS: Educational objectives for a junior psychiatry clerkship: development and rationale. Acad Psychiatry 21:179–204, 1997. Available at: http://www.admsep.org/academic.html. Accessed June 11, 2004.

Brodkey AC, Sierles FS, Spertus IL, et al: Clerkship directors' perceptions of the effects of managed care on medical students' education. Acad Med 77:1112–1120, 2002

Burkholder L, Migeon M, Paauw D: Creating a clerkship curriculum, in Internal Medicine Clerkship Guide. Edited by Paauw D, Burkholder L, Migeon M. St Louis, MO, Mosby, 1999

Callahan CA, Erdmann JB, Hojat M, et al: Validity of faculty ratings of students' clinical competence in core clerkships in relation to scores on licensing examinations and supervisors' ratings in residency. Acad Med 75 (suppl):S71–S73, 2000

Carroll JG, Monroe J: Teaching clinical interviewing in the health professions: a review of empirical research. Eval Health Prof 3:21–45, 1980

Case SM, Swanson DB: Constructing Written Test Questions for the Basic and Clinical Sciences, 2nd Edition. Philadelphia, PA, National Board of Medical Examiners, 1998

Case SM, Swanson DB, Becker DF: Verbosity, window dressing and red herrings: do they make a better test item? Acad Med 71 (suppl):S28–S30, 1996

Case SM, Ripkey DR, Swanson DB: The effects of psychiatry clerkship timing and length on measures of performance. Acad Med 10 (suppl):S34–S36, 1997

Clegg KA: Combined clerkships. Paper presented at the annual meeting of the Association of Directors of Medical Student Education in Psychiatry, Jackson Hole, WY, June 14, 2003

Cohen PA: Student ratings of instruction and student achievement: a meta-analysis of multisection validity studies. Review of Educational Research 51:281–309, 1981

Costin F, Greenough WT, Menges RJ: Student ratings of college teaching: reliability, validity and usefulness. Review of Educational Research 41:511–534, 1971

Craig JL: Retention of interviewing skills learned by first-year medical students: a longitudinal study. Med Educ 26:276–281, 1992

Devera-Sales A, Paden C, Vinson DC: What do family medicine patients think about medical students' participation in their health care? Acad Med 74:550–552, 1999

Dielman TE, Hull AL, Davis WK: Psychometric properties of clinical performance ratings. Eval Health Prof 3:103–117, 1980

Edwards JC, Kissling GE, Brannan JR, et al: Study of teaching residents how to teach. J Med Educ 63:603–610, 1988

Ende J, Pozen JT, Levinsky NG: Enhancing learning during a clinical clerkship: the value of a structured curriculum. J Gen Intern Med 1:232–237, 1986

Ferrell BG: Demonstrating the efficacy of the patient logbook as a program evaluation tool. Acad Med 66 (suppl):S49–S50, 1991

Fincher RME: The clerkship director, in Guidebook for Clerkship Directors. Edited by Fincher RME. Washington, DC, Association of American Medical Colleges, 2000a, pp 1–4

Fincher RME (ed): Guidebook for Clerkship Directors. Washington, DC, Association of American Medical Colleges, 2000b

Gay TL, Himle JA, Riba MB: Enhanced ambulatory experience for the clerkship: curricular innovation at the University of Michigan. Acad Psychiatry 26:90–95, 2002

Gold WL, McArdle P, Federman DD: Should medical school faculty see assessments of students made by previous teachers? Acad Med 77:1096–1100, 2002

Goldney RD, McFarlane AC: Assessment in undergraduate psychiatric education. Med Educ 20:117–122, 1986

Greenfield D: Organizing psychiatric training around "firm models." Newsletter of the American Association of Directors of Psychiatry Residency Training, Fall 1995

Griffith CH 3rd, Wilson JF, Haist SA, et al: Relationships of how well attending physicians teach to their students' performances and residency choices. Acad Med 72 (suppl):S118–S120, 1997

Griffith CH 3rd, Wilson JF, Haist SA, et al: Do students who work with better housestaff in their medicine clerkships learn more? Acad Med 73 (suppl):S57–S59, 1998

Gronlund NE: Stating Behavioral Objectives for Classroom Instruction. London, Macmillan, 1970

Hafferty FW, Franks R: The hidden curriculum, ethics teaching and the structure of clinical education. Acad Med 69:861–871, 1994

Hall MJ, Adamo G, McCurry L, et al: Use of standardized patients to enhance a psychiatry clerkship. Acad Med 79:28–31, 2004

Halpern R, Lee MY, Boulter PR, et al: A synthesis of nine major reports on physicians' competencies for the emerging practice environment. Acad Med 76:606–615, 2001

Harden RM, Gleeson FA: Assessment of clinical competence using an objective structured clinical examination. Med Educ 13:41–54, 1979

Hemmer P: Descriptive evaluation, in Guidebook for clerkship directors. Edited by Fincher RME. Washington, DC, Association of American Medical Colleges, 2000, pp 70–147

Hemmer PA, Markert RJ, Wood V: Using in-clerkship tests to identify students with insufficient knowledge and assessing the effect of counseling on final examination performance. Acad Med 74:73–75, 1999

Hodges B: Interactions with the pharmaceutical industry: experiences and attitudes of psychiatry residents, interns, and clerks. CMAJ 153:553–559, 1995

Hodges B, Regehr G, Hanson M, et al: An objective structured clinical examination for evaluating psychiatry clerks. Acad Med 72:715–721, 1997

Hodges B, Hanson M, McNaughton N, et al: Creating, monitoring, and improving a psychiatry OSCE: a guide for faculty. Acad Psychiatry 26:134–161, 2002

Hubbard JP: Measuring Medical Education: The Tests and the Experience of the National Board of Medical Examiners, 2nd Edition. Philadelphia, PA, Lea & Febiger, 1978

Hull AL: Medical student performance: a comparison of house officer and attending staff as evaluators. Eval Health Prof 5:89–94, 1982

Hundert EM, Hafferty F, Christakis D: Characteristics of the informal curriculum and trainees' ethical choices. Acad Med 71:624–633, 1996

Hunt DD, Scott C, Zhong S, et al: Frequency and effect of negative comments ("badmouthing") on medical students' career choices. Acad Med 71:665–669, 1996

Irby DM, Milam S: The legal context for evaluating and dismissing medical students and residents. Acad Med 64:639–643, 1989

Jozefowicz RF, Koeppen BM, Case SM, et al: The quality of in-house medical school examinations. Acad Med 77:156–161, 2002

Kassebaum DG, Eaglen RH, Cutler ER: The objectives of medical education: reflections in the accreditation looking glass. Acad Med 72:647–656, 1997

Katzelnick DJ, Gonzales JJ, Conley MC, et al: Teaching psychiatric residents how to teach. Acad Psychiatry 15:153–159, 1991

Kay J, Silberman EK, Pessar LF (eds): Handbook of Psychiatric Education and Faculty Development. Washington, DC, American Psychiatric Association, 1999

Kessler RC, Berglund PA, Zhao S, et al: The 12-month prevalence and correlates of serious mental illness, in Mental Health, United States, 1996 (DHHS Publ No [SMA] 96-3098). Edited by Manderscheid RW, Sonnenschein MA. Washington DC, U.S. Government Printing Office, 1996, pp 59–70

Konner M: Becoming a Doctor: A Journey of Initiation in Medical School. New York, Viking, 1987

Kuhn TW, Cohen MJM, Polan HJ, et al: Standards for psychiatry clerkship directors. Acad Psychiatry 26:31–37, 2002

Leach DC: A model for GME: shifting from process to outcomes. A progress report from the Accreditation Council for Graduate Medical Education. Med Educ 38:12–14, 2004

Leamon MH, Servis ME, Canning RD, et al: Student and resident evaluations of faculty—how dependable are they? A comparison of student evaluations and faculty peer evaluations of faculty lectures. Acad Med 74 (suppl):S22–S24, 1999

Leamon MH, Fields L, Cox PD, et al: Medical students in jail: the psychiatric clerkship in an outpatient correctional setting. Acad Psychiatry 25:167–172, 2001

Leichner P, Sisler GC, Harper D: A study of the reliability of the clinical oral examination in psychiatry. Can J Psychiatry 29:394–397, 1984

Leichner P, Sisler GC, Harper D: The clinical oral examination in psychiatry: the patient variable. Ann R Coll Physicians Surg Can 19:283–284, 1986

Levine RE, O'Boyle M, Haidet P, et al: Transforming a clinical clerkship with team learning. Teach Learn Med 16:270–275, 2004

Liaison Committee on Medical Education: Functions and Structure of a Medical School: Standards for Accreditation of Medical Education Programs Leading to the M.D. Degree. Washington, DC, Association of American Medical Colleges, 2004. Available at: http://www.lcme.org/functions2004oct.pdf. Accessed June 10, 2005.

Links PS, Foley F, Feltham R: The educational value of student encounter logs in a psychiatry clerkship. Med Teach 10:33–40, 1988

Littlefield JH, Harrington JT, Anthracite NE, et al: A description and four-year analysis of a clinical clerkship evaluation system. J Med Educ 56:334–340, 1981

Litzelman D, Sierles FS, Skeff K, et al: Clerkship evaluation: clinical teachers and program elements, in Guidebook for Clerkship Directors. Edited by Fincher RME. Washington, DC, Association of American Medical Colleges, 2000, pp 148–186

Lofchy J: The clerk crisis clinic: a novel educational program. Acad Psychiatry 27:82–87, 2003

Long DM: Competency-based residency training: the next advance in graduate medical education. Acad Med 75:1178–1183, 2000

Loschen EL: Using the Objective Structured Clinical Examination in a psychiatry residency. Acad Psychiatry 17:95–104, 1993

Loschen EL: The OSCE revisited: use of performance-based evaluation in psychiatric education. Acad Psychiatry 26:202–204, 2002

Luoma JB, Martin CE, Pearson JL: Contact with mental health and primary care providers before suicide: a review of the evidence. Am J Psychiatry 159:909–916, 2002

Magarian GJ: Determining and assigning the grade, in Guidebook for Clerkship Directors. Edited by Fincher RME. Washington, DC, Association of American Medical Colleges, 2000, pp 99–101

McDermott JF Jr, Tanguay PE, Scheiber SC, et al: Reliability of the Part 2 board certification examination in psychiatry: inter-examiner consistency. Am J Psychiatry 148:1672–1674, 1991

Melchiode GA, Puryear DA, Babick M: The emergency room as a clerkship site. Am J Psychiatry 140:894–897, 1983

Metheny WP: Limitations of physician ratings in the assessment of student clinical performance in the obstetrics and gynecology clerkship. Obstet Gynecol 78:136–141, 1991

Monaghan MS, Galt KA, Turner PD, et al. Student understanding of the relationship between the health professions and the pharmaceutical industry. Teach Learn Med 15:14–20, 2003

Murray CJ, Lopez AD (eds): The Global Burden of Disease: A Comprehensive Assessment of Mortality and Disability From Diseases, Injuries, and Risk Factors in 1990 and Projected to 2020. Cambridge, MA, Harvard University Press, 1996

Newble DI, Entwistle NJ: Learning styles and approaches: implications for medical education. Med Educ 20:162–175, 1986

Newble DI, Swanson DB: Psychometric characteristics of the objective structured clinical examination. Med Educ 22:325–334, 1988

Norquist GS, Regier DA: The epidemiology of psychiatric disorders and the de facto mental health care system. Annu Rev Med 47:473–479, 1996

Olson SF: Neurology Clerkship Joint Statement. St. Paul, MN, American Academy of Neurology, March 26, 2004

Pangaro L, Ainsworth M, Albritton TA, et al: Evaluating and grading students, in Guidebook for Clerkship Directors. Edited by Fincher RME. Washington, DC, Association of American Medical Colleges, 2000, pp 70–147

Pangaro L, Bachicha J, Brodkey A, et al: Expectations of and for clerkship directors: a collaborative statement from the Alliance for Clinical Education. Teach Learn Med 15:217–222, 2003

Papadakis MA, Hodgson CS, Teherani A, et al: Unprofessional behavior in medical school is associated with subsequent disciplinary action by a state medical board. Acad Med 79:244–249, 2004

Pessar LF: Ambulatory care teaching in the psychiatry clerkship. Acad Psychiatry 24:61–67, 2000

Phalen S, Magrane D: The clerkship director as manager and change agent, in Guidebook for Clerkship Directors. Edited by Fincher RME. Washington, DC, Association of American Medical Colleges, 2000, pp 201–212

Purdy S, Plasso A, Finkelstein JA, et al: Enrollees' perceptions of participating in the education of medical students at an academically affiliated HMO. Acad Med 75:1003–1009, 2000

Raghoebar-Krieger HMJ, Sleijfer D, Bender W, et al: The reliability of logbook data of medical students: an estimation of inter-observer agreement, sensitivity and specificity. Med Educ 35:624–631, 2001

Regier DA, Farmer ME, Rae DS, et al: One-month prevalence of mental disorders in the United States and sociodemographic characteristics: the Epidemiologic Catchment Area Study. Acta Psychiatr Scand 88:35–47, 1993

Risucci DA, Lutsky L, Rosati RJ, et al: Reliability and accuracy of resident evaluations of surgical faculty. Eval Health Prof 15:313–324, 1992

Robins E, Guze SB: Establishment of diagnostic validity in psychiatric illness: its application to schizophrenia. Am J Psychiatry 126:107–111, 1970

Rosenthal RH, Levine RE, Carlson DL, et al: The "shrinking" clerkship: characteristics and lengths of clerkships in psychiatric undergraduate education. Acad Med 29:47–51, 2005

Sachdeva AK, Blair PG, DaRosa DA: Directing a clerkship over geographically separate sites, in Guidebook for Clerkship Directors. Edited by Fincher RME. Washington, DC, Association of American Medical Colleges, 2000, pp 213–239

Schulz R, Drayer RA, Rollman BL: Depression as a risk factor for non-suicide mortality in the elderly. Biol Psychiatry 52:205–225, 2002

Serby M, Schmeidler J, Smith J: Length of psychiatry clerkships: recent changes and their relationship to recruitment. Acad Psychiatry 26:102–104, 2002

Shem S: The House of God. New York, Dell, 1978

Sierles FS: Medical school factors and career choice of psychiatry. Am J Psychiatry 139:140–142, 1982

Sierles FS, Magrane D: Psychiatry clerkship directors: who they are, what they do, and what they think. Psychiatr Q 67:153–162, 1996

Sierles FS, Taylor MA: Decline in medical student career choice of psychiatry and what to do about it. Am J Psychiatry 152:1416–1426, 1995

Sierles FS, Fichtner CG, Garfield DAS, et al: The "firm model" of patient care and postgraduate and undergraduate training in psychiatry at a Veterans Affairs medical center, in Proceedings of the 48th Institute of Psychiatric Services of the American Psychiatric Association, Chicago, IL, October 18, 1996. Washington, DC, American Psychiatric Association, 1996, p 166

Sierles FS, Daghestani A, Weiner CL, et al: Psychometric properties of ABPN-style oral examinations administered jointly by two psychiatry residencies. Acad Psychiatry 25:214–222, 2001

Sierles FS, Dinwiddie SH, Patroi D, et al: Factors affecting medical student career choice of psychiatry from 1999 to 2001. Acad Psychiatry 27:260–268, 2003a

Sierles FS, Yager J, Weissman SH: Recruitment of U.S. medical graduates into psychiatry: reasons for optimism, sources of concern. Acad Psychiatry 27:260–268, 2003b

Skeff K, Mutha S: Role models—guiding the future of medicine. N Engl J Med 339:2015–2017, 1998

Skochelak S, Albanese M: Teaching strategies and methods, in Guidebook for Clerkship Directors. Edited by Fincher RME. Washington, DC, Association of American Medical Colleges, 2000, pp 44–69

Stagnaro-Green A, Barrett S, Alexis M, et al: Effective implementation of continuous quality improvement methodology to expedite clerkship grade submission. Teach Learn Med 11:34–38, 1999

Stern DT, Williams BC, Gill A, et al: Is there a relationship between attending physicians' and residents' teaching skills and students' examination scores? Acad Med 75:1144–1166, 2000

Stillman RM: Pitfalls in evaluating the surgical student. Surgery 96:92–95, 1984

Tonesk X: Clinical judgment of faculties in the evaluation of clerks. J Med Educ 58:213–214, 1983

Tonesk X: AAMC program to promote improved evaluation of students during clinical education. J Med Educ 61(9 Pt 2):83–88, 1986

Tremonti LP, Biddle WB: Teaching behaviors of residents and faculty members. J Med Educ 57:854–859, 1982

U.S. Department of Health and Human Services: Mental Health: A Report of the Surgeon General. Rockville, MD, Substance Abuse and Mental Health Services Administration, Center for Mental Health Services, 1999

Whitman NA: A Handbook for Group Discussion Leaders: Alternatives to Lecturing Medical Students to Death. Salt Lake City, University of Utah School of Medicine, 1982a

Whitman NA: There Is No Gene for Good Teaching: A Handbook on Lecturing for Medical Teachers. Salt Lake City, University of Utah School of Medicine, 1982b

Wilkerson L, Feletti G: Problem-based learning: one approach to increasing student participation, in The Department Chairperson's Role in Enhancing College Teaching (New Directions for Teaching and Learning, No 27). Edited by Lusas A. San Francisco, CA, Jossey-Bass, 1989, pp 51–60

Withy K: An inexpensive patient-encounter log. Acad Med 76:860–862, 2001

Young AS, Klap R, Sherbourne CD, et al: The quality of care for depressive and anxiety disorders in the United States. Arch Gen Psychiatry 58:55–61, 2001

APPENDIX 2–A

MEDICAL STUDENT INTERVIEW EVALUATION FORM

Modified from Brodkey AC, Sierles FS: "Psychiatric Clerkships," in *Handbook of Psychiatric Education and Faculty Development.* Edited by Kay J, Silberman EK, Pessar LF. Washington, DC, American Psychiatric Press, 1999, pp. 256–257.

Student: _____   Date: _____

Instructor (signature): _____

	Yes	No
In beginning the interview, did the student		
Introduce himself/herself appropriately?	❏	❏
Explain why he/she was here?	❏	❏
Elicit patient concerns regarding the purpose of the interview, privacy, and physical comfort?	❏	❏
Establish rapport by asking the patient about himself/herself?	❏	❏
In the initial phase of the interview, did the student	❏	❏
Allow the patient to tell his/her story of the present illness?	❏	❏
Use open-ended questions?	❏	❏
Use the patient's statements to guide the flow of the interview?	❏	❏
During the interview, did the student appropriately utilize		
Nonverbal communications?	❏	❏
Facilitating, supportive, and empathic comments?	❏	❏
Interviewer silence?	❏	❏
Acknowledgment and acceptance of the patient's feelings?	❏	❏
Appropriate reassurance?	❏	❏
Summary statements?	❏	❏
Open- and close-ended questions?	❏	❏
Confrontation and clarification?	❏	❏
The patient's own words (and clarify their meanings)?	❏	❏
Techniques to structure hyperverbal patients?	❏	❏
Techniques for asking difficult/embarrassing questions?	❏	❏
During the interview, did the student avoid		
Interrupting the patient inappropriately?	❏	❏
Asking long, complex questions?	❏	❏
Asking questions suggesting the answer that he/she wanted?	❏	❏

	Yes	No
Asking directive or yes/no questions too early or too often (interrogation-like manner)?	❏	❏
Sudden, inappropriate changes of topic?	❏	❏
Asking the patient for information that he/she had already provided?	❏	❏
Using jargon?	❏	❏
Judgmental, patronizing, overly familiar, disdainful, or otherwise unprofessional attitudes?	❏	❏

In ending the interview, did the student

Indicate a few minutes ahead that the interview was going to end?	❏	❏
Provide feedback and summation and inform the patient about what's next?	❏	❏
Ask whether the patient had anything further to mention?	❏	❏

In general, did the student

Follow up verbal and nonverbal leads offered by the patient?	❏	❏
Handle emotionally laden material well?	❏	❏
Communicate ideas clearly?	❏	❏
Delineate the psychosocial setting associated with onset or exacerbation of the illness?	❏	❏
Demonstrate respect, concern, empathy, sensitivity, and responsiveness?	❏	❏
Identify and analyze strengths and weaknesses in his/her own interviewing skills?	❏	❏

History, mental status exam, and diagnosis: Did the student demonstrate

Familiarity with the symptoms commonly associated with the patient's condition?	❏	❏
The ability to elicit necessary and relevant historical data, including the chief complaint, history of the present illness, and past personal and psychiatric history?	❏	❏
An understanding of the key features of the mental status exam, including the cognitive exam?	❏	❏
The ability to reason clinically from the data to a differential diagnosis and plan of assessment and treatment?	❏	❏

How difficult was the patient to interview? (circle one)

Very easy	Easy	Moderately hard	Hard	Very hard

Overall rating of the interview (circle one)

Outstanding	Good	Adequate	Inadequate

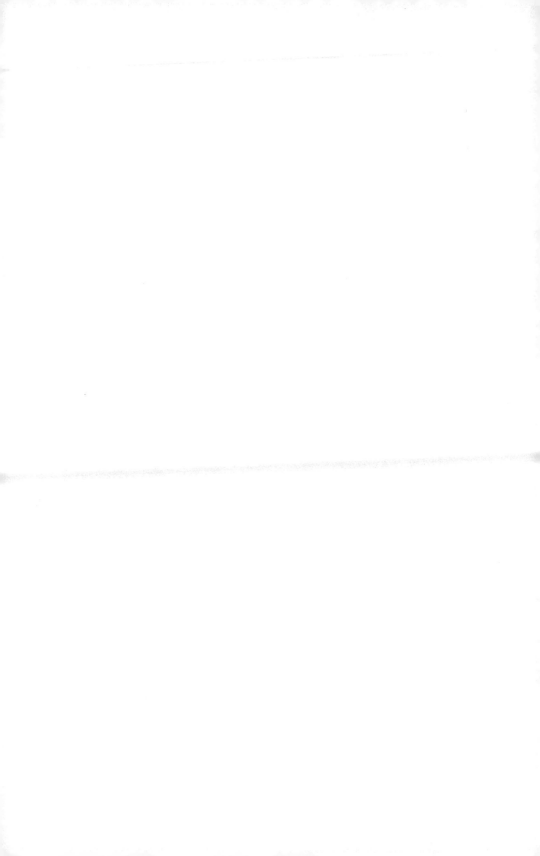

CHAPTER 3

UNDERGRADUATE ELECTIVES

Theodore B. Feldmann, M.D.

This chapter focuses on the importance of psychiatric electives and other educational programs in medical school education. These activities complement the required core curriculum and help to stimulate student interest in psychiatry. The development and implementation of these programs are discussed, and guidelines for their creation are presented.

Curriculum reform is occurring at many medical schools. Core basic science courses are increasingly being replaced by multidisciplinary courses with significant independent study components. Psychiatry clerkships are also being modified at many schools. In some instances clerkship length is being decreased, whereas in others combined psychiatry and neurology rotations are being created.

Given the changes occurring in the required psychiatry curriculum, why is it important for psychiatric educators to develop medical student electives and other special activities? The answer to this question lies in an examination of the characteristics of successful medical student programs in psychiatry (Table 3–1). These programs all share certain characteristics (Feldmann 1994). Obviously, curriculum strength is essential. The quality and variety of teaching programs enable students to gain a positive view of psychiatry as a medical specialty and career choice. All courses must have a strong clinical emphasis, accentuating what psychiatrists do with patients. As a result, students get a realistic view of psychiatry that helps to overcome

TABLE 3–1.   Characteristics of successful medical student programs in psychiatry

A strong core curriculum
Commitment to education
Diversity of educational experiences
High visibility within the medical school
Aggressive outreach to students
Projection of a positive view of psychiatry
An emphasis on what psychiatrists do
Personalized contacts and mentoring
Tracking of interested students
Special activities for students

the stigma of mental illness and the students' discomfort with emotional and behavioral problems. The hands-on experience that students receive increases their awareness of the effectiveness of psychiatric therapies. The importance of seeing psychiatrists every day cannot be underestimated in terms of shaping students' attitudes about psychiatry as a viable medical specialty. Thus, maintaining a high visibility within the medical school is also important. This in turn creates an atmosphere in which students feel they have access to the department. The result is that personalized contacts and mentoring relationships are established. When students are identified as having an interest in psychiatry, an aggressive outreach to them helps to solidify their commitment. The tracking of interested students may make a difference in their career choices. Although these areas overlap to a great degree, the common thread is that students gain an in-depth exposure to psychiatric educators not just as teachers but as people who are interested in their well-being and professional future.

The development of high-quality electives and special programs allows psychiatry departments to address many of the areas listed above. One of the greatest strengths of psychiatry is its diversity. Unfortunately, it is often difficult to present this diversity to students within the constraints of pre-clinical core courses and clerkships with limited time. The development of electives and other special programs helps students to gain a better appreciation of the field. This in turn heightens students' educational experience and improves the perception of psychiatry. Thus the goals of both education and recruitment are fostered (Weissman 1993).

Support for psychiatric education must literally come from the top. It is therefore essential that the department chair establish an environment

TABLE 3–2.   Roles of the director of medical student education

Determines the educational philosophy of the medical student curriculum

Organizes and coordinates the curriculum

Balances student needs versus educational needs (i.e., makes sure the curriculum is both student friendly and academically sound)

Works with residency training director on recruitment issues

Acts as liaison between students and the department

conducive to and supportive of psychiatric education. This support encompasses much more than simply encouraging faculty and residents to teach students. The chair must also be willing to actively participate in student teaching and other special activities (Pardes 1989). An example is Chair's Rounds, a regularly scheduled activity during the clerkship in which the chair meets with students for a case conference and discussion. The chair should also be available to talk with students who are interested in psychiatry. Taking the time to meet with students makes a powerful impression and often makes a critical difference in recruitment.

A key person in the development of a quality program is the director of medical student education (Table 3–2). This is the person who sets the overall tone for the psychiatric medical student curriculum. He or she is also the person who has the most consistent contact with medical students. This person must be dynamic, outgoing, and able to foster an atmosphere in which students feel comfortable coming forward with their educational and career concerns. It is also imperative that this person possess the organizational skills required to develop and implement a high-quality curriculum.

Another important person in the medical student curriculum is the residency training director. As emphasized earlier, as more senior faculty are involved in teaching, students come to see them as mentors and role models. This evaluation enhances the perception of psychiatry as a vibrant and expanding specialty and also projects the image of psychiatrists as being concerned about medical education. Involvement of the residency training director in teaching activities serves two additional functions. Students who are interested in psychiatry will naturally have many questions about residency programs. The training director is in the best position to provide information that is useful to students. At the same time, direct contact with students allows the residency director to get to know the students who wish to pursue psychiatric training. It also gives the training director an opportunity to identify and track students who display an aptitude for psychiatry.

It is essential that the residency training director and the director of medical student education work together closely. These two positions have much in common, but they often work in isolation due to time constraints, pressure for clinical service, or "turf" issues. When this occurs, the department chair should intervene to maximize communication and cooperation between the two offices.

Finally, the importance of the involvement of residents in student teaching cannot be underestimated. Residents often get to know medical students before faculty members do. The common bond between residents and students of being in training often allows students to feel more comfortable approaching residents about academic or career issues. There is also less formality between residents and students, leading to more of a peer relationship. Therefore, residents are a tremendous asset in the recruitment of medical students into psychiatry. As such, departments should actively encourage teaching by residents and should provide the training and resources (e.g., the American Psychiatric Association (2002) pamphlet "Psychiatric Residents as Teachers: A Practical Guide") necessary for residents' involvement.

DEVELOPMENT OF ELECTIVES IN PSYCHIATRY

Diversity of educational experiences is an important component in the overall quality of a psychiatric curriculum. Although the preclinical core courses and the third-year clerkship form the foundation of a department's educational programs, electives also play an important role. Electives serve several important functions. First, they increase students' awareness of the diverse nature of the specialty. Electives also expose students to specialized areas of psychiatry that are not necessarily covered in core courses. Furthermore, electives allow students to pursue study in their own areas of special interest. They foster creativity in education through nontraditional methods of instruction. Finally, electives allow for an interface between psychiatry and other clinical specialties; examples include behavioral medicine electives taught jointly by psychiatrists and family physicians, and consultation-liaison rotations.

Although there is considerable variability in curriculum structure from one medical school to another, most schools in the United States offer elective time at both the preclinical and clinical levels. A variety of strong courses aimed at students through all four years of medical school will increase the overall quality of the curriculum. The goal, once again, is to

TABLE 3–3. Concerns of preclinical students

Passing required courses
Adjusting to the medical school environment
Developing new study habits
Forming and maintaining peer relationships
Developing a professional identity

provide students with the broadest possible exposure to psychiatric issues and practice. This in turn will contribute to increased interest in psychiatry and may result in increased recruitment into psychiatry residency programs (Weintraub et al. 1996).

PRECLINICAL ELECTIVES

The target audience for preclinical electives consists of first- and second-year medical students. To develop electives for this group, it is necessary to understand the unique needs of preclinical students (Table 3–3). One of the most important concerns for students at this level is mastery of the extensive basic science material presented in the core curriculum. Another involves adjusting to life in medical school and the pressures that go along with medical education. Medical school is quite different from college; to be successful, students must adjust to these differences. The development of a strong peer support system is essential for students to achieve academic success. Beginning students also struggle with identity issues in becoming a physician. Finally, each student begins his or her medical education with unique individual and interpersonal issues. These personal variables must be acknowledged and addressed for the student to maximize the educational experience.

With these needs and concerns in mind, it is possible to identify three broad categories of preclinical psychiatric electives: 1) those that integrate psychiatry into the basic sciences, 2) courses presenting an introduction to clinical psychiatry, and 3) examinations of lifestyle issues that influence health and illness (Table 3–4). Electives can easily be developed to address each of these areas.

TABLE 3–4. Categories of preclinical electives

Basic science correlation
Clinical and professional issues
Interpersonal issues in health

TABLE 3–5.   Sample electives to integrate basic science

The Brain and Behavior: Clinical Neuroscience
Research Advances in Psychiatry
Behavioral Medicine: The Mind-Body Connection

Two areas of psychiatry lend themselves particularly well to the interface of psychiatry and basic science: neuroscience and behavioral medicine (Table 3–5). Many schools now have clinical neuroscience courses as part of the core curriculum. Although they are valuable educational experiences, these courses often present a large volume of material in relatively short time frames. Students may have difficulty absorbing this material and also feel pressure to pass a core course. Electives in neuroscience allow students to examine this material in depth in a more relaxed environment. These elective courses help to integrate basic science material such as anatomy, biochemistry, and pharmacology into a clinical framework. Given the tremendous advances in current knowledge of the brain and behavior, neuroscience electives provide an exciting and stimulating environment in which students can apply their basic science knowledge to clinical situations. Behavioral medicine electives facilitate a better understanding of the interaction of anatomy, physiology, and pathology in disease processes. Health and wellness issues are also emphasized through behavioral medicine.

Electives focusing on an introduction to clinical psychiatry serve a variety of functions (Table 3–6). They help students to view psychiatrists as physician mentors and role models, clinicians, and medical specialists. In addition, they contribute to the development of students' professional identity as physicians. Not only do these courses provide introductory clinical material, they also give students a better understanding of what psychiatrists do. Examples include electives on the physician-patient relationship, courses focusing on clinical issues (e.g., depression), and courses on subspecialty areas such as child development and forensic psychiatry.

TABLE 3–6.   Electives introducing clinical issues

The Doctor–Patient Relationship
Advanced Interviewing Skills
Acquired Immunodeficiency Syndrome (AIDS) and the Health Care Provider
Behavioral Science and the Law

TABLE 3–7. Electives dealing with lifestyle issues

Physicians and the Arts
Health Awareness Workshop
The Psychology of Women and Men
Substance Abuse

Perhaps the most diverse and creative electives are those related to lifestyle issues (Table 3–7). These electives are more likely to address the personal concerns or interests of students. Included in this group are stress management courses, electives dealing with human immunodeficiency virus (HIV) and acquired immunodeficiency syndrome (AIDS), social and cultural issues in medical practice, the psychology of women and men, and substance abuse. Students should also be encouraged to pursue their own creative interests during medical school. At the University of Louisville, for example, an elective called "Physicians and the Arts" allows students to develop special projects based on their own personal and creative interests.

Special Considerations in Preclinical Electives

A number of elements must be taken into consideration in the development of preclinical electives. These include course structure, evaluation, faculty recruitment, and involvement of residents.

The traditional lecture or seminar format can be applied to any preclinical elective. It must be remembered, however, that these formats are how most basic science courses are taught. Students often look for something different in their electives. An innovative approach, then, may make an elective more attractive. Small-group discussions of preassigned readings; problem-based learning exercises; preceptorships in clinical settings; and independent study, research, or computer-based learning are some of the alternative instructional methods that can be utilized.

The evaluation of student performance in preclinical electives is often problematic. The most important initial consideration is the fact that these courses are electives. Students view them quite differently than the core courses. Course requirements and evaluation procedures must be set up with more flexibility than those of the core courses. Faculty members must also be aware of the pressure and time constraints of the core curriculum. The bottom line is that students will not sign up for electives that are perceived as being too intense or time-consuming compared with the core courses. Although all educators like to think that their courses are the most important, that is an extremely unrealistic view. It also demonstrates a lack of empathy with the students' experience.

With these considerations in mind, the instructor must find inventive methods of evaluation, preferably those that involve the active participation of the student. Final examinations are to be discouraged. Student evaluations can be based on completion of a special project, independent study program, brief research paper, learning objective checklist, experiential report, or other evaluation instrument (Kay 1981). Self-evaluation by students is another useful method. Again, the more creative the evaluation methodology, the greater the overall educational experience. Whatever method is chosen, however, it should be remembered that electives have a relatively low priority for students compared with anatomy, physiology, and other major courses.

Faculty Recruitment for Electives

Recruitment of faculty to teach electives usually occurs in one of two ways. Most often, individual faculty members submit proposals for electives based on their particular academic interests. At other times, the director of medical student education or the department's education committee may identify a particular educational need. Faculty members are then recruited to develop the course. Regardless of the method, however, the essential requirements are that the instructor be enthusiastic and committed to developing a top-flight course. A dynamic and charismatic teacher can often make the difference between the success and failure of an elective. Clearly, someone who simply lectures and does not attempt to actively engage students will not attract a great deal of interest. Students expect to have fun in electives in addition to acquiring a body of knowledge or skills. With that in mind, it is important to remember one of the cardinal rules of good teaching: *Whatever you do, don't be boring!*

CLINICAL ELECTIVES

At most medical schools, students take clinical electives during the fourth year. These students have very different concerns than their preclinical colleagues. Most senior students select electives to broaden their clinical knowledge base in a specific area. Others look for rotations that will help them to clarify their career choice. Finally, there are many students who want to pursue areas of special interest regardless of residency plans. Clinical electives should be developed with sufficient diversity to meet the needs of all three groups (Table 3–8).

Most clinical electives are composed of intensive clinical experiences, such as adult inpatient, outpatient, consultation-liaison, or emergency psychiatry. Specialized rotations may also be developed, including rotations in child, adolescent, or forensic psychiatry. Each of these areas gives students

TABLE 3–8. Key elements of clinical electives

Diversity of clinical settings
Exposure to subspecialties
"Acting-intern" level of responsibility
Intensive supervision

an in-depth look at psychiatry, helps to clarify career goals, and acquaints students with what a psychiatry residency is really like.

In addition to clinical electives in traditional academic settings, a wide range of alternative practice environments should be included (Table 3–9). Medicine is increasingly moving away from the traditional hospital-based practice. Today's students will find themselves working more in ambulatory care settings, in rural and underserved areas, in community psychiatry, and in managed care (Gabbard 1992). Therefore, electives with private psychiatrists or in rural mental health clinics, for example, are useful in broadening the training experiences of the students. Finally, electives combining two or more clinical activities, such as emergency psychiatry and consultation-liaison psychiatry, are effective in maximizing the student's educational experience.

Successful clinical electives incorporate a high degree of clinical responsibility coupled with intensive supervision. Senior students should be expected to perform at an acting-intern level. They should also participate in seminars and case conferences along with first-year residents. This added level of responsibility not only challenges students to acquire advanced clinical skills but also helps students entering psychiatry residencies to get a head start on the first postgraduate year. Supervision must be available on two levels: daily clinical supervision and regular process supervision. The latter form, ideally occurring twice a week throughout the rotation, allows for more in-depth examination of psychodynamic issues and also provides an opportunity for the student to reflect on his or her experience with patients.

TABLE 3–9. Examples of clinical electives

Advanced inpatient rotations
Child psychiatry
Ambulatory care electives
Rotations in community mental health centers
Forensic psychiatry
Rotations in rural or underserved areas
Combined clinical rotations

Evaluation of student performance is generally done according to a standardized instrument used by the medical school. Additional feedback from supervisors about strengths and weaknesses is invaluable for senior students. The fourth year of medical school is really a transitional period bridging the gap between required medical school courses and residency. An open and candid relationship with supervisors is important in maximizing the educational benefit of the elective. An alternative and useful evaluation tool involves having the student keep a daily log of patient encounters, psychodynamic impressions, and general observations. The contents of the log will often serve as a useful discussion point for process-oriented supervision. If the elective involves research work, a brief summary paper also provides an effective evaluation method.

A final type of clinical elective is the senior honors program in psychiatry. This format has been used by other specialties, particularly surgery, to provide in-depth clinical experience for senior students. These programs are generally longer (e.g., 8–12 weeks) and more intensive than other clinical electives and are designed primarily for students who are interested in pursuing academic careers. A variety of formats can be utilized in developing honors programs. One method involves designating two tracks for the rotation: clinical and research. The student then chooses one track in consultation with the faculty advisor or program director. The clinical track involves more extensive responsibility and supervision than other electives, whereas the research track allows the student to work on established research with a faculty member or develop research activities suited to the student's particular interest. The honors program ideally is a selective rather than an elective course, with the director of medical student education interviewing students to determine their suitability for the rotation. Honors programs are exciting ways for students interested in psychiatry to prepare for residency training.

PARTICIPATION IN MULTIDISCIPLINARY COURSES

Multidisciplinary courses are being developed with increasing frequency at medical schools across the country. Many of these courses are part of the core curriculum at both preclinical and clinical levels. These courses also provide interesting and unique elective experiences for medical students. Regardless of whether these courses are part of the core or elective curriculum, they offer both rewards and challenges for psychiatric educators.

There are a number of benefits to be derived from participation in multidisciplinary electives. First, the visibility of psychiatry to students and within the medical school is increased. As a result of psychiatrists' work in these courses, students gain a better understanding of what psychiatrists do.

By working with other specialties such as neurology or primary care, psychiatrists are seen as practitioners of an important medical specialty rather than of a remote or esoteric profession. Multidisciplinary electives bring unique resources and expertise to the curriculum that cannot be provided by a single department.

Multidisciplinary electives can include specialized neuroscience courses. Courses of this type may be preclinical, research based, or clinical. Another example is outpatient consultation to primary care or specialty clinics. This activity differs from traditional hospital-based consultation-liaison rotations because it occurs in an ambulatory care setting (a major area of emphasis in medical schools).

Despite the positive features associated with multidisciplinary electives, several problems or difficulties may be encountered. To achieve success, the departments involved in these courses must have common goals. It is essential to identify what students should learn from the experience. Educational goals and learning objectives must be carefully prepared before the course begins. All participating departments must play equal roles in teaching and administration. The course director, regardless of the department he or she represents, is responsible for ensuring that the educational needs of the students take precedence over the needs of any particular department. The course director must also work closely with all faculty and departments to prevent departmental turf issues or biases from interfering with the educational mission of the course. Core faculty in each department must be identified; these faculty members must be willing to work together and share in responsibility for the success of the course.

Whether multidisciplinary courses are part of the core or the elective curriculum, their development and implementation are labor intensive. When designed in a thoughtful and innovative manner, however, they are extremely rewarding for faculty and students alike.

SPECIAL ACTIVITIES FOR MEDICAL STUDENTS

Although the academic curriculum constitutes the most important facet of the medical student program in psychiatry, a number of other activities can be developed to give the specialty greater exposure. There are two major objectives of these special activities. The first is to provide students with a better understanding of what psychiatry is, free of the constraints of traditional academic courses. A second, related outcome is to increase recruitment. Although there is always tension between education and recruitment—and many psychiatric educators feel that recruitment is unrelated to education—it is nevertheless naive to think that these areas are mutually exclusive. The survival of psychiatry depends not only on educating physicians but also on recruiting the best medical students into the ranks of the specialty.

PSYCHIATRY CLUBS

The campus psychiatry club is an organization for medical students who have an interest in psychiatry, psychology, mental health issues, or human behavior (Kay 1984). Such clubs generally have monthly meetings during which presentations or panel discussions on important issues in psychiatry are held. Meetings should be informal and open to any students wishing to attend; students should be told that interest in a psychiatric career is not a prerequisite for participation. Food and soft drinks are usually served at each meeting.

The club serves as a source of information for students who are interested in psychiatry as a career or for students who simply have an interest in the study of human behavior. It also functions to assist students in learning more about psychiatry and provides an opportunity to become acquainted with faculty members and residents. The emphasis of the club is collegial, with frequent social events designed to acquaint students with the department. New friendships and lasting professional relationships will be one result of membership in the club. A newsletter can also be published every month or whenever there is important news or information about the club or the department. Computer technology can be utilized to create a Web page or e-mail list for students participating in the club.

A faculty member who is responsible for all of the group's activities initially organizes the club. Active participation by residents should also be encouraged. Eventually, however, students must be encouraged to take ownership of the group, including the election of student officers or the creation of a steering committee to oversee activities. It must be remembered that a successful psychiatry club requires a great deal of nurturing by the department. The demands on medical students for time are very great; therefore, the faculty advisor must be willing to make a commitment to keep the club going even if student interest is slow to develop.

HEALTH AWARENESS WEEK: THE UNIVERSITY OF LOUISVILLE PROGRAM

A unique student activity, the Health Awareness Week, was developed by Joel Elkes and Leah Dickstein at the University of Louisville (Dickstein and Elkes 1987). Although the founders of this program have retired, it remains a central component of the medical school's orientation for first-year students. The program consists of a week-long series of events designed to assist students in making the transition to medical school. Programs are aimed at maintaining a healthy lifestyle while dealing with the rigors of medical school, managing stress effectively, developing effective study habits, and initiating the development of a professional identity. Many social activities are also planned for students and their spouses or partners. These facilitate the acquisition of a strong social support system. Community outings are held to familiarize students with the city. Included are trips to the zoo, picnics, a riverboat cruise, and exposure to the area's cultural and recreational activities. The final day of Health Awareness Week includes the formal medical school orientation. Thus, first-year students receive exposure to psychiatry from the first day of medical school.

A great many faculty members and residents are involved in this activity. One of the unique aspects of the program, however, is that second-year students help to coordinate and organize most of the events. They thus serve as mentors who share their own experiences and insights into medical school. Each freshman unit lab of approximately 16 students is assigned 2 second-year advisors along with 2 faculty advisors. Regular contact is maintained throughout the academic year by monthly lunches with each unit lab. This ongoing contact helps to ensure that first-year students feel supported and serves to diminish feelings of isolation.

LITERATURE AND FILM SEMINARS

Another interesting and useful type of activity is literature or film seminars focusing on medicine-related themes (Fritz and Poe 1979; Schneider 1977; Sondheimer 1994). These sessions may utilize a variety of sources—including films, novels, short stories, or plays—to illustrate behavioral, affective, or cognitive aspects of human behavior. For example, the film *The Doctor* is a useful vehicle for exploring reactions to illness as well as issues of empathy and physician sensitivity. The story focuses on a physician, played by William Hurt, who develops throat cancer. As a result of his own experiences, the doctor learns much about illness and what it is like to be a patient. There are countless literary and cinematic works that lend themselves to this type of seminar. The seminar can be offered either as an elective for academic credit or as a department-wide activity. Faculty facilitators may be chosen to lead the group discussion, or outside speakers from other departments (e.g., drama) or local theatrical companies may be invited to participate. Sessions may be held on campus or at faculty members' homes. The overall goal is to stimulate thought and discussion about human behavior in a nontraditional format while also fostering a sense of camaraderie and collegiality between students and the department.

STUDENT PARTICIPATION IN DEPARTMENTAL FUNCTIONS

A relatively easy, yet important, component of a psychiatric curriculum for medical students involves inviting them to special departmental activities. These include parties, picnics, grand rounds, journal clubs, and special seminars or conferences (Yager et al. 1991). For the latter two activities, students should be offered a reduced registration fee or, ideally, the fee should be waived completely. Doing this allows students with an interest in psychiatry to maintain contact with the department. This type of outreach is very important, but it is one that psychiatrists have been slow to adopt. Other specialties, such as surgery, have been much more aggressive in identifying potential residents early in medical school and then linking them up with faculty in an ongoing way throughout medical school. Announcements of special activities can be made in the psychiatry club newsletter, by the director of medical student education, from the chair's office, or on the department's Web site.

UTILIZING THE AMERICAN PSYCHIATRIC ASSOCIATION

Finally, resources from the American Psychiatric Association (APA) should be utilized and made available to medical students. The benefits of student membership in the APA should be explained at psychiatry club meetings, in behavioral science courses, and at the beginning of each clerkship. Membership forms can easily be distributed to all interested students. The APA Office of Education is also an important resource for educational materials or information about careers in psychiatry. Coordination of special seminars or activities with the APA district branch is another useful activity. Mentoring programs, for example, connect interested students with psychiatrists in the community and give students a different perspective about psychiatric practice outside an academic environment.

SUMMARY

A comprehensive program of medical student electives in psychiatry, coupled with special activities such as a psychiatry club, greatly increases the strength of a department's curriculum. Students come to see psychiatry as a diverse and vibrant specialty and gain a greater appreciation of the psychiatrist's role as a physician. Students entering psychiatry residencies also have a greater knowledge base as a result of elective experiences. Finally, diverse exposure to the field stimulates student interest in psychiatry, ultimately fostering recruitment efforts.

REFERENCES

American Psychiatric Association, Committee on Graduate Medical Education 2001–2002: Psychiatric Residents as Teachers: A Practical Guide (2nd Revision 4/02). Washington, DC, American Psychiatric Association, 2002 (also available at: http://www.psych.org/edu/res_fellows/psychresidentguide.pdf)

Dickstein L, Elkes J: Extraordinary program prepares students for stresses of medical school. Psychiatric Times 4(6):24, 1987

Feldmann TB: The generalist initiatives: a challenge for psychiatric educators. Association of Directors of Medical Student Education in Psychiatry Newsletter 6(1):3–4, 1994

Fritz GK, Poe RO: The role of a cinema seminar in psychiatric education. Am J Psychiatry 136:207–210, 1979

Gabbard GO: The big chill: the transition from residency to managed care nightmare. Acad Psychiatry 16:119–126, 1992

Kay J: The independent psychiatry project: a model exercise in student learning. J Med Educ 56:347–351, 1981

Kay J: The psychiatry club: enhancing career choice of psychiatry. J Med Educ 59:62–63, 1984

Pardes H: Educating psychiatrists for the 1990s. Acad Psychiatry 13:3–12, 1989

Schneider I: Images of the mind: psychiatry in the commercial film. Am J Psychiatry 134:613–620, 1977

Sondheimer A: The literature and medicine seminar for medical students: a potential recruitment tool. Acad Psychiatry 18:38–41, 1994

Weintraub W, Plaut SM, Weintraub E: Medical school electives and recruitment into psychiatry: a 20-year experience. Acad Psychiatry 20:220–225, 1996

Weissman SH: Recommendations from the May 1992 conference to enhance recruitment of U.S. medical graduates into psychiatry. Acad Psychiatry 17:180–185, 1993

Yager J, Linn LS, Winstead DK, et al: Characteristics of journal clubs in psychiatric training. Acad Psychiatry 15:18–32, 1991

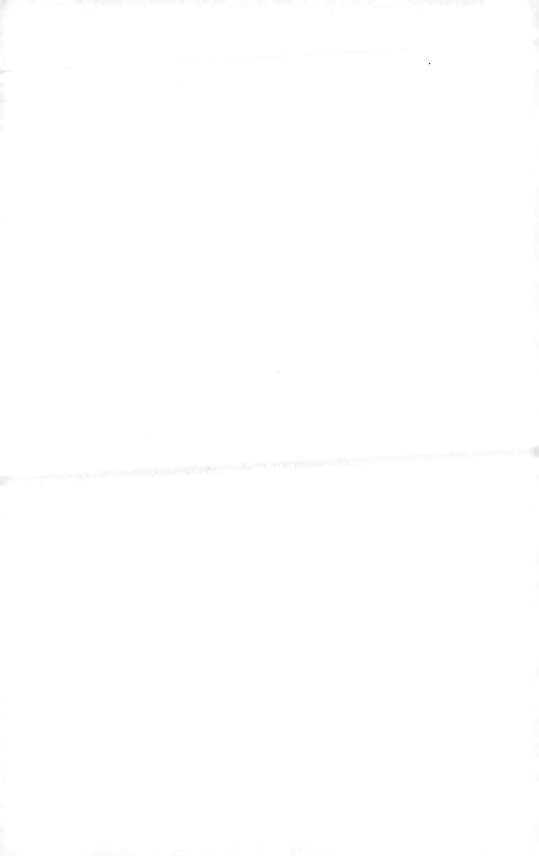

CHAPTER 4

EVALUATION OF STUDENTS

Bryce Templeton, M.D., M.Ed.

DEVELOPING AN EVALUATION PROGRAM

After determining programmatic objectives and designing a curriculum, the instructor's next task is to develop an evaluation program. The goals of the evaluation program involve both assessing student progress and also determining the effectiveness of the training program. Recommendations regarding evaluating student progress are outlined in this chapter.

An effective evaluation program must be linked to the educational objectives. Educators have spent considerable effort in attempting to create some structure or outline for objectives. Important outcomes of these efforts have included a system involving three *taxonomies* or *domains:* a cognitive domain (e.g., knowledge, problem solving), an affective domain (primarily focusing on attitudinal changes), and a less well-developed psychomotor domain (e.g., a woodworker's or sculptor's skills, driving and flying skills, surgical skills). For application to medical education, these domains have been slightly altered as follows: knowledge, problem-solving ability, technical skills (a combination of cognitive and psychomotor skills, such as the performance of a physical examination), interpersonal skills, and day-to-day performance (which includes attitudinal and related performance outcomes). Each of these terms has been operationally defined (Templeton 1980).

In the case of medical education, another important dimension concerns a series of physician tasks that include obtaining a history, conducting a physical examination (including mental status assessment), ordering and interpreting ancillary studies, developing diagnostic hypotheses, planning a course of treatment, and following a course of patient management.

The design of an effective and comprehensive evaluation program can be achieved by creating a two-dimensional matrix with the above domains on one axis and the list of physician tasks on another axis. Table 4–1 illustrates such an approach (Templeton and Selarnick 1994). The rows contain the list of physician tasks that are applicable to most clinical specialties. The columns represent the medically applicable modification of the cognitive–affective–psychomotor division of educational objectives.

Knowledge and problem-solving skills are most efficiently assessed with written examinations; problem-solving skills in this context refer to analyses of clinical vignettes to assess diagnostic and management skills. Psychiatry has few if any technical skills in terms of attributes having a strong psychomotor component (e.g., examining the fundus of the eye, utilizing an endoscope, or performing surgical tasks). The evaluation of interpersonal skills such as interviewing technique typically requires the time-consuming observation of students by experienced clinicians and therefore is expensive to conduct. Work habits and attitudes are best assessed by day-to-day observation of student performance on inpatient and ambulatory settings in a student's work with patients, their families, faculty, residents, and other staff.

CONCEPTS AND TERMINOLOGY

In discussing evaluation procedures, there are a number of useful terms (Thorndike 1971). For example, *formative evaluation* refers to ongoing assessments that are typically used to help guide the trainee and/or the course director such as in the use of mid-clerkship reviews of a student's progress. By contrast, *summative evaluation* is designed to make major decisions about a student—for example, the determination of readiness for progression from one year to the next or for receiving a license to practice. Quizzes may be used as part of summative assessment, if the scores are incorporated into the course grade, or as a formative assessment if they are not so incorporated.

Reliability

Another set of terms concerns reliability and validity. *Reliability* is essentially the reproducibility of a measurement and is usually specified as a correlation coefficient ranging from 1.0 (perfect correlation) to 0.0 (random correlation) to −1.0 (extreme negative correlation). Thus, if a written exam were to have a reliability of 1.0, giving the same exam to a student 2 or 3 weeks later would result in an identical score. Interrater reliability is used

TABLE 4–1. Task and abilities matrix: a program of medical student evaluation

Tasks	Knowledge and understanding	Problem solving and judgment	Technical skills	Interpersonal skills	Work habits and attitudes
Taking a history	Intramural exams & Steps 1 & 2	Intramural exams & Steps 1 & 2	NA	OSCEs or other direct observation	Attending and resident ratings
Performing physical and mental status examinations	Intramural exams & Steps 1 & 2	Intramural exams & Steps 1 & 2	NA	NA	Attending and resident ratings
Using diagnostic aids	Intramural exams & Steps 1 & 2	Intramural exams & Steps 1 & 2	NA	NA	Attending and resident ratings
Defining problems	Intramural exams & Steps 1 & 2	Intramural exams & Steps 1 & 2	NA	NA	Attending and resident ratings
Managing therapy	Intramural exams & Steps 1 & 2	Intramural exams & Steps 1 & 2	NA	OSCEs or other direct observation	Attending and resident ratings
Keeping records	Intramural exams & Steps 1 & 2	Intramural exams & Steps 1 & 2	NA	NA	Attending and resident ratings
Employing special sources of information	Intramural exams & Steps 1 & 2	Intramural exams & Steps 1 & 2	NA	NA	Attending and resident ratings
Monitoring patient care	Intramural exams & Steps 1 & 2	Intramural exams & Steps 1 & 2	NA	OSCEs or other direct observation	Attending and resident ratings

Note. NA=not applicable; OSCE=objective structured clinical examination.

in discussing observers' judgments about performance such as interviewing skills or responses in an oral exam.

Validity

The term *validity* concerns the degree to which an assessment procedure measures what it is intended to measure. Important forms of validity include the following: 1) *face validity*, that is, how valid the evaluation appears to be in the eyes of a faculty member or student (testing experts and the courts give it little credence because it is unsystematic and too subjective; however, if an examination lacks face validity in the eyes of students, it can have a demoralizing impact on them); 2) *content validity*, that is, how well the assessment systematically samples from a well-designed content outline or from a listing of important skills; 3) *criterion validity* or predictive validity, that is, how well the assessment of clinical skills during an examination setting predicts performance with patients in other settings in the weeks or months to come; and 4) *construct validity*, a more complex concept that in medical training is usually measured by demonstrating a growth in evaluation ratings during the course of training (e.g., a gradual gain in in-training examination scores during residency training).

Evaluation procedures must be reliable and valid to have credibility with students, colleagues, and (if necessary) the courts (Helms and Helms 1991). The latter take on great importance when a student fails a course or clerkship, especially if the course or clerkship failure results in dismissal from medical school for poor academic performance, which often precipitates a lawsuit on the part of the dismissed student.

With increasing cutback of funds to support medical education, the need to operate evaluation programs in a more cost-effective manner will be increasingly important. Methods of reducing costs include sharing evaluation materials among academic centers and being sure to delegate evaluation responsibilities to the least costly staff member who can carry out the task effectively.

Evaluation must be employed within a setting of *due process*, which requires that a school describe in writing what is required of a student, how a student is to be evaluated, and, if a student fails to meet performance standards, how and to whom the student may appeal (Irby et al. 1981). Generally, due process procedures are determined by the dean's office in collaboration with attorneys and are described in the school's student handbook. Educators should keep a copy of the current student handbook close to their desk and should be familiar with their school's due process guidelines.

Useful Resources

In developing an evaluation program for their medical students, educators can make use of a number of resources that are available within every institution: 1) an office of medical education, 2) the clerkship directors in the other major disciplines, and 3) the residency training directors. Those fortunate enough to teach in a school with an office of medical education can find out who has the best expertise in various aspects of evaluation, such as multiple-choice testing, assessing interviewing skills, and assessing day-to-day performance. Other useful resources include many good monographs (Muslin et al. 1974; Neufeld and Norman 1985; Templeton 1980) and articles in various educational journals, including *Academic Medicine, Academic Psychiatry, Medical Education* (a British journal), *Medical Teacher,* and *Teaching and Learning in Medicine.*

A great deal of useful information can be obtained by attending the annual meetings of the Association of Directors of Medical Student Education in Psychiatry (ADMSEP), the Association for Academic Psychiatry (AAP), and the American Association of Directors of Psychiatric Residency Training (AADPRT) and the regional and national meetings of the Group on Medical Education of the Association of American Medical Colleges (AAMC).

WRITTEN EXAMINATIONS

Written exams are very helpful in tracking a student's acquisition of essential knowledge and, despite various critics, will continue to prove useful to both instructors and trainees (Hubbard 1978; Weaver et al. 1979). For most medical schools, a class size of more than 50 students will require the instructor to make use of multiple-choice examinations. Essay questions or other non-multiple-choice formats are simply too time-consuming to grade for such large classes. Essay tests too often suffer from insufficient sampling of the course content. Grading of essay tests is time-consuming, and careful studies of essay grading typically demonstrate major problems with reliability. The use of frequent quizzes during preclinical courses and, if logistically feasible, during the clerkship can help keep students up to date on their reading and can help students become better prepared for intramural finals as well as the United States Medical Licensing Examination (USMLE).

An important question for each department concerns the decision to develop its own examinations versus using the *subject examinations* provided by the National Board of Medical Examiners (NBME). Use of the NBME subject exams (often called shelf exams) provides a reliable assessment of students' knowledge of the field and also provides information that helps the department compare its own students with those from other medical schools. In addition, use of shelf exams helps maintain credibility of the course among other departments and may help students feel better prepared for Step 1 and Step 2 of the USMLE. The major disadvantage of the NBME exams is their cost, which might run $3,000–$5,000 per year. Advantages of administering self-developed intramural examinations include ensuring a close link between one's teaching objectives and the assessment and the relative ease of retesting the student who fails the first test. Major disadvantages include the enormous amount of time required to create at least two or three versions of an end-of-clerkship exam; the difficulty of developing equivalent versions of an exam; and the lack of data showing how one's own students perform in comparison with students at other medical schools. As of 2004, approximately 84% of medical schools in the United States use the NBME subject exams during the clinical years, and a growing number are making use of more recently developed subject exams for first- and second-year students. The NBME Web site (http://www.nbme.org) can provide additional details.

How should subject exams be incorporated into a final clerkship grade? Most clerkship directors feel that the major component of a clerkship grade should be the attending physician's assessment. Many clerkships use various formulas to weigh the attending physician's assessment with the subject exam score. Our faculty have been concerned about a few instances in which a student has been rated by an attending physician to receive honors; then later, a review of end-of-clerkship subject exam scores places the same student in the lowest twentieth percentile. As a result, we have set subject-exam hurdles for each overall clerkship grade that a student must achieve to obtain that grade (e.g., currently an NBME subject raw test score of 78 [i.e., 71st percentile] to receive honors).

WRITING MULTIPLE-CHOICE TEST ITEMS

The best way to become a proficient preparer of multiple-choice examinations is to get some training. Several types of training are available. The first is to become a member of a test committee for one of the major testing groups: the NBME, the American College of Psychiatrists (which administers the Psychiatry Resident In-Training Examination [PRITE]), or the American Board of Psychiatry and Neurology. Another form of training is to attend workshops on exam preparation such as those held at national education meetings (e.g., those held by ADMSEP, the AAMC, or the AAP).

Medical schools will occasionally sponsor such item-writing workshops. Finally, the use of written manuals can be extremely helpful. Examples include the booklet of sample questions provided by the NBME.

LINKING OBJECTIVES AND EXAMS

To establish a link between the course objectives and the content of the examination, the instructor must prepare a content outline. Various approaches are used. Probably the simplest approach involves taking the units of instruction (e.g., the assigned chapters or the scheduled lectures) and preparing a given number of test items per unit of instruction to achieve an examination of sufficient length (e.g., 144 test items divided by 16 class sessions = 9 items per session). If the instructor has sufficient time, it might be advisable to review the content of an examination from the perspective of a series of dimensions, each of which contains mutually exclusive components (Muslin et al. 1974). For example, for a second-year or end-of-clerkship examination in clinical psychiatry, it would be useful to assess the student's knowledge of various physician tasks (e.g., use of the patient's history, results of the physical examination, mental status examination, and ancillary studies; differential diagnosis; and various forms of therapy). In addition, it would be useful to review the exam content from the perspective of various diagnoses to be certain that the exam samples from a wide variety of important clinical disorders. Other important content dimensions include the age of the patient and etiological factors.

FORMATTING TEST ITEMS

The three formats that are most widely used today are one best answer, a/b/both/neither, and full matching set. Although the one-best-answer format is very useful, in the hands of inexperienced writers it is associated with the largest number of inadvertent clues to the correct answer. Among the most common errors that help give away the correct answer are the following:

1. Making many of the correct answers the longest of the options.
    (A) xxxxxx xx xxxxxx xxx xxxx   <— Correct answer
    xxxx x xxxxxx xxxxxxx xxxx
    (B) xxxxx xxxxx xxxxxx   <— Length of all other options
2. Making the correct answer different in some manner, such as being the only option containing an eponym or the only option containing both a generic and a brand name.

DSM-IV-TR criteria for schizophrenia include

	A	B	C	D	E
Avolition			X		X
Delusions	X	X	X	X	X
Disorganized speech		X	X	X	
Hallucinations	X	X	X	X	X
Indifference to praise				X	X
Odd beliefs	X	X		X	X

Answer = C (American Psychiatric Association 2000, p. 312).

FIGURE 4–1. Chart-option format for exam questions.

> (A) xxxxxxxx (Xxxxxx Xxxxxx)   <— Correct option
> (B) xxxxxxx xxxxxxxxxxx xxx   <— Incorrect option
> (C) xxxxxxxxxxx xxxxxxxxxxx   <— Incorrect option

A useful design of multiple-choice exam questions has been to include questions with *stems* stating, for example, "Characteristics of disorder X include..." or "Complications of drug Y include...." At one time, these questions worked well with the so-called K-type item (a multiple true–false format), which is no longer used by the NBME. One alternative to the K-type approach is to write an "except" stem, such as "Each of the following is a DSM-IV-TR characteristic of disorder X *EXCEPT*..." or "Each of the following is a complication of drug Y *EXCEPT*...." As a second alternative, I have devised a *chart-option* format, which is illustrated in Figure 4–1.

The chart-option technique is a one-best-answer format that lends itself well to making multiple equivalent forms, so-called item modeling. In my view, retaining the use of "except" test items vastly increases the instructor's ability to test a variety of important topics. Although the NBME has discontinued the use of EXCEPT questions, these questions perform well in terms of item statistics (described below); and the author has found no peer-reviewed publications that document their lack of utility.

INTERPRETING TEST STATISTICS

Most medical schools have an optical-scan scoring machine that provides a method of efficiently scoring multiple-choice examinations. Test developers should find out who runs the system and should learn how to make the best use of the system. These machines will sometimes provide valuable information about the overall test and will generate *item statistics*, which give crucial information about the effectiveness of individual questions. When these data come from an end-of-clerkship examination involving only 15–25 students, their utility will be very limited. But if the data come from a full class of 100–250 students, the resulting information will be quite valuable. For example, the mean percentage correct, usually identified for the overall examination, tells the instructor the number of test items typically answered correctly by the average student. These data can be evaluated as follows:

- Mean percentage correct for a specific exam:
  85%–100%: Exam is too easy; the reliability of resulting scores will be less certain.
  70%–85%: Exam is just about right; students will feel they are being tested on things they need to know.
  <70%: Students will feel the exam is too difficult, has too much minutiae, etc.
- Other important data concerning individual test items include the P value, that is, the percentage of students who answered the item correctly.
  95%–100%: Items are probably too easy for the level of student being tested.
  70%–95%: Satisfactory level of difficulty.
  50%–70%: Items are a bit difficult but should not be thrown out.
  <50%: Items are probably too difficult; they should be saved for a higher-level trainee or discarded.
- For each test item, the instructor will also receive an r value, which essentially is a correlation coefficient that indicates how well the item differentiates between the top group of examinees (e.g., top 25%) in comparison to the bottom group (e.g., bottom 25%). The derivation of the r value is more complicated. These data should be interpreted as follows:
  >0.15: A good item (the higher the r value the better, but it will rarely go above 0.30–0.40).
  0.05–0.15: The item is not helping very much in obtaining reliable scores; it should probably be modified or discarded from the pool.
  <0.00: Any item with a negative r value should probably be discarded before final scoring.

Pass–fail judgments require an examination with adequate reliability. A number of different formulas are available. The Kuder-Richardson Formula 20, employed in the past by the NBME, has been hypothesized to mathematically compare a multiplicity of split-half test scores to estimate the overall reproducibility of the final score (for more details, see Schumacher 1978).

The reliability of a written exam used for pass–fail purposes should probably be above 0.80. The reliability of an exam can be estimated in two ways. First, many school optical-scan scoring systems will provide an estimate of the overall reliability of each exam. The reliability of an examination is highly correlated with its length: the longer the examination, the more reliable the score. If the reliability of a final exam is less than 0.80, its length should be increased at its next administration. If the machine scoring system does not provide such an estimate or if the final grade is determined by adding up the results of a series of exams, an alternative approach is to simply include a sufficient number of items to ensure a reasonably reliable examination. The use of 130–140 multiple-choice test items to generate a pass–fail score will typically provide reasonable reliability.

Ensuring that pass–fail judgments are based on a sufficient number of test items can be achieved in one of two ways: 1) by giving one or more short quizzes and a longer final exam and adding up the scores for each test to obtain the final grade (quiz 1, 45 items; quiz 2, 45 items; final exam, 54 items; total, 144 items), or 2) by having a single final examination of more than 140 questions.

To keep the examination secure so that it can be used again, each exam book needs to be labeled with a student's name taken from a class roster, and then exam papers must be passed out by name to the appropriate student. The instructor must be certain to receive an examination booklet from each student before each student leaves the exam room. Despite doing this, repeatedly using the same examination will eventually cause major problems when a group of students complains to the dean that some students had prior access to major portions of the exam and others did not.

During administration of the exam, students should receive guidelines about how to communicate comments or concerns about specific test items. If students are permitted to keep the exam, posting one copy and requesting that all comments be placed on the posted copy within 48 hours will provide the easiest method of reviewing student concerns. If the exams are collected after administration, students can be asked to write comments on the exam and to write a note about each page of concern on the first page.

After completion of the examination, the answer sheets are sent for preliminary scoring. While the test is being scored, the instructor should review the students' written complaints and make tentative decisions about whether or not to keep the items that received complaints based on a review of the assigned text or consultation with other faculty members. The item statistics should then be reviewed, and special attention should be given to items with a P value of less than 30% and items with negative r values. It is important to make sure that the latter are correctly keyed. Based on a synthesis of these factors, the instructor should then decide which items should be deleted from final scoring. As part of the request for final scoring, it is important to ask for a histogram showing the distribution of raw scores.

Testing experts have had a long-standing debate about the utility of *norm-referenced* testing, in which the instructor looks at the bell curve and fails a percentage of the lowest scorers; and *criterion-referenced* testing, in which the instructor sets a pass–fail standard in advance of the exam. Although I am very sympathetic with the arguments in favor of criterion-referenced testing, I do not think it is practical. I tend to de-emphasize the word *failure* and simply notify students that those who do not achieve a certain score must undergo remediation and be reexamined. In my view, passing 100% of students before requiring some to undergo remediation is unwise. I find that a pass rate of 92%–96% keeps the course credible in the eyes of the students; with this failure rate, the students conclude that they must study the material to satisfy the departmental requirements. In addition, this type of standard-setting approach also helps keep students, as a group, from performing poorly on the USMLE Step 1 and Step 2 examinations.

Credibility of a written examination in the eyes of students can be enhanced by the following: letting students know about the nature of the assessment (format and content) at the very beginning of the course or rotation; ensuring broad sampling among the information presented; ensuring that the difficulty level is appropriate (see comments about the mean percentage correct at the beginning of this subsection); and avoiding a we-never-fail-anyone philosophy. A sloppy approach to testing can have a major adverse effect on a class's view of the course and the department. Anecdotal reports suggest that frequent (possibly weekly) quizzes combined with an NBME shelf examination work very well.

For remediation, I have employed two approaches. For the behavioral science course, I have developed two forms of a short-answer exam containing a randomly selected list of about 30 terms covered in the course for which students must write definitions. The exams also include a series of one-paragraph vignettes for which the student must select the correct diagnosis from a moderately comprehensive list of diagnoses printed on the examination. In view of the fact that remediation usually involves fewer than 10 students, I have graded these papers by hand. The pass–fail determination was initially very subjective. However, by keeping a record of scores of previous students undergoing remediation, I have gradually acquired a more confident basis for what is still a fairly subjective judgment. This practice has helped maintain reasonable performance on the Step 1 examination. In the case of remediation for the end-of-clerkship NBME shelf exam, students are required to retake NBME shelf exams until they meet the department's required percentile score.

Medical student directors would benefit greatly from two types of test-item banking. A number of relatively inexpensive software packages that are available for test-item storage and for test generation are described in Chapter 7, "New Teaching Technologies and Approaches for Medical Students and Residents." In addition, at one time, ADMSEP helped to sponsor such a bank. It is unfortunate that an effective system for sharing test questions is currently lacking. Perhaps the growing use of NBME shelf examinations will reduce the need for such a resource.

The USMLE Step 1 and Step 2 examinations can have an important impact on one's instructional program and on one's job. If an instructor's students receive mean scores on the Step 1 Behavioral Science component or the Step 2 Psychiatry component that fall much below the mean scores for the other discipline scores obtained by those students (e.g., the mean scores for Biochemistry or Internal Medicine), the psychiatry chair will receive a note from the dean's office, and the instructor, in turn, will be called in to see the department chair. The instructor can plead for more curriculum time, but this approach often falls on deaf ears. An instructor with low mean scores who wishes to retain his or her job had better change something: review or revise the curriculum; meet with or get some new lecturers; set up more quizzes; make the pass–fail level somewhat higher; try to instill more enthusiasm into both classroom teachers and the students; and so on.

The *Hawthorne effect*, a concept drawn from industrial psychology, was derived from a study in which both increases and decreases in industrial lighting produced more worker productivity as long as the changes appeared to be designed to help the workers. The instructor needs to find a way to carry out whatever instructional changes that are employed with enough enthusiasm to ensure that the Hawthorne effect will work in his or her favor and will help bring the Step 1 and 2 scores up to a level that will be acceptable in the eyes of the chair and the dean.

EVALUATING INTERVIEWING SKILLS

Evaluation of interviewing skills represents one aspect of the assessment of abilities that have noncognitive attributes. Departments vary greatly in the extent to which they participate in interviewing instruction (Lipkin et al. 1995). The range of approaches varies from schools in which the department's role may be primarily directed (during the third year) to the mental status examination and related aspects of a psychiatric assessment, to other schools in which the department may take a major role in the school's over- all medical interviewing instruction.

In any case, evaluating interviewing skills is difficult (Kalet et al. 1992). It is often difficult to get a sufficient number of faculty members to observe just one interview by each medical student. Some instructors resist the use of any structured evaluation forms and prefer to simply watch an interview and provide the trainee with verbal feedback in an unsystematic manner. Many programs rely on the use of global rating scales by a single instructor who observes a single student with a patient; these forms include items such as "Followed leads appropriately" and "Used language that was appropriate to the patient's level of education." Both the unstructured approach and the use of global rating forms by an instructor are associated with relatively low reliability (Templeton and Allen 1990).

Checklists appear to provide more reliable data. Checklists usually fo- cus primarily on the data requested and collected by students. But some checklists also try to focus on certain process measures—for example, whether the student introduced himself or herself in an acceptable manner (see, for example, the Brown Interview Checklist [Novack et al. 1992]). Fig- ure 4–2 illustrates a generic checklist that can be used in assessing a medical student's initial interview with a psychiatric inpatient or outpatient. If the checklist data are to be used for formal evaluation, the faculty needs to de- termine how many items reflect meeting minimal standards.

STANDARDIZED PATIENTS

Standardized patients, formerly called simulated patients, are individuals who are hired to portray a patient and the patient's medical or psychiatric problems at a specific point in the patient's life. Some are trained just for history-taking skills, whereas others help train both history and physical examination skills. A growing number of schools are developing standard- ized patient programs for teaching and evaluating medical interviewing and physical examination skills. These programs are usually administered by an office of medical education or the dean's office, have their own budget, and have personnel with considerable sophistication in training standardized patients and in devising methods of evaluating student performance in a re- liable and valid manner.

Tape #:_____   Date of Taping:_____

Date of Coding:_____20_____   Reviewer's Initials:_____

Patient Age:_____   Patient Sex: M   F

Interview Length:_____minutes.

[Instructions: Check each item reflecting an inquiry by the physician trainee and/or giving of information by the patient.]

PRESENT ILLNESS

____ Onset, time of

____ Symptoms (Ss)

____ Course of Ss (sudden onset, intermittent, steadily worse, etc.)

____ Did some event precipitate hospitalization/ambulatory visit?

PAST MEDICAL HISTORY

____ Allergies

____ Drug reactions

____ Medications, recent/current

____ Past illnesses (nonsurgical)

____ Past operations

____ Other hospitalizations

____ Alcohol use/abuse

____ Substance use/abuse, other

FAMILY MEDICAL HISTORY

____ Mother (living vs. dead; L/D)

____ Mother, state of health

____ Nature of relationship or feelings about

____ Father (L/D)

____ Father, state of health

____ Nature of relationship or feelings about

____ Siblings (L/D)

____ Siblings, state of health

____ Nature of relationship or feelings about (mention of one or more)

____ Marital status

____ Nature of relationship or feelings about spouse (if married)

____ Children, state of health

____ Nature of relationship or feelings about (mention of one or more)

____ Family members do/don't have same problem as patient's admission

____ Diabetes in other family members

____ Hypertension in other family members

____ Heart disease, other type, in other family members

____ Kidney problems in other family members

____ Liver problems in other family members

____ Psychiatric problems in other family members

____ Seizures/epilepsy in other family members

REVIEW OF SYSTEMS

____ GEN   Fever

____ GEN   Weight change

____ SKIN   Bruising

____ HEAD   Headaches

____ HEAD   Passing out

____ EYES   Double vision

____ EYES   Other impairment

____ EARS   Pain

____ NOSE   Nosebleeds

____ NOSE   Sinus problems

____ MOUTH   Any problems

____ NECK   Thyroid/node enlargement

____ CV   Chest pain

____ CV   Palpitations

____ CV   Edema (ankles, hands, etc.)

____ CV   Murmurs

____ CV   Shortness of breath

____ RESPT   Asthma/wheezing

____ RESPT   Cough

____ RESPT   Coughing up blood

____ RESPT   Sputum

____ GI   Swallowing difficulty

____ GI   Nausea/vomiting

____ GI   Abdominal pain

____ GI   Food intolerance

(continued)

FIGURE 4–2.   Initial interview evaluation—generic checklist.

REVIEW OF SYSTEMS (continued)

____	GI	Gallbladder attacks
____	GI	Diarrhea/constipation
____	GI	Blood in bowel movements
____	GI	Black bowel movements
____	GU	Increased frequency
____	GU	Urinating at night
____	GU	Blood in urine
____	GU–Male	Pain
____	GU–Male	Discharge (VD)
____	GU–Male	Prostate problems
____	GU–Male	Urinary stream
____	GU–Female	Pain
____	GU–Female	Discharge
____	GU–Female	Menstrual pattern
____	GU–Female	Venereal disease
____	GU–Female	Contraception use
____	GU–Female	Obstetrical history
____	GU–Female	Recent breast exam
____	MUSC	Joint pain
____	NMUSC	Joint swelling
____	NMUSC	Weakness of extremities
____	UMUSC	Circulation problems

MENTAL STATUS

____ Assaultive feelings

____ Date of month (orientation)

____ Day of week (orientation)

____ Delusions

____ Depressed mood

____ Highs (euphoria, racing thoughts, etc.)

____ Nervousness

____ Hallucinations

____ Suicidal thoughts

____ Homicidal thoughts

PSYCHOSOCIAL

____ Childhood: loved or abused

____ Education

____ Held a job

____ Close personal relationship

____ Recent life crisis (past decade)

____ Housing, current satisfaction with

____ Financial status

____ Major surgery, reaction to

____ Major illnesses, reaction to

____ Sleep patterns

____ Sexual life/problems

____ Hobbies; other pleasurable activities

CLOSURE OF INTERVIEW

____ Warned patient >1 minute before ending interview

____ NotiÞed patient of ending

____ Provided some note of encouragement (e.g., "I hope things go well with...")

____ Thanked patient

FIGURE 4–2. Initial interview evaluation—generic checklist *(continued).*

OBJECTIVE STRUCTURED CLINICAL EXAMINATIONS

An objective structured clinical examination (OSCE) is an evaluation procedure involving a series of 8–12 *stations*, each of which requires the student to demonstrate some form of clinical performance. At each OSCE station, a student is usually required to perform some aspect of the medical history, the physical examination, or patient education. Usually each station includes a standardized patient. OSCEs provide another mechanism of assessing some noncognitive attributes under fairly standardized conditions.

In a school that has a standardized patient program and/or an OSCE program, instruction in and evaluation of interviewing skills might be most efficiently accomplished through collaboration with the standardized patient program. The goals should then be to ensure that the bank of cases employed in the program include an appropriate number of well-designed psychiatric cases (e.g., the assessment of patients with alcoholism, anxiety, bereavement, or somatoform disorders), that the evaluative instruments include attention to important aspects of psychiatry as it applies to medical student instruction, and that psychiatric instructors are able to obtain feedback about how the students handle the aspects of interviewing that are of special importance to the department.

VIDEO EXAMINATIONS

A few instructors become enamored of video examinations in which a patient is portrayed for 1–8 minutes and then students are asked to answer written questions, usually multiple-choice, about the patient portrayed in the video. From my experience reviewing a number of these video examinations, usually only 5% of the questions require the accompanying video. Another 10%–35% of questions could be answered with a printed text of the interview. Typically, 65%–90% of video-based questions do not require a video or text presentation. In addition, problems in case-to-case variability make sampling and therefore content validity a major problem; limitations of this chapter, however, preclude detailed explanation. In my view, an instructor is best advised not to employ video examinations.

EVALUATING STUDENTS DURING SMALL-GROUP INSTRUCTION

Many departments include small-group instruction as part of the course in behavioral science or introductory psychiatry during the first 2 years of medical school. These groups are usually designed to include discussion about topics related to lectures or readings. Instructors who serve as group leaders are often able to provide meaningful evaluations of certain noncognitive attributes for students at the extremes of performance: 1) students who are especially good participants, who take leadership roles in the group, who appear very knowledgeable, and who are thorough and timely in assignments; and 2) the few students who stand out because they are excessively shy or inhibited, come late or miss sessions, do not relate to or get along well with peers, and so on. However, instructors often feel at a loss in grading the remaining students, even if the group has met weekly for 4–9 months. To maintain the valuable data about the two outlier groups, I encourage faculty members to simply record, for the remaining students, "Performed acceptably within the group" without much additional detail and then provide the relevant narrative detail about the high and low performers. Including senior residents or senior medical students as co-leaders is an effective method of providing these trainees with some hands-on instruction in teaching and evaluating students.

ORAL EXAMINATIONS

Studies of question-and-answer oral examinations generally show the following deficiencies: most of the questions require primarily recall of information and not "problem solving," as many examiners contend; sampling of content varies widely among examiners unless the exam is highly structured; oral examiners have difficulty achieving good interrater reliability; and the hidden cost per student examined is very high. Based on available research, the popularity of this technique among some instructors seems unfounded.

PERFORMANCE ASSESSMENT OF NONCOGNITIVE TRAITS

Assessing students' day-to-day performance provides an important approach in evaluating many noncognitive characteristics and is an important aspect of student evaluation, especially during the clinical assignments of the third and fourth year. Here again, problems of poor interrater reliability are rampant. For example, McLeod (1987) demonstrated the wide variation in faculty judgments regarding medical student case write-ups. Most medical schools have adopted clinical skills rating forms that each department is required to use.

In our school, the office of medical education in conjunction with the clerkship directors created a form with anchors that is required to be used

TABLE 4–2. Methods of ensuring effective assessment of day-to-day performance

Conduct an end-of-clerkship group meeting of instructors and ancillary personnel.

Have photographs available at the above sessions.

Synthesize information for each student from several sources: instructors, residents, and ancillary personnel.

Collect the evaluation forms within 10 days of the end of the clerkship.

within all clerkships. Some rating form elements are more appropriate than others. Based on a vote by clerkship directors, our school continues to include a rating of the student's fund of knowledge; this rating item has been retained despite the fact that all clerkships utilize shelf examinations and intramural data suggest that faculty ratings of students' fund of knowledge lack reliability. When given the assignment to develop a departmental clerkship rating form, an instructor should get some names of other clerkship directors from the ADMSEP membership directory and ask to review what other departments are using.

Recommendations regarding how these forms can be employed in the most reliable, valid, and cost-effective manner are outlined in Table 4–2.

Some faculty members are substantially tougher or easier graders than their colleagues, which causes morale problems among students; providing faculty members, every year or so, with a summary of their distribution of grades and the distribution of the grades for the department may help to bring outliers closer to the mean.

Some schools encourage departments to avoid inflating grades by strictly limiting the number of students who may receive honor grades. Although there are good reasons to comply with the dean's office request, if a department's distribution of grades falls too far to the left of other clinical departments, students may become unduly critical of the department for adhering too strictly to schoolwide policies. In my own experience, when the psychiatry department assigned 50%–60% of students a satisfactory grade (when most other departments had only 20%–35% in this category) and the exam component came from intramurally developed exam material, student resentment was substantial. When the department adopted NBME shelf exams and the distribution of overall grades was substantially influenced by the students' ability or inability to obtain a shelf exam score above the departmentally set hurdle, the resentment toward the department and the director disappeared.

TRAINING FACULTY AND RESIDENTS TO GIVE FEEDBACK TO STUDENTS

The effectiveness of the faculty and residents in evaluating students can probably be enhanced through both formal and informal mechanisms. In an informal approach, maintaining contact with the faculty and residents to be aware of their concerns about all aspects of the teaching program will help to maintain their interest in providing thoughtful and valid feedback about student performance. More formal approaches include meeting periodically with faculty or residents. Alternative approaches include devoting a regular faculty meeting to review of these concerns or periodically attending divisional meetings (e.g., divisional meetings of the inpatient service or the consultation service). One might also consider distributing copies of the most recent edition of the American Psychiatric Association (2002) brochure "Psychiatric Residents as Teachers: A Practical Guide."

PROMOTIONS COMMITTEE PARTICIPATION

Serving on a basic science or clinical science promotions committee is an important faculty responsibility and provides an opportunity to get to know other faculty members and to learn how other departments handle their teaching and evaluation responsibilities. Based on my experience, it is surprising that these committees often find themselves struggling with a difficult summative decision about an individual student about whom relatively little is known other than that he or she is in academic difficulty. Although the committee may request psychiatric evaluation for a particular student, there may be value in attempting to obtain a relatively standard database on each student having academic difficulty, including such information as presence of interfering medical problems, a recent death in the family or some other family crisis, evidence in the student of alcohol or substance abuse, and possible loss of motivation for continuing medical studies.

If a formal psychiatric consultation is requested, questions that should be posed by the committee to the consultant should include the following: Are there any reasons why the student should be discouraged from continuing medical school on a temporary or long-term basis? Does the consultant recommend some form of ongoing treatment? Are there any other suggestions for the committee that might help the student succeed? The student may feel a greater degree of comfort with issues of confidentiality if the assessment is carried out by a non-full-time faculty member and if the student is aware of the specific questions the consultant has been asked to answer (as opposed to expecting the consultant to submit a very detailed history containing private information that the committee does not really need).

LICENSURE AND THE ASSESSMENT OF CLINICAL SKILLS

In 1998, the Educational Commission for Foreign Medical Graduates (ECFMG) instituted the Clinical Skills Examination (Whelan et al. 2002). The examination was required of all graduates of foreign medical schools seeking graduate medical training in the United States. This clinical exam consisted of approximately 10–11 stations in which an examinee spent time with a standardized patient. The tasks at each station typically included undertaking a focused patient history, selective aspects of the physical examination, and a write-up of each encounter. All examinees were required to go to the examination site in west Philadelphia. This facility has a central video recording studio, about 24 exam rooms with one-way mirrors, and cameras built into each exam room. The scoring of each encounter was based on the following: a data checklist of relevant aspects of the patient history and physical examination tasks accomplished; a judgment of English language proficiency by the standardized patients who were trained for this task; an assessment of the examinee's interpersonal skills; and a global rating of the examinee's write-up of each encounter by one of a panel of physician reviewers. A number of quality control procedures were employed to help ensure a reliable and valid assessment of each examinee (Boulet et al. 2003). Several studies of various aspects of this clinical examination have been published (Ayers and Boulet 2001; Boulet et al. 2001; Chambers et al. 2000; Whelan et al. 2001).

The USMLE program instituted a comparable clinical skills examination, Step 2 CS, beginning in June 2004. The USMLE licensure program is jointly administered by the NBME and the Federation of State Medical Boards of the United States (FSMB). Step 2 CS will replace ECFMG's Clinical Skills Examination and will be required as part of the USMLE licensure system. This examination will be required of all trainees graduating from United States medical schools in 2005 or thereafter as well as all international medical graduates planning to come to the United States for residency training. The examination is given at five Clinical Skills Evaluation Centers located in Atlanta, Georgia; Chicago, Illinois; Houston, Texas; Los Angeles, California; and Philadelphia, Pennsylvania. Additional details about the examination are available through the NBME Web site (http://www.nbme.org).

CONCLUSION

Evaluation plays an important role in medical education. If performed in a reliable manner with valid techniques, it allows educators to determine the readiness of students to progress in training and to judge the overall effectiveness of their educational efforts. For evaluation to work successfully, psychiatric educators must apply the same degree of care exercised in diagnosing and treating patients to the selection and application of evaluative procedures in their work with students.

REFERENCES

American Psychiatric Association: Diagnostic and Statistical Manual of Mental Disorders, 4th Edition, Text Revision. Washington, DC, American Psychiatric Association, 2000

American Psychiatric Association, Committee on Graduate Medical Education 2001–2002: Psychiatric Residents as Teachers: A Practical Guide (2nd Revision 4/02). Washington, DC, American Psychiatric Association, 2002 (Also available at: http://www.psych.org/edu/res_fellows/psychresidentguide.pdf)

Ayers WR, Boulet JR: Establishing the validity of test score inferences: performance of 4th-year U.S. medical students on the ECFMG Clinical Skills Assessment. Teach Learn Med 13:214–220, 2001

Boulet JR, van Zanten M, McKinley DW, et al: Evaluating the spoken English proficiency of graduates of foreign medical schools. Med Educ 35:767–773, 2001

Boulet JR, McKinley DW, Whelan GP, et al: Quality assurance methods of performance-based assessments. Adv Health Sci Educ Theory Pract 8:27–47, 2003

Chambers KA, Boulet JR, Gary NE: The management of patient encounter time in a high-stakes assessment using standardized patients. Med Educ 34:813–817, 2000

Helms LB, Helms CM: Forty years of litigation involving medical students and their education, I: general educational issues. Acad Med 66:1–7, 1991

Hubbard JP: Measuring Medical Education: The Tests and the Experience of the National Board of Medical Examiners, 2nd Edition. Philadelphia, PA, Lea & Febiger, 1978, pp 1–17

Irby DM, Fantel JI, Milam SD, et al: Legal guidelines for evaluating and dismissing medical students. N Engl J Med 304:180–184, 1981

Kalet A, Earp JA, Kowlowitz V: How well do faculty evaluate the interviewing skills of medical students? J Gen Intern Med 7:499–505, 1992

Lipkin M Jr, Putnam SM, Lazare A (eds): The Medical Interview: Clinical Care, Education, and Research. New York, Springer-Verlag, 1995

McLeod PJ: Faculty assessments of case reports of medical students. J Med Educ 62:673–677, 1987

Muslin HL, Thurnblad RJ, Templeton B, et al (eds): Evaluative Methods in Psychiatry. Washington, DC, American Psychiatric Association, 1974

Neufeld VR, Norman GR: Assessing Clinical Competence. New York, Springer, 1985

Novack DH, Dube C, Goldstein MG: Teaching medical interviewing. A basic course on interviewing and the physician-patient relationship. Arch Intern Med 152:1814–1820, 1992

Schumacher CF: Scoring and analysis, in Measuring Medical Education: The Tests and the Experience of the National Board of Medical Examiners, 2nd Edition. Edited by Hubbard JP. Philadelphia, PA, Lea & Febiger, 1978, pp 59–67

Templeton B: Evaluation in the continuum of psychiatric education, in Comprehensive Textbook of Psychiatry, 3rd Edition. Edited by Kaplan HI, Freedman AM, Sadock BJ. Baltimore, MD, Williams & Wilkins, 1980, pp 2181–2189

Templeton B, Allen MM: Interrater reliability in evaluating trainee interviewing skills. Acad Psychiatry 14:188–196, 1990

Templeton B, Selarnick HS: Evaluating consultation psychiatry residents. Gen Hosp Psychiatry 16:326–334, 1994

Thorndike RL: Educational Measurement, 2nd Edition. Washington, DC, American Council on Education, 1971

Weaver FJ, Ramirez AG, Dorfman SB, et al: Trainees' retention of cardiopulmonary resuscitation. How quickly they forget. JAMA 241:901–903, 1979

Whelan GP, McKinley DW, Boulet JR, et al: Validation of the doctor-patient communication component of the Educational Commission for Foreign Medical Graduates Clinical Skills Assessment. Med Educ 35:757–761, 2001

Whelan GP, Gary NE, Kostis J, et al: The changing pool of international medical graduates seeking certification training in US graduate medical education programs. JAMA 288:1079–1084, 2002

CHAPTER 5

ADMINISTRATION OF THE RESIDENCY PROGRAM

David Bienenfeld, M.D.

The biopsychosocial model of human behavior, with which all psychiatrists are familiar, is a special application of *general systems theory*. General systems theory provides a framework for the derivation of administrative systems and the understanding of administrative dynamics (Figure 5–1). In this model, all systems are 1) *sets of interrelated objects* in 2) *an environment* 3) *Inputs* from the environment enter the system and are utilized in 4) *processes* that perform the work of the system, yielding 5) *output*. The effect of that output on the environment provides 6) *feedback*. Viewing the residency training program as such a system allows for a coherent picture of its administration (Mann 1975).

The structure and function of the system are most productively determined by looking first at its output. The output of a residency program is well-trained and well-educated psychiatrists. With that goal in mind, the training director can analyze, design, implement, and assess the training process; the structure necessary to implement that process; the resources and ingredients on which the process operates; the environment that must be accommodated; and the feedback mechanisms of quality control.

THE PROCESS

The education of residents is a venture that demands flexibility, responsivity, and collaboration. Because there are numerous participants and stake-

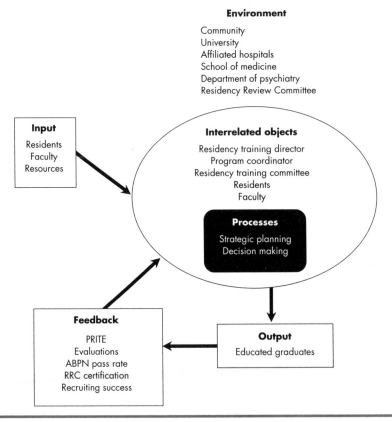

FIGURE 5–1. General systems outline of residency training.

Note. ABPN=American Board of Psychiatry and Neurology; PRITE=Psychiatry Resident In-Training Examination; RRC=Residency Review Committee.

holders in the educational process, and because the pressures and demands on the system are in constant flux, change and adaptability are essential characteristics of the successful program. Training directors, however, must be wary of losing sight of the program's broader purposes in the face of acute pressures. They must discriminate between the processes of *planning* and *governance*, between goal setting and problem solving.

Strategic planning is the process of setting long-range goals for the organization. The training program that has a clear and constant sense of mission will be best suited to accommodating short-term issues. Arriving at long-term goals requires consensus among the major participants: residents, faculty, and administrators. Typically, the derivation of a mission statement occurs in the setting of a program or departmental retreat. Usually such a retreat is a daylong event, held away from the everyday work environment, utilizing methods such as brainstorming and nominal group technique, often with the assistance of an outside facilitator.

The organizational mission statement should reflect the underlying purpose of the program, with enough specificity to be meaningful and enough latitude to accommodate change over a period of years. The mission then defines the nature and number of residents selected for training, the content of the curriculum, the sites and services used in the program, the dimensions of resident evaluation, and all the other aspects of implementation. These factors are the objects of the governance of residency training; they are the products of the decision-making or problem-solving process.

External certifying agencies, including the Accreditation Council for Graduate Medical Education (ACGME) and the American Board of Psychiatry and Neurology (ABPN), dictate a number of criteria for the structure, function, and curriculum of the program (see "The Environment," below). In setting standards to guarantee training quality across the country, these criteria may threaten the "local color" of individual programs. It is no mean feat to regard the meticulous certification criteria as minimal requirements and to build a program's unique character on top of them, but it is a task that quality programs undertake. Although every program is required to provide some basic training in research methods, an individual program may decide that education and experience in scientific investigation are its primary pedagogical mission. A different program may find the certification standards for psychotherapy inadequate and define its mission to include in-depth training in the psychotherapies.

Where strategic planning reflects constancy, decision making embodies the change that is required to maintain the survival of the mission. Both individuals and organizations are inherently resistant to change, and the effective leader is one who facilitates change with the least disruption and conflict. The most important dimension of organizational decision making is that it is participatory; voices of all relevant constituencies are heard. Although the department chair may delegate authority to the residency training director, the power to implement policy requires the participation and collaboration of all parties.

Certainly there are disadvantages to participatory decision making. It is time-consuming and is not useful for response to immediate crises. With the diffusion of responsibility, it becomes difficult to assign either credit or blame for the outcomes. The process may lead to the leader's being viewed as weak. It requires special leadership skills to attain consensus, if not unanimity.

Nonetheless, the advantages clearly outweigh the disadvantages. According to Floyd (1985), participatory decision making provides the following:

- Greater understanding and acceptance of decisions by the involved parties
- Greater identification with the decisions and more commitment to them
- Better morale within the program
- Consistency with the needs of mature faculty and residents for autonomy and achievement
- Group pressure on dissenters to comply
- Cooperation and team identification
- Availability of the particular skills of individuals to the entire organization

INTERRELATED OBJECTS

The contingency theory of management maintains that there is no single best way to organize. The organizational structure must relate to both the purpose and the environment (Lawrence 2001). The participatory processes of strategic planning and decision making require an organizational structure that represents its constituencies yet maintains the centrality and continuity of the program's mission.

Residency training directors (or *program directors*) function as both leaders and managers. They "carry the flag" of the educational mission and serve as its most consistent advocates, and they also coordinate the individuals and committees, the faculty, and the residents in making the daily work of teaching and learning possible. Some of the optimal character traits for a program director are listed in Table 5–1.

Program coordinators (or administrative assistants) are responsible for implementation of the actions and decisions of the training director and the residency training committee. The ideal candidate for this position shares many of the same characteristics as the optimal training director (see Table 5–2). Much more than secretaries, coordinators maintain resident files and contracts, arrange applicant interviews, schedule special activities such as oral examinations and graduation, facilitate curriculum scheduling, compile material for communication to agencies such as the state medical board and the ABPN, and solicit timely evaluations, among a host of other duties. The training director and program coordinator should ideally maintain a calendar of repeating events to allow for sufficient preparation (Table 5–3).

The program coordinator's role is vital to the success of the program.

TABLE 5–1. Characteristics of the ideal program director

Charisma—The ability to project a credible image of leadership and inspire residents and faculty

Affability—Warmth and candor that make residents comfortable approaching the director

Availability—Willingness to provide ready access to trainees and educators

Flexibility—The capacity to accommodate to an ever-changing environment

Creativity—The ability to craft innovative solutions to educational challenges

Integrity—Honesty, professionalism, trustworthiness

Equanimity—Internal sense of balance and confidence to buffer the many assaults on the director's self-esteem

Meticulousness—Willingness to attend to the countless details necessary to maintain and improve the program

Energy—Vigor and enthusiasm to develop and expand the curriculum and perform its daily tasks

TABLE 5–2. Characteristics of the ideal program coordinator

Dependability—Trustworthiness to carry the responsibilities delegated by the training director

Thoroughness—An exacting attention to detail, particularly regarding documentation necessary for program accreditation

Efficiency—The ability to handle multiple tasks simultaneously and meet deadlines

Warmth—A personal style that makes applicants feel welcomed and that allows residents to approach with issues they may be reluctant to bring directly to the program director

Accessibility—An open door to residents and faculty

Balance—The ability to maintain both empathy with resident problems and appropriate boundaries between himself/herself and the residents

Coordinators are the first contact with applicants and with residents within the program who have issues for the training director. In practice, the administrative coordinator provides a nurturing and sustaining role that far transcends the administrative job description.

The *associate* (or *assistant*) *training director* has a role more idiosyncratically defined in each program. In smaller programs, there may be none at all. In others, there may be one assistant director for the entire program. Or there may be several, with each associate director being responsible for education at one affiliated institution and for a particular curriculum element such as consultation-liaison psychiatry or psychotherapy.

TABLE 5–3.   Annual calendar—residency training

Month	Program coordinator	Residency training director
July	New residents begin.	New residents begin.
August	Schedule semiannual reviews; send reminder to each resident about 3 weeks ahead. Schedule live patient oral examinations. Send each resident reminder plus description/instruction sheet. Resident picnic. Review recruitment materials.	Begin receiving and screening applications for residency.
September	Schedule Psychiatry Resident In-Training Examination (PRITE). Clear with clinical sites; get room and preceptors. Schedule Residency Selection Committee meetings. Begin scheduling applicant interviews. Send evaluation forms for July–September.	Fall Components Meeting, American Psychiatric Association (APA).
October	PRITE.	PRITE. Begin interviews with resident applicants.
November		Dean's letters released.
December	Holiday party. Send evaluation forms for October–December.	Holiday party.
January	Request American Board of Psychiatry and Neurology (ABPN) results of graduates.	

TABLE 5–3. Annual calendar—residency training (*continued*)

Month	Program coordinator	Residency training director
February	Recruiting dinner for local applicants. National Resident Matching Program (NRMP) Match list due.	NRMP Match list due.
March	Send appointment letters to newly matched residents. Start scheduling audiovisual oral exams for April: recruit examiners, notify sites and residents. Send evaluation forms for January–March. Send post-Match questionnaires to applicants who matched elsewhere.	American Association of Directors of Psychiatric Residency Training (AADPRT) annual meeting. NRMP results announced. After-Match recruiting, if necessary.
April	Audiovisual oral exams. Mailings to incoming residents.	Prepare rotation and seminar schedules for July–June. Assign psychotherapy supervisors. Submit budget requests to hospitals. Chief residents selected.
May	Graduation plans.	APA annual meeting. Review and revise orientation manual.
June	Prepare certificates of completion of postgraduate year 1 and residency for graduating residents for ABPN. Send evaluation forms for April–June. Prepare contracts for new residents. Graduation. Orient new residents.	Chief residents' national conference. Graduation. Orient new residents.

The *residency training committee*, also called the *educational policy committee*, serves as the major collaborative planning and decision-making body in the training program. Its composition should reflect those with the greatest investment in the educational process. Typically, membership includes the residency training director as chair, the associate training director(s), chiefs of relevant divisions or services (such as forensic and child psychiatry), other faculty members who are integral to the curriculum, and resident representatives. The training committee is responsible for designing, evaluating, and refining the curriculum; determining policy; allocating the resident workforce; disseminating information; and evaluating residents in academic difficulty.

Task forces and *work groups* may be delegated by the training director or the residency training committee to accomplish specific tasks that are of limited duration or require special expertise. Such tasks may include proposing specific didactic curricula, designing evaluation instruments, researching solutions adopted at other programs to a particular problem, or organizing a postgraduate year 1 mentorship program.

The chief resident occupies a nebulous space between residents and faculty. He, she, or they may be elected by fellow residents or appointed by faculty. Almost always, the chief resident sits on the residency training committee. If the chief is elected by peers, his or her job is usually political, as liaison between trainees and department. If he or she is appointed by faculty, the job is generally more educational or administrative. Each program will define the chief's authority and responsibility differently, but potential roles include any of the following:

- Junior faculty, teaching less-experienced residents
- Coordinator of call schedules
- Clinical chief for a selected service, such as a resident clinic
- Special clinical responsibilities, such as screening medical students for therapy
- "Student body president," representing resident sentiments to the program director and faculty

INPUT

The ingredients that ultimately yield classes of educated and trained psychiatrists are the residents themselves, the faculty, and the resources available to both. Our focus here is on the administrative integration of these elements into the training program.

Once the results of the National Resident Matching Program are announced or once a resident and training program have otherwise committed to each other, a contract must be finalized. The elements of the contract will vary across institutions but should always include the identities of the parties, the exact nature of the position, the salary and benefits, the duration of the contract and terms of its renewal and cancellation, and the obligations and responsibilities of the parties (Table 5–4). There must be a "due process" policy in place at the institutional or program level to clarify procedures and alternatives when a resident has academic or professional difficulties. Most commonly, this policy is contained in a resident policy manual, to which reference may be made in the contract. Minimal elements of the contract are dictated and monitored by the ACGME (Accreditation Council for Graduate Medical Education 2003).

The resources used by the training program include clinical facilities, clerical and administrative services, and, of course, money. Clarification of the nature of these commitments allows for optimum strategic planning. Although contracts and agreements with clinical facilities are generally conducted at the department level or higher, the residency training director should have familiarity with their content and, ideally, input into their provisions (Wilson and McLaughlin 1984). Such agreements should specify the following:

- Clinical facilities and services committed
- Staff and personnel committed
- Terms of financial exchange
- Lines of authority and responsibility
- Individual and institutional liability coverage
- Mechanisms of quality review and quality control

ENVIRONMENT

Thus far, we have considered primarily the *participants* in the educational program: the training director, his or her committees, the program coordinator, the faculty, and the residents. These figures operate in a complicated context, and their choices and behavior are shaped powerfully by nonparticipant *stakeholders*. Stakeholders are the individuals, groups, and institutions that affect and are affected by the policies and products of the training program (Srivastva 1983). The missions of the department, the school of medicine, the affiliated hospitals, and the university must all be accommodated in training program decisions. Political, social, and economic elements of the community and the society at large have a powerful influence. Decisions in organizations are reached as often on the basis of environmental exigencies as on internal logic and desirability (Griffith 1979).

TABLE 5–4. Elements of the resident contract

I. Parties to the contract
    A. Hospital, university, school of medicine
    B. Resident
II. Duration of contract: beginning and ending dates
III. Title or name of position
IV. Salary
    A. Amount
    B. Payment schedule
V. Benefits
    A. Insurance
        1. Health
        2. Life
        3. Disability
    B. Perquisites
        1. Travel funds
        2. Book funds
        3. Moving expenses
        4. Uniforms, laundry
        5. Meals
VI. Professional liability coverage
VII. Leaves of absence
    A. Vacation
    B. Sick leave
    C. Disability leave
    D. Other
VIII. Duty hours
IX. Moonlighting policy
X. Counseling services
XI. Physician impairment policy and resources
XII. Sexual harassment policy
XIII. Resident obligations
    A. Satisfactory academic and clinical performance
    B. Conformance to applicable procedures and bylaws
    C. Ethical and professional behavior
XIV. Conditions and procedures for termination of contract
XV. Grievance procedures and due process provisions

TABLE 5–5.   Stakeholders and conflicts

Stakeholder	Common conflict of values with training program
Community	Wish for clinical services that would drain program resources
University	Promotion and tenure standards inconsistent with program philosophy
School of medicine	Need for relationship with clinical entity incompatible with program's mission
Affiliated hospital	Desire for more bed and call coverage by residents
Department chair	Need for budgetary restraint

Training directors often operate at the boundaries of the program and its environment. They are the chief spokespeople for the training program. In this position, it is advisable that the training director reach consensus with the stakeholder about goals and missions. The position rarely carries enough authority for the training director to be a parochial advocate for the program's interests in opposition to those of the department, the college, or the hospital (Wilson and McLaughlin 1984). Cultivation of relationships with stakeholders is part of the ongoing maintenance of the program's effectiveness. Table 5–5 lists typical conflicts between training programs and stakeholders.

Outside the local environment, a host of entities operate to influence the function of each residency training program. This jumble of acronyms is decoded in Table 5–6 (Strauss and Preven 1991).

The training director's relationship with the department chair is worthy of particular attention. In successful programs, the training director has the authority to define the objectives of the programs and to implement curricula to achieve those ends. He or she must have a strong voice in the selection of residents and faculty. Establishment and enforcement of performance standards for residents must be under the domain of the program director (and his or her assistants and committees). Political and fiscal exigencies make it inevitable that departmental realities and training ideals will come into conflict. The training director and the chair must have an effective mechanism for communication and negotiation. Options for this function include open-door access to the chair, regular and frequent meetings, and scheduled performance reviews. If communication is effective, conflicts in values can usually be resolved or accommodated; otherwise, the results will range from problematic to disastrous.

TABLE 5–6. Organizations influencing functions of the training program

AADPRT—American Association of Directors of Psychiatric Residency Training. Includes the training directors of nearly all training programs in the United States. Also includes associate directors and fellowship directors. Provides education and advocacy for training directors.

AAP—Association for Academic Psychiatry. An organization of psychiatric educators providing education and camaraderie for teachers of students and residents.

ABPN—American Board of Psychiatry and Neurology. The organization that administers written and oral examinations to postgraduate physicians and certifies their safety and competence.

ACGME—Accreditation Council for Graduate Medical Education. Sponsored by the American Board of Medical Specialties, the American Hospital Association, the American Medical Association, the Association of American Medical Colleges, and the Council of Medical Specialty Societies. Certifies that institutions have met standards for accreditation of their residency training programs. See also *RRC*.

APA—American Psychiatric Association. The chief professional organization of American psychiatry. Represents the political, economic, and educational interests of its 40,000 members. The APA's Office of Education provides information, consultation, assistance, and liaison with other wings of the APA. Within the component structure of the APA, the Committee on Graduate Education deals specifically with residency issues and reports to the Council on Medical Education and Career Development.

ECFMG—Educational Commission for Foreign Medical Graduates. Provides certification of graduation from non-U.S. medical schools and administers examinations of readiness of international medical graduates to enter residency training in the United States.

HCFA—Health Care Financing Administration. The regulatory agency that sets and administers policy for distribution of Medicare funds, the largest single source of residency stipend money.

NRMP—National Resident Matching Program. The official cooperative plan for appointments to graduate medical education. Each spring the NRMP operates the Match, which constitutes the primary vehicle for U.S. medical graduates to enter residency training programs.

PRITE—Psychiatry Resident In-Training Examination. Sponsored by the American College of Psychiatrists, this 5-hour written examination is administered each fall. Results are for internal use only.

RRC—Residency Review Committee. A subgroup of the ACGME that reviews programs in each respective specialty. The RRC for Psychiatry certifies psychiatric training programs.

USMLE—United States Medical Licensing Examination. The three-step examination required for licensure eligibility in the United States. Replaces the former Federal Licensing Examination and National Board of Medical Examiners examination. Non-U.S. medical graduates must first pass an examination of English proficiency.

FUNDING

Possibly the most pressing element of the residency environment is financing the program. Without dollars, there is no training. And in all systems, the source of the money will expect something in return. The program director bears the dual tasks of maintaining support for his or her residency program and protecting its academic integrity.

It is a surprise to those unfamiliar with graduate medical education that the single largest source of residency training funds in the United States is Medicare. The federal program created to pay for medical care for the elderly and disabled also pays for more residency education than all other sources combined. When Medicare reimburses a hospital for clinical care, the payment includes supplements for educational expenses if the hospital is a teaching institution. The supplements are in three categories:

1. Direct medical education reimbursement (DME) pays for resident salaries and a fraction of the expenses for faculty and administrative costs.
2. Indirect medical education reimbursement (IME) pays for the added cost of providing care in a teaching institution. Medicare acknowledges that patients in teaching hospitals may stay longer, receive more diagnostic procedures, and/or suffer more complications than patients in nonteaching institutions, and it reimburses hospitals accordingly.
3. Disproportionate share adjustment (DSH) goes to many, but not all, teaching hospitals. Because teaching hospitals may provide care to more indigent patients than are served by other hospitals in the area, Medicare compensates the hospital for part of the extra cost of this care (Magen 2004).

The second largest source of residency funding is the Department of Veterans Affairs (VA). VA medical centers with teaching programs may directly employ and pay residents. State psychiatric hospitals, though they have been shrinking for decades, are another major source of funding for psychiatric residencies.

It stands to reason that hospitals providing stipend support will want resident labor in return. At the same time, psychiatric education requires experiences in settings that generate few or no funds. Community psychiatry, psychotherapy, and child and adolescent psychiatry are notoriously poorly funded and can usually offer little or nothing in the way of financial support. Didactics and supervision generate no revenues. The training director is thus in a position of needing to protect the integrity of the curriculum while managing to pay his or her residents. Each program director finds his or her own combination of diplomacy, flexibility, creativity, and audacity to strike the best balance possible in his or her environment.

In a system where different residents in the same program get paychecks and benefit packages from different sources, the training director is faced with a particularly precarious balancing act to prevent, or at least manage, jealousies and competition among trainees. It is also crucial for the training director to have some degree of certainty about the availability of stipends for the coming year before finalizing recruitment and the Match. There are few circumstances more regrettable than matching more residents than one can pay.

FEEDBACK

Maintaining and improving quality education requires "closing the loop," constantly assessing the process and the product. Such evaluation should take place at two levels: First, the program measures the skills and knowledge of the individual residents. Second, the director and his or her committee look at the overall effectiveness of the curriculum and the program.

Measuring the progress of individual residents requires a sound identification of the educational objectives against which the trainee will be measured (Bienenfeld et al. 2000). The outcomes should have *content* validity (i.e., they actually measure what they are intended to measure) and either *predictive* validity (i.e., they correlate with future competence) or *concurrent* validity (i.e., they measure qualities possessed by those of known summative competence). They should be objective, specific, and reliable (i.e., reproducible across evaluators). It is important to distinguish *formative* competencies (i.e., those accumulated on the road to expertise) from *summative* competencies (i.e., those expected at the conclusion of the training) (Yager and Bienenfeld 2003).

Typical measures used to evaluate individual resident progress include the Psychiatry Resident In-Training Examination (PRITE), clinical skills examinations ("mock boards"), and checklists of specific skills, comparable to procedure logs in surgical residencies. Supervisors' ratings are an obvious source of performance assessment. Less commonly used are more proximate measures of the results of residents' work, such as patient outcomes and satisfaction surveys. Evaluation of residents is covered more specifically in Chapter 10, "Evaluation of Residents." The training director should use all these measures in providing feedback to residents, and he or she is required by the certifying agency for psychiatry residents (the Residency Review Committee [RRC]) to do so at least twice yearly.

The evaluation of program quality may use some of the same measures but constitutes a separate process. For this purpose, the program examines its qualities against accepted standards and measures the performance of its trainees and graduates in the aggregate.

The Residency Review Committee (RRC) for Psychiatry of the ACGME undertakes regular evaluations of training programs for the purpose of certification. This ACGME accreditation, however, certifies only that minimum standards have been met and does not constitute a true measure of quality. By the time RRC certification is in danger, there have generally already been serious deficits in program quality.

Success at recruiting new residents is a measure of the program's quality as perceived by applicants. Group mean scores on the PRITE allow cognitive gains to be followed from year to year. The ABPN provides records of the test results of a program's graduates. More direct, but more difficult to obtain, are evaluations of graduates' performance by their employers or colleagues. Similarly, recent graduates can be surveyed or interviewed about the relevance of their training to the needs of their careers (Andrews and Lomax 1999; Bienenfeld et al. 2003; Langsley 1986).

Within the program, evaluations of rotations, seminars, and teachers by the residents can provide a picture of their perceived value. Such evaluations must be tempered by the realization that popularity and quality are separate dimensions; an unpopular rotation or an uncharismatic teacher may wind up providing the knowledge and skills that will ultimately prove most useful to the graduate physician.

Vehicles for obtaining this feedback from residents include the following:

- Standard evaluation forms (written or online)
- Semiannual reviews with residents
- Regular attendance at resident meetings
- Informal contact and inquiry (e.g., over lunch)

When the faculty member is an employee of the department, the training director should provide results of faculty evaluation to the chair for use in annual performance reviews. When the faculty member is a volunteer, the mechanism of feedback is much more fluid, depending on the relationships among the training director, the faculty member, the associate training director for the site of the rotation, and the department chair. In such circumstances, even more constant vigilance and more active nurturance of the relationship are required than is the case with salaried full-time faculty. Similarly, rotations at fully affiliated institutions can be reviewed by the training committee, on which the associate training director or site supervisor is likely to sit. When a rotation is at an administratively disconnected institution (e.g., a rural community mental health center), the training

director must work diplomatically, often outside formal channels, to identify the nature of any problem and to attempt to remediate it.

In the end, evaluation is an ongoing process. It is among the most important functions of the residency training committee. Determining the
desired outcomes allows the committee to have in mind its benchmarks as
it assesses the quality of the training program.

STRATEGY AND TACTICS

The schema outlined so far in this chapter places the administration of the
residency training program into a conceptual context. The implementation
of these philosophies occurs in an environment of varied and ceaseless pressures and demands, conflicting expectations, and unanticipated complications. The program director is always faced with the challenge of juggling
multiple priorities. Techniques from the corporate world translate well to
the domain of psychiatric education.

The first objective in facing a task is to identify both its importance and
its urgency. *Importance* is the relevance of a task to the ultimate mission of
the organization, in this case advancing the quality of the training program.
Urgency is the need for a task to be performed immediately. Contrary to
intuition, importance and urgency are not the same. Writing a chapter on
administration of the residency program, due to the editor in 6 months,
raises the profile of the residency; it is important but not urgent. Signing a
delinquent discharge summary to avoid losing hospital privileges is urgent,
but not important to the residency. Stephen Covey (Covey et al. 1994), a
corporate consultant, has arrayed importance and urgency to define four
quadrants of priority for tasks and projects: high or low importance and
high or low urgency (Figure 5–2).

The most productive program director will spend most of his or her energy
on Quadrant II activities, those of high importance and low urgency. To do so,
he or she must minimize the demands in the other three quadrants. Quadrant
III and IV activities, those of low importance to the educational mission, should
be delegated as much as possible. Although the training director may enjoy creating spreadsheets to document resident attendance at conferences, such a
project is not a good use of his or her valuable time and energy. What is unim-
portant for the program director may well be important for the program coordinator, a chief resident, or a hospital volunteer. Quadrant I activities are the
nightmares of training directors. A program information form required for
program accreditation is critically important; if it is due in 2 days, it is urgent.
Most Quadrant I activities are Quadrant II tasks that have been allowed to
become urgent, often by procrastination.

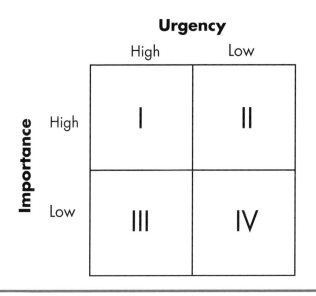

FIGURE 5–2.   Priority matrix.

Organizing the daily "To Do" list according to these priorities allows the director to allocate time and effort. He or she can schedule time to accomplish the fruitful Quadrant II jobs rather than trying to squeeze them into the cracks between lower-importance tasks. He or she can also identify those jobs that can be delegated and can prevent Quadrant II opportunities from becoming Quadrant I headaches.

To avoid such an outcome, the program director should keep track of all the projects on his or her agenda, evaluate their priorities, and then establish a task calendar for each project. Every large project can be broken down into multiple smaller tasks, some of which are sequential and some of which can be accomplished simultaneously in parallel. Assigning a deadline to each task (and sticking to it) allows the director to coordinate elements of the project, delegate pieces to those who can perform them best and/or most efficiently, and keep a Quadrant II project from becoming a Quadrant I emergency.

REFERENCES

Accreditation Council for Graduate Medical Education: Institutional Requirements. Chicago, IL, Accreditation Council for Graduate Medical Education, 2003. Available at: http://www.acgme.org. Accessed June 26, 2004.

Andrews LA, Lomax JW: Developing and monitoring the curriculum, in Handbook of Psychiatric Education and Faculty Development. Edited by Kay J, Silberman EK, Pessar L. Washington DC, American Psychiatric Press, 1999, pp 363–380

Bienenfeld D, Klykylo W, Knapp V: Process and product: development of competency-based measures for psychiatry residency. Acad Psychiatry 24:68–76, 2000

Bienenfeld D, Klykylo W, Lehrer W: Closing the loop: assessing the effectiveness of psychiatric competency measures. Acad Psychiatry 27:131–135, 2003

Covey SR, Merrill AR, Merrill RR: First Things First: To Live, to Love, to Learn, to Leave a Legacy. New York, Simon & Schuster, 1994, pp 75–103

Floyd CE: Rationale for faculty participation, in Faculty Participation in Decision Making: Necessity or Luxury? Washington, DC, Association for the Study of Higher Education, 1985, pp 1–10

Griffith F: Decision-making, in Administrative Theory in Education: Text and Readings. Edited by Griffith F. Midland, MI, Pendell, 1979, pp 233–244

Langsley DG: Evaluation during residency, in How to Evaluate Residents. Edited by Lloyd JS, Langsley DG. Chicago, IL, American Board of Medical Specialties, 1986, pp 11–30

Lawrence PR: The contingency approach to organizational design, in Handbook of Organizational Behavior. Edited by Golembiewsky RT. New York, Marcel Dekker, 2001, pp 7–18

Magen J: Graduate Medical Education Financing: The Basics. Available at: http://www.aadprt.org/training/GME/GME_Financing_Summary.rtf. Accessed May 20, 2005.

Mann D: Problems of organizational calculation, in Policy Decision-Making in Education: An Introduction to Calculation and Control. New York, Teachers College Press, 1975, pp 53–83

Srivastva S: Common themes in executive thought and action, in The Executive Mind: New Insights on Managerial Thought and Action. Edited by Srivastva S. San Francisco, CA, Jossey-Bass, 1983, pp 1–14

Strauss GD, Preven DW: Administering the residency program, in Handbook of Psychiatry Residency Training. Edited by Kay J. Washington, DC, American Psychiatric Association, 1991, pp 1–16

Wilson MP, McLaughlin CP: Organizational relationships and leadership roles, in Leadership and Management in Academic Medicine. San Francisco, CA, Jossey-Bass, 1984, pp 78–114

Yager J, Bienenfeld D: How competent are we to assess residents' competence in psychotherapy? Acad Psychiatry 27:174–181, 2003

CHAPTER 6

WHAT AND HOW TO TEACH IN THE RESIDENCY PROGRAM

Ronald O. Rieder, M.D.

Lisa A. Mellman, M.D.

Residency training directors have so much to do to keep a program running that they do not often grapple with their own views about what to teach and how to optimize learning. Their own primary educational goals and their own beliefs about how residents will successfully learn the essential elements of being a psychiatrist are often only partially developed. In this chapter, the two of us, with 35 years of experience as training directors, pose these questions to ourselves. We believe, however, that considering the "what" and "how" should be done with full recognition of the restrictions and resources that always impinge on our inclinations, so we have included reference to these as well. We believe that training directors can substantially shape their own program, especially if they have defined their own goals, and we provide some advice regarding how to deal with the obstacles. We also believe that training directors can create an environment where positive identification of residents with the training director and other faculty members is fostered, and teaching and learning are modeled. In this environment, questioning and openness will flourish.

Our overall aim is to help training directors shape their own programs, but we feel it is useful in that regard to give specifics of the directions we have taken at our own Columbia University program. Programs differ substantially across the country, and obviously our own decisions would not fit all, but we believe that by giving these details we will alert training directors to problems that need to be addressed, as well as opinions to be considered.

We have organized this chapter into two main sections: "What to Teach," which focuses on developing a set of program goals, and "How to Foster Learning," which focuses on creating a positive, constructive learning environment. We have not, however, kept to a strict separation between the what and the how.

WHAT TO TEACH: SETTING GOALS

WHO SETS THE GOALS

Those appointed as residency training directors usually imagine that one of the key aspects of their job will be to establish the educational direction of their residency program. They may envisage themselves as a captain setting the bearings of their ships on faraway lands. It comes as an abrupt awakening, then, to discover the many forces that constrain and influence the program director's freedom in this regard. Primary among these are the 33 pages (as of 2004) of Accreditation Council for Graduate Medical Education (ACGME) program requirements for residency training in psychiatry (available from the ACGME Web site: http://www.acgme.org or http://www.acgme.org/downloads/RRC_progReq/400pr101.pdf).

It may provide no solace that one of the requirements is in fact "the preparation of a written statement outlining the educational goals of the program with respect to knowledge, skills and other attributes of residents at each level of training and for each major rotation or other program assignment," because the document goes on to specify, under "Objectives of Training," 30 specific requirements ranging from being able to perform a complete history and physical examination to teaching psychiatry to medical students. The requirement for competence in psychotherapy, recently added by the ACGME, is another example of outside forces steering the content of residency education.

In addition to the ACGME, others are likely to have a view of what the program's goals should be. The department chairs and faculty members are likely to believe that the residency program should serve the needs and objectives of the department and its divisions—for example, provide clinical care in a variety of settings, such as the inpatient units and the emergency room, especially for evening and weekend patient care. However, it could be that they are most concerned about applications for the research fellowship, or specific subspecialty programs such as the psychoanalytic institute, or the child and adolescent psychiatry residency. If so, they will make the case for the importance of these experiences in residency training and even for the selection of residency applicants interested in these areas. Residents themselves are also likely to formulate and push for their own goals, in an individualized or at times collective manner. Their aim is often, understandably, to prepare themselves for clinical practice and, often, to resist activities that would add additional hours to their day.

Even other groups outside the department have claims with regard to psychiatry residency training. A recent example is the Institute of Medicine report initiated by the National Institute of Mental Health, which called for more research training during residency. Similar recommendations have been put forth to expand training in ethics, minority issues, psychiatry related to human immunodeficiency virus (HIV) infection, group therapy, forensic psychiatry, and the treatment of the chronically ill.

WHAT GOALS SHOULD BE SET

Given this "magnetic field" that is certainly likely to influence or even wreak havoc with any training director's compass, what can we recommend? First, that residency training directors become well acquainted with all the ACGME requirements and the extent to which they are being met or could be met by the program. In fact, many of these requirements give training directors some autonomy and can be satisfied with a wide array of responses. Training directors should also catalog the local and national forces that have made claim on the residency, as described under "Who Sets the Goals," above.

All these requirements can be impediments to the aims of the program director. However, as discussed below, they can also be of substantial help in implementing one's own agenda. The most important task is the process of deciding on one's own goals. It begins with asking the questions *"What knowledge and skills are most essential to the practice of psychiatry?"* and *"What knowledge and skills are most needed to continue to learn and practice in the future?"*

Alternative questions that could be asked are "What type of training is most attractive to resident applicants?" or "What knowledge and skills are desirable in the marketplace (e.g., managed care organizations)?" Such questions orient the goals around others' desires and perceptions. If residency directors are to arrive at their own goals through a process of self-examination and decision making, the first set of questions in the previous paragraph are the most relevant. We prefer the questions that require the residency training director to grapple with his or her beliefs and ideals about psychiatry and psychiatrists, now and in the future. We believe that out of the arising conviction will come the commitment and energy to implement the goals and, equally importantly, at times to change one's own direction when it is appropriate.

Alternatively, instead of asking such questions, there are other ways of proceeding—for example, taking as goals the six competencies of residency training promulgated by the ACGME (Accreditation Council for Graduate Medical Education 1999):

a. **Patient Care** that is compassionate, appropriate, and effective for the treatment of health problems and the promotion of health
b. **Medical Knowledge** about established and evolving biomedical, clinical, and cognate (e.g., epidemiological and social-behavioral) sciences and the application of this knowledge to patient care
c. **Practice-Based Learning and Improvement** that involves investigation and evaluation of [one's] own patient care, appraisal and assimilation of scientific evidence, and improvements in patient care
d. **Interpersonal and Communication Skills** that result in effective information exchange and teaming with patients, their families, and other health professionals
e. **Professionalism,** as manifested through a commitment to carrying out professional responsibilities, adherence to ethical principles, and sensitivity to a diverse patient population
f. **Systems-Based Practice,** as manifested by actions that demonstrate an awareness of and responsiveness to the larger context and system of health care and the ability to effectively call on system resources to provide care that is of optimal value

One objection we have to establishing these competencies as goals is that they are too broad and too general to focus program directors, residents, and faculty members on a mission to establish a quality education. The competencies are much more focused on measurement rather than teaching. They are also, like the ACGME's program requirements, imposed by a regulatory agency, not chosen and "owned" by the program director. The natural response to the six competencies is a "fill in the blank" response—in other words, to find some way that the current program promotes and measures these competencies. We believe that only by setting their own goals will program directors have the commitment necessary to push their goals to substantially better the program, and obtain the satisfaction that comes from doing so. However, after one's goals are set, the ACGME competencies can be useful in examining and categorizing what one has set out to do.

What Knowledge and Skills Are Most Essential to the Practice of Psychiatry?

We believe that the core knowledge and skills for the practice of psychiatry are interviewing, diagnosis, psychopharmacology, psychotherapy, and working effectively with others in systems of care. In focusing on these areas, specific problems and decisions arise.

Interviewing. Finding out about the patient is not an easy task, nor is it self-evident what is necessary to develop this skill. We have found that residents need strong encouragement to establish specific objectives in evaluation interviews and to be able to ask patients the specific questions that will provide information such as the degree of suicidality. In other words, residents need to learn to be in charge of the interview. This means having an interview goal that is being pursued, which could be done by passive listening but also can require interrupting patients and not accepting "I don't know" as an answer. Residents need to learn to elicit important phenomenology, to explore areas of pain and shame in their patients, and to understand the person and life behind the symptoms. Videotaping residents' interviews and having attending physicians conduct live or videotaped interviews of patients "blind" (i.e., without first being presented a lengthy case description) are useful strategies. Interviewing through an interpreter is also a key skill.

Diagnosis. Two problems are frequently encountered: 1) residents eliciting only information that is relevant to diagnoses—in other words, being overly reverential to DSM-IV-TR (American Psychiatric Association 2000) and especially to Axis I, which is more frequently seen on inpatient units; and 2) residents ignoring a rigorous diagnostic process, which is more likely to be seen in outpatient settings where psychotherapy is practiced.

Psychopharmacology. The issue with psychopharmacology is whether to focus on the first-line treatments, applying evidence-based medicine, or to set a goal of having residents treat nonresponsive cases and expect residents to initiate combined or unique treatments that have less available research backing. We believe both are important but especially the latter, because so much primary psychopharmacology is being administered by primary care physicians.

Psychotherapy. Decisions in the area of psychotherapy are often the most difficult to make and the hardest to defend. There has been serious debate as to whether residents should be extensively trained in psychotherapy. One

answer is that such training is required by the Residency Review Committee (RRC) for Psychiatry of the ACGME, but for us the compelling reasons
are that psychotherapy has an increasing body of evidence regarding its efficacy in a number of formats for a number of disorders (Nathan and Gorman 2002) and that it offers residents an opportunity to understand the
cognitive and emotional psychopathology of psychiatric disorders. In other
words, in psychotherapy sessions residents can learn from patients the de-
spair, fears, memories, impulses, attachments, and repetitions that are as
important as—or even more important than—the observable signs and
more easily reported symptoms of psychiatric disorders. All psychotherapies offer opportunities in this regard, but we believe that psychodynamic
psychotherapy leads to the broadest and perhaps deepest explorations of
these matters.

Residency program directors must decide how to allocate the time
available for psychotherapy training among the various psychotherapies.
The RRC has emphasized psychodynamic, cognitive, supportive, and brief
psychotherapy along with integrated psychotherapy and psychopharmacological treatment. As a result, interpersonal therapy, group therapy, family
therapy, and others seem to be given lower status. We recommend that residency programs set a goal of real competence in supportive psychotherapy
and in one or two of the other psychotherapies rather than attempting to
distribute emphasis equally across many modalities. Learning specific
forms of psychotherapy well requires extensive resources from the department in the form of didactic teaching, individual supervision, and access to
suitable patients for substantial periods of time. Supervision and the treatment of suitable patients are particularly important for developing these
skills. Most residencies do not have the resources to teach more than two
or three forms of psychotherapy, and some residencies stretch to teach even
one. Our own choice has been to emphasize psychodynamic psychotherapy,
with cognitive therapy a strong second and substantial training in supportive psychotherapy often being used in conjunction with medications.

In addition to the type of psychotherapy, programs must decide on the
length of psychotherapeutic experiences they offer. Here we have come to
believe something paradoxical, that to train residents to do brief therapy it
is very useful to begin with longer-term experiences. Brief therapy involves
more activity and is best done by sure-footed clinicians. Residents should
not learn by "shooting from the hip." Whether they are doing psychodynamic or another form of psychotherapy, the program should allow them in
the early years to go at a slow pace and heavily utilize supervision between
sessions to understand what they are doing. Also, we believe that longer-
term experiences with patients lead to the trusting therapeutic alliance that

allows the resident to hear the patient's own narrative about his or her illness and a chance to grasp the importance of this point of view before attempting psychotherapy to change it. It also allows for the opportunity to witness change in the patient resulting from psychotherapy.

Working in systems of care.   Historically, outpatient psychiatry has often been conducted on a model of one physician–one patient at a time, but today psychiatrists are much more involved in working in complex environments, including families, co-therapists, managed care regulators, ward staff, and utilization review personnel. Because physicians are trained to have substantial authority, residents—especially those who have recently been working on a medical or surgical service—may find it difficult to share authority and responsibility with nonmedical colleagues. They also must switch their focus from phenomena within a patient to phenomena between themselves and other individuals. These interpersonal skills are so closely related to personality attributes that it may seem hard to approach them the way that the other skills listed above are taught. However, we have found that residents can learn such skills when they are put into these situations and when they are given frank feedback about, for example, a dismissive attitude or an inability to conceptualize their impact on a system. Sometimes this learning appears to be a set of remembered rules rather than internalized change, but that may be only the beginning stage of learning. We look for those with deficits in this area and push them to make progress.

What Knowledge and Skills Are Most Needed to Continue to Learn and Practice in the Future?

Our answer to this second question for program directors is 1) neurobiology, 2) the ability to read the psychiatric literature, and 3) a commitment to evidence-based practice.

Neurobiology.   We include in the term *neurobiology* neuroanatomy, neurochemistry, neurocircuitry, brain imaging, psychiatric genetics, and other brain sciences. Perhaps we have been influenced by working at a medical center with a Nobel laureate in this area (Dr. Eric Kandel), but to us it seems evident that the neural mechanisms underlying higher mental processes are now being understood and that the identification and manipulation of those mechanisms will be the focus of psychiatric diagnosis and therapeutics for the near and distant future. What is not evident are the educational goals that should be currently pursued in this area for psychiatric residents. We think that, at minimum, there needs to be 1) some level of fluency about neural structures; 2) understanding of the data and concepts regarding how behaviors (such as those seen in anxiety and depression) are the result of the flow of information through circuits that connect neural structures; 3) recognition of how current medications have both therapeutic effects and unwanted side effects through actions on these circuits, which can, to some extent, be understood, predicted, and even utilized in drug design; and 4) recognition of how current medications affect gene transcription, not just receptors, and how the genetic predisposition to illnesses results from the additive action of many genes that affect neural functioning.

Ability to read the psychiatric literature and commitment to evidence-based psychiatry.   These two goals are linked but are better achieved if they are differentiated. During the past 10 years there has been an unheralded but extremely discouraging development: psychiatric journals have achieved a level of sophistication that makes it almost impossible for residents (and probably most psychiatrists) to comprehend essential elements, such as the nature of the measurements, the statistics used, and even the rationale for drawing the conclusions from the data. This difficulty is especially true for reports of brain imaging and genetic studies, which have the most significance for understanding the etiopathogenesis of psychiatric disorders. The therapeutics literature is somewhat easier to comprehend, but in this area the influence of pharmaceutical companies, which can often be subtle and unnoticed, can lead to unwarranted conclusions (Safer 2002). The obstacles to this goal are therefore substantial. We do not have a perfect solution, but we recommend the following: 1) the difficulty of reading the literature needs to be acknowledged; 2) faculty members should not expect residents to be prepared to read and comprehend the literature; and 3) strong didactic courses should be offered that discuss how various types of psychiatric research are done, how the data are derived, and the kind of statistics that tend to be used and that provide practice in reading and critiquing both good and poor papers. Residents have to be encouraged to be skeptical of conclusions but not be dismissive of research; they need to learn to review the literature, even if they cannot always fully understand the articles. It is a narrow line to walk. Having residency training directors teach or co-teach such courses is excellent modeling, as discussed below under "Program Directors as Models."

A commitment to evidence-based psychiatry is developed not in the classroom, nor even from reading the psychiatric literature, but rather in the day-to-day supervision that residents receive for their patient care. The essential ingredients are a commitment to providing the most effective care possible, an expertise in obtaining information that could be applied to a specific clinical situation, a willingness to learn from others (including other types of psychiatrists, other universities, and other countries), a critical attitude toward faddish theories and claims, and a willingness to believe that what psychiatrists do could often be improved. It is fortuitous that immediate Internet access to evidence-based summaries such as the Cochrane Reviews (http://www.cochrane.org) is now available. Reviewing the literature was once a problem, but it is now often the easiest element to acquire. Changing the attitudes and teaching approaches of supervisors is more difficult. One route to achieving this goal is to enlist the support of powerful figures in the department, such as the chair, to model the commitment and process; this approach seems to have been successful in some programs.

Becoming a Psychotherapist

Helping residents develop as psychotherapists involves additional issues beyond the decisions regarding psychotherapy teaching discussed in the subsections above. The major question is whether the development of psychotherapeutic competence requires personal reflection, insight, and sometimes even substantial personal change in areas such as empathy, awareness and tolerance of affect and intimacy, and moralistic attitudes. Certainly psychoanalysis as a discipline has decided that personal psychoanalysis and change are essential. In most residency programs, psychodynamic psychotherapy is taught by psychoanalysts or others with this interest, and from them there is often encouragement to enter personal psychotherapy. However, there is no consensus among training directors on this issue, and there are no data that would help in making programmatic decisions. Our own belief is that conducting effective psychodynamic psychotherapy does involve professional capabilities that are personal, such as empathy and the ability to sense the feelings of patients. These are extremely difficult to teach through the usual methods of didactic teaching and clinical supervision, which suffice for other psychiatric skills. We do believe that personal psychotherapy is very important and perhaps essential in this regard. However, we believe that there are ways that such change can be fostered in residency training itself.

The major instrument for such training is the detailed supervision of the resident's psychotherapy sessions with patients. Traditionally this supervision has been conducted through the review of process notes—nearly verbatim notes recorded by the resident during the session. We are also beginning to review videotaped sessions, although they pose some additional challenges to the psychotherapy itself, such as increased anxiety (in the resident perhaps even more than in the patient). In either case, this type of supervision is extremely time intensive; 1 hour of supervision will usually only cover 1 or 2 hours of resident psychotherapy. This level of detail is necessary because it must reveal specific unhelpful interactions of the resident with the patient. Frequently noted among these are interactions in which the resident 1) failed to comprehend what the patient was in some way expressing, 2) experienced an unrecognized affect or impulse with regard to the patient that prompted a defensive or otherwise unhelpful response, or 3) expressed in some form a directive to the patient that came from the therapist's needs rather than those of the patient. To make these kinds of interactions clear, we give the following respective examples: a resident 1) does not recognize sadness or guilt; 2) is sexually excited by the patient, which leads him or her to change the topic; or 3) tells the patient to "try harder" to find a relationship. Other important psychotherapeutic errors are derived from residents' beliefs, defenses, conflicts, affects, and impulses; we describe these because we have found them to be common and basic.

When supervisors have access to detailed notes or videotapes of sessions, they have the opportunity to explore these problematic interactions (and the reasons behind them) with the resident. The process folio, a series of process-oriented write-ups described by Yager and Kay (2003), also provides access to the resident's detailed conceptual thinking about cases. This exposure is not so different from psychotherapy itself, and at times residents can feel anxious or resentful. However, a good supervisor has the equivalent of a therapeutic alliance with the resident: a supervisory alliance, in which what the resident feels and does is subject to correction but not rebuke (Ende et al. 1995). The supervisor models empathy and openness for the resident in the process of illuminating the subtle influence of the resident's fluctuating feelings during the session. Review of process notes or videotaped sessions in supervision also allows supervisors to point out and reinforce instances in which the resident demonstrated understanding of the patient and interventions that facilitated the treatment. This combination of positive reinforcement, modeling, and fine focus on process can very substantially enhance the resident's capabilities of performing psychotherapy and can lead residents to identify strongly with their supervisors in their psychotherapeutic roles. Our views on this matter have been prompted by the reports to us of many residents over many years. We emphasize this issue because we believe that the detailed supervision of resident psychotherapy is endangered by financial pressures, and we wish to give a rationale for its continuation.

Beyond Knowledge and Skills

Teaching goals are usually divided into knowledge, skills, and attitudes. In this section we have focused on knowledge and skills, but there are many attitudes that need to be considered in psychiatric residency training. These cut across all medical disciplines, and most can be considered part of the ACGME competence of professionalism. We wish to focus on what we regard as the most important of these attitudes: responsibility to patients, and the program director's role in motivating residents to contribute to the field of psychiatry.

Responsibility to patients has long been embedded into medical education, and that is still the case. However, we believe that it is endangered, or at least diminished, by the new, strictly enforced rules regarding work hours for residents promulgated by the ACGME (Steinbrook 2002) and by the message of managed care that only necessary (i.e., approved rather than optimal) treatment should be provided. In the practice of medicine, it is sometimes necessary to provide more time or energy for patients than one expected to provide, and at times there is great benefit to be derived from going the extra mile. Models of expending this extra effort have always been provided during residency, but the new ACGME rules focus on institutional responsibility to patients, not personal responsibility, and in managed care settings residents see patient care administered with more attention being given to time and cost than to quality. We think that program directors should look for opportunities to model and promote commitment to patients and to the finest patient care possible. The impact of this new environment should be openly discussed with residents.

We also believe that program directors and other faculty members have an opportunity to inspire residents, again usually by modeling. The field of psychiatry needs leaders to help it develop in many ways—new understanding of psychiatric disorders, new treatments, new ways to deliver treatment to those in need, and carrying the humanistic perspective into political issues. The field needs great clinicians, educators, researchers, and administrators. There are legends about how department chairs in the past inspired our current leaders to make their contributions. Now chairs are often so busy with financial and other administrative matters that they hardly know the residents. Program directors may feel that they are not viewed with the same respect and do not have the same level of influence. We encourage them to try to exert their influence, because most residents have ambitions to tap. Discovering these ambitions—and supporting them with both encouragement and practical advice—is all that is needed. It may even make the training director into a bit of a legend.

WHAT RESIDENCY DIRECTORS CONFRONT IN ATTEMPTS TO ACCOMPLISH THEIR GOALS

MACHIAVELLI AND THE TRAINING DIRECTOR

Although residency education does not often have high status or large financial resources, it nevertheless attracts interest and debate from a variety of sources in the department. This attention can be very threatening and demoralizing to program directors, who can feel that they are in fact not in charge of anything other than colossal paperwork tasks. We recommend somewhat Machiavellian strategies to deal with this situation. First one must know the desires and ambitions of the oppositional forces.

Perhaps surprisingly, we list the residents themselves as the first of these opposing groups. Of course we know that there is significant overlap between the aims of program directors and the needs of the residents, as is evident in the preceding section. Programs become better by paying close attention to residents' feedback and responding with changes. However, residents—especially early during the residency—often lack perspective and are preoccupied with learning what is immediately applicable to the care of their patients. This is usually the practical management of patients, such as details of pharmacological management, some interviewing "gems," and diagnostic rules, along with how to obtain tests, consultations, and so forth. They also often do not want to spend time away from their patient duties, because to do so means that they will have to work longer hours when they return. The question must be asked, "Should residents be taught only what they want to learn?" Our answer is "No." The practical knowledge should certainly be imparted, but much of this should be left to the clinical supervisors. We respect a tradition of academic medicine, which involves long ward rounds, with more focus on discussion of disease mechanisms than on patient management. The program director must proclaim and achieve the goal of having residents learn the facts and theories of psychiatry (albeit while sitting down rather than standing up). Although this information could be imparted by supervised practice, we believe there is good reason to have a strong didactic program wherein, for example, neurobiological and psychodynamic principles are taught systematically, and to begin this effort during the early years of the residency.

Often service chiefs are more senior and politically powerful in a department of psychiatry than the program director, and service chiefs see residents, more or less, as a physician workforce. With the tremendous financial belt-tightening that has been and is still occurring, hospitals aim for productivity, which translates into wanting residents to treat greater numbers of patients. Program directors, and residents, feel that this can become burdensome and counterproductive educationally because residents have less time to discuss, read about, or even talk to or think about their patients. There is no easy solution to this problem, but program directors must confront it. They will need strategies and allies, as discussed below under "Strategies for Implementing the Training Director's Goals" and "Faculty Resources." However, they need to have a vision or goal as well. This should not be conceptualized as "limit the service delivery." It should be to "integrate teaching into everyday life." This means making each case a learning case, and it means making each service chief and supervising attending physician into a teacher. It may mean making nurses and social workers teachers, symbolized by faculty appointments. It certainly means setting expectations that one of the most important aims of a clinical service is the education of residents, and instituting a process by which the quality of the education is evaluated and publicized.

In the first few subsections under "What to Teach: Setting Goals" in this chapter, we described the numerous forces that can and often do impinge on residency training. In this paragraph we discuss how program directors can utilize, rather than be buffeted by, these forces. We refer to Machiavelli (1513) to bolster the resolve of program directors to think of themselves as potentially powerful princes within the politics of their department. A few of Machiavelli's principles do apply. Certainly this one:

> The princes [program director] should…avoid anything which would make him hated and despised…. When a prince has the goodwill of the people [residents] he should not worry about conspiracies…. From this can be drawn another noteworthy consideration: that princes should delegate to others the enactment of unpopular measures and keep in their own hands the distribution of favors. (Machiavelli 1513, XIX, pp. 102–106)

And perhaps even the following:

> You must realize that a prince, and especially a new prince, cannot practice all those things which give men a reputation for virtue…. He should not deviate from what is good, if that is possible, but he should know how to do evil, if that is necessary. (Machiavelli 1513, XVIII, p. 1001)

By these, we mean that program directors should not remain above the fray and hope that they can institute their goals by proclaiming their virtue. We suggest they consider the strategies listed in the following subsection.

STRATEGIES FOR IMPLEMENTING THE TRAINING DIRECTOR'S GOALS

1. It is important to know the RRC regulations thoroughly. They can often be selectively quoted to defend what one wishes to institute.
2. The long-term practical benefits to the department of good residency training should be emphasized. These include retaining well-trained psychiatrists who become faculty members, attracting better and better

applicants, and enhancing the reputation of the department by being seen as doing well in the Match and a good place to train.

3. The department chair is important and is always a potential ally. It is important that he or she know what the training director is doing and is trying to accomplish. The training director should seek the chair's advice on problems and should alert him or her to difficulties; the chair should not find out about such things through other channels. It is desirable to find out what the chair's educational policy and priorities are and to try to get him or her to be an active teacher or supervisor. The chair should be encouraged to have social interactions with residents at informal activities. Every small victory—for example, a fellowship awarded to one of the residents, some good results on the Psychiatry Resident In-Training Examination (PRITE)—should be reported to the chair. The training director should ask to be included on important committees where service issues are discussed.

4. Faculty members need to be courted, especially those who do not have a natural alliance with the residents. They need to receive feedback about their teaching—not only when it is deficient. They need to get praise, and public praise if there is opportunity to do so—for example, initiating a request for academic promotion. They should be asked to voice their opinions regarding education without being put in charge of it. Educational retreats are very useful for this purpose, even brief retreats on an evening or weekend to plan or review a part of the program.

5. Residents are the program director's most important allies but are also the most dangerous ones. The most essential thing is for program directors to be well known by and in frequent contact with the residents. If this is not the case, the residents will fix the negative transferences that inevitably emerge, including paranoid ones, on the program director. They too have to know what the program director is trying to accomplish, and the frustration in not being able to effect these goals. Program directors often worry that they will be seen as splitting or as being too allied with the residents, but residents know that realities are such that not all their wishes can be effected. They are usually satisfied that the program director shares their goals and their frustrations. If this strong connection can be made, then the residents can be used to good advantage. For example, a polite appeal from residents made directly to the chair is very difficult to reject.

FACULTY RESOURCES

We end this section with a discussion of dealing with not having the funding or faculty resources to put educational goals into effect. This is quite commonly a problem. We have learned, however, that there may be untapped resources, and we offer these suggestions:

1. Faculty appointments are a type of currency. They are prestigious, and at times they are helpful or even necessary for becoming part of networks or group plans for insurance, and the like. Program directors who are interested in developing a new program or in increasing the amount of supervision should seek permission to recruit voluntary faculty members with those skills or to upgrade the titles of those involved.
2. The extent of clinical income that is generated by resident activity, or educational resources coming to the hospitals via the Medicare graduate medical education funding streams, should be discovered by the program director and should be used to make a case that educational innovations be funded.
3. It might be possible to trade resources in ways that would vary from program to program, depending on the extent to which the program director has control over the resident lines. Unused lines are especially useful for this purpose. For example, it might be possible to use one for a non-accredited fellowship in emergency room psychiatry or for research, and to receive in return the funds that would have gone for this purpose, and these might be available for use in flexible ways such as buying computers.
4. Finally, there is of course the possibility of access to pharmaceutical grants for educational purposes. These are controversial, but most hospitals allow them in the way the American Psychiatric Association accepts them—as unrestricted educational grants that are designed by the recipients, not by company personnel, and do not include direct advertising or access to residents. For example, we accept pharmaceutical support for our Grand Rounds program, but not, however, for any one speaker. Rather, we receive support for the costs of a month of Grand Rounds. We thus remain in control of whom we choose as speakers and give an equal honorarium regardless of the speaker or topic. Finding a way to configure educational projects that meet one's own standards and are still appealing to the companies requires some ingenuity and at times some tough bargaining, but it is quite possible.

HOW TO FOSTER LEARNING

THE LEARNING ENVIRONMENT

One of the most important goals of a program director should be to establish an environment where learning is embedded in the daily life of the resident. By this we mean inspiring residents to want to learn, expect to learn, enjoy learning, and see teaching and learning going on around them. This results from a set of attitudes conveyed by the program director and faculty in a variety of ways (Hafferty 1998; Pinsky et al. 1998).

A constructive learning environment develops when the approach to patient care, and to discussions about psychiatric knowledge, involves questioning, experimentation, and excitement. There is no question that residents want to be taught a body of knowledge that will allow them to make clinical decisions with relative confidence; we do not suggest that faculty take on an extremely skeptical attitude that nothing is really known. There is a growing evidence base for psychiatry that is relatively accessible, and this evidence base should be incorporated into clinical decision making. However, the first action in seeking this information is to define a question, and the evidence that is found in such a search should not be taken as "The Answer" to this question. Questioning should continue with, for example, the question of whether the data available are applicable to the patient at hand. Many of the treatment studies in psychiatry have been conducted with patient samples that are not reflective of the patients seen, even patients with the same diagnosis, because these clinical trials seek patients with no comorbid conditions or who have not been treatment resistant. This continued questioning leads to a "let's try and see" attitude, in which both the resident and the supervisor take each case as a clinical experiment wherein the outcome is not at all certain but the expectation is that something will be learned by it. It is useful to introduce residents to the case reports that are published in the *American Journal of Psychiatry* and other journals to illustrate how clinical treatments can be reported as experiments with $N=1$. Encouraging and assisting residents to write up such a case is an extremely potent means of conveying this message.

WAYS OF LEARNING

Two general principles of learning have been well studied and can be described as models of positive versus negative reward, or of reinforcement versus aversive conditioning. Both can lead to substantial behavioral change. We apply the concepts of identification and intimidation to residency education in a similar way. The intimidating teacher or supervisor instills shame for errors and fear of humiliation or embarrassment that lead students to try to learn what it takes to avoid such outcomes. Intimidation is an extremely potent tool for learning, and we expect that most readers can recall a specific bit of knowledge that became emblazoned in their minds through this process when they made an error and received such a response. This is likely to have occurred in medical school; it is our impression that intimidation is still widely used there.

It would be very possible to construct a residency that uses intimidation to promote learning. Posting PRITE scores, for example, could be a means of doing so. However, we do not recommend it, because it is not conducive to the task of learning the most important aspects of psychiatry. Psychiatric residents do have to learn specific bits of data, but even more they need to learn how to interact with psychiatric patients. This interaction requires engagement, warmth, openness, flexibility, clear communication, reward, and optimism. We believe that the learning environment should provide positive identification with affirming, generative, thoughtful teachers as the primary basis of learning these capabilities. We want residents to come to admire their teachers and supervisors so much that they are inspired to develop their own knowledge and skills and become like these admired figures. To promote this it is necessary to 1) have long-term relationships between faculty members and residents, 2) have faculty members be admirable individuals who take a genuine interest in their students, 3) make sure that faculty members are indeed openly and consistently valued by the program directors and other departmental administrators, and 4) make sure that problematic supervisor-resident pairings get attention and that destructive ones, if they emerge, are addressed and even terminated.

PROGRAM DIRECTORS AS MODELS

Program directors should take the lead in exemplifying this learning environment. This could be done through supervising and mentoring residents. A cautionary note is the risk of getting close with some residents and not others, which can generate jealousy and resentment. We encourage program directors to teach often in the didactic program. Specific courses we recommend teaching are 1) courses for the development of skills such as interviewing, formulating mental status, diagnosis, or teaching; 2) courses preparing residents for careers, such as "Career Options" or "Office Practice"; and 3) courses that evaluate the literature, such as a course in journal reading or the journal club itself. In each of these courses, teachers have the opportunity to demonstrate their own knowledge and directly convey their commitment to helping residents be successful psychiatrists. Some of the courses listed above are self-evident; perhaps "Career Options" and "Office Practice" are not. In "Career Options" we ask faculty members practicing a variety of psychiatric careers (e.g., community psychiatry, child psychiatry, psychoanalysis, research) to speak openly about the advantages and disadvantages of their subspecialty, even openly discussing their incomes, with the program director helping with the interview and discussion. In "Office Practice" we give residents practical tips on how to rent an office, set fees, get on panels, obtain referrals, and so forth.

In all courses or conferences led by program directors the values of questioning and open seeking of truth should be modeled. This involves getting residents to participate in the discussions rather than allowing them to be passive listeners. Sometimes it involves what is called "pimping"—the direct questioning of residents regarding their opinions or knowledge. This technique risks the intimidation that educators try to guard against, but when it is done without instilling shame and humiliation, it can be an excellent illustration of the learning environment. Residents' opinions must be taken very seriously; program directors must admit what they do not know. Residents must learn that asking questions and admitting one's lack of knowledge are appreciated (Irby et al. 1991).

RESIDENT TEACHING

Resident teaching is also a key element in establishing an atmosphere for learning. It can take a variety of forms, ranging from resident presentations in a seminar-type class or journal club to residents being the primary course director or clinical supervisor for medical students or junior residents. We have found that pairing residents in a seminar course, asking for a joint presentation on a topic, is effective in maximizing the residents' efforts to arrive at a high-quality product. We have elective opportunities to teach but also require all residents to teach medical students. Courses taught by the residency and medical student training directors on how to teach and supervise include such topics as lecturing, performing a literature review, and obtaining trainee participation. Taking teaching seriously in this way, and getting residents to reflect on it, can change the residents' involvement in their own education. Having resident teaching awards, some selected by the medical students and some by the faculty, similarly enhances serious attention to both teaching and learning.

PASSING MUSTER

In the beginning of the chapter we suggested that to determine the appropriate goals for the residency, training directors should ask themselves two questions—"What knowledge and skills are most essential to the practice of psychiatry?" and "What knowledge and skills are most needed to continue to learn and practice in the future?"—and not begin with the stated requirements of the ACGME. Although the answers to these questions will reflect the program's view of a psychiatrist and the philosophy of the individual department, there is always a risk that these ideas would be unrelated to any accepted vision of residency education, such as that embodied in the ACGME general competencies. In fact, in a balanced program, the goals set by the training director will probably easily fit the ACGME core competencies as well. Some goals will represent several competencies. For example, the goals we have described for our program of interviewing, diagnosis, psychopharmacology, and psychotherapy are also examples of patient care. In addition, interviewing is considered part of medical knowledge and of interpersonal and communication skills (Table 6–1). We recommend that once training directors have determined their own goals, they reconfigure them under the headings of the ACGME competencies. If all six core competencies are well represented, the priorities set by the training director will likely also pass muster with the ACGME.

SUMMARY

Program directors should take advantage of the opportunities they have to shape the content and nature of their programs, being aware that they will encounter many obstacles, mostly in the form of interested parties. We recommend taking as goals the most essential elements of psychiatry residency training, rather than attempting to institute in some way each and every one of the many disparate elements in the ACGME program requirements or the broadly stated ACGME competencies. The focus should be on "What knowledge and skills are most essential to the practice of psychiatry?" and "What knowledge and skills are most needed to continue to learn and practice in the future?" Psychotherapy and the learning necessary to become a psychotherapist deserve special thought and planning. Program directors should also be very attentive to the development of a positive atmosphere in the residency. We term this the *learning environment* and recommend that training directors play a major role themselves in modeling and developing it. To be successful at such lofty goals, against such formidable odds, we recommend knowledge of certain Machiavellian principles and thinking of oneself as able to affect generations to come.

TABLE 6–1. How recommended goals can fulfill the ACGME general competencies

Our goals	Patient care	Medical knowledge	Practice-based learning	Interpersonal and communication skills	Professionalism	Systems-based practice
Interviewing	X	X		X		
Diagnosis	X	X				
Psychopharmacology	X	X	X			
Psychotherapy	X	X		X		
Working in systems of care				X	X	X
Neurobiology		X				
Ability to read the literature						
Commitment to evidence-based psychiatry		X	X			
Responsibility for patients			X		X	
The learning environment			X	X	X	
Questioning			X			
Resident teaching			X		X	

Note.   ACGME = Accreditation Council for Graduate Medical Education.

REFERENCES

Accreditation Council for Graduate Medical Education: Minimum Program Requirements Language. Chicago, IL, Accreditation Council for Graduate Medical Education, 1999. Available at: http://www.acgme.org/outcome/comp/compMin.asp. Accessed June 27, 2004.

American Psychiatric Association: Diagnostic and Statistical Manual of Mental Disorders, 4th Edition, Text Revision. Washington, DC, American Psychiatric Association, 2000

Ende J, Pomerantz A, Erickson F: Preceptors' strategies for correcting residents in an ambulatory care medicine setting: a qualitative analysis. Acad Med 70:224–229, 1995

Hafferty FW: Beyond curriculum reform: confronting medicine's hidden curriculum. Acad Med 73:403–407, 1998

Irby DM, Ramsey P, Gillmore GM, et al: Characteristics of effective clinical teachers of ambulatory care medicine. Acad Med 66:54–55, 1991

Machiavelli N: The Prince (1513). Translated by Bull G. New York, Penguin, 1975

Nathan PE, Gorman JM: Treatments That Work. New York, Oxford University Press, 2002

Pinsky LE, Monson D, Irby DM: How excellent teachers are made: reflecting on success to improve teaching. Adv Health Sci Educ Theory Pract 3:207–215, 1998

Safer D: Design and reporting modifications in industry-sponsored comparative psychopharmacology trials. J Nerv Ment Dis 190:583–592, 2002

Steinbrook R: The debate over residents' work hours. N Engl J Med 347:1296–1302, 2002

Yager J, Kay J: Assessing psychotherapy competence in psychiatric residents: getting real. Harv Rev Psychiatry 11:109–112, 2003

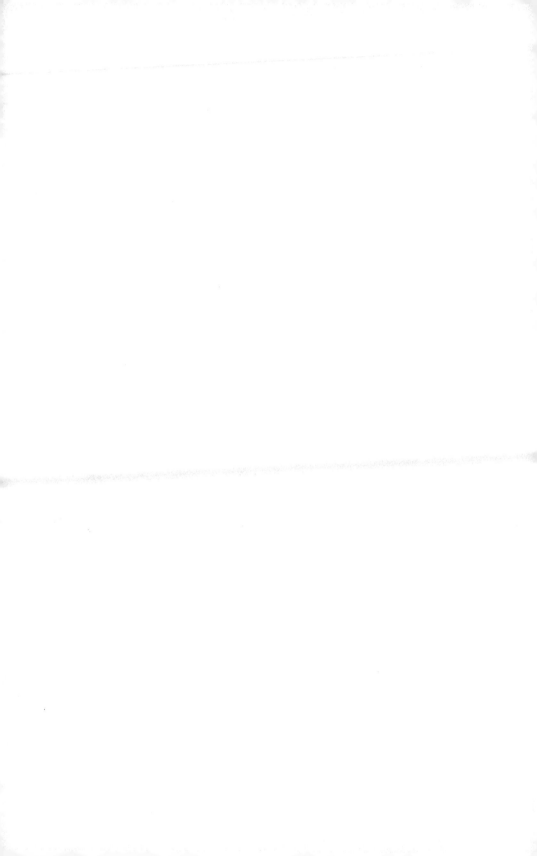

CHAPTER 7

NEW TEACHING TECHNOLOGIES AND APPROACHES FOR MEDICAL STUDENTS AND RESIDENTS

Greg Briscoe, M.D.

Carlyle H. Chan, M.D.

Information in medicine is expanding at an ever-greater rate. Today's psychiatric educators, residents, and medical students must grapple with an incredibly large volume of medical knowledge. Many physicians and students welcome assistance in managing this swelling ocean of data, and contemporary technologies can help in this regard. For example, trainees and educators in psychiatry can review information from digital reference materials and educational sources (on personal digital assistants [PDAs], CD-ROMs, and the Internet). Moreover, the same parties can enhance and streamline their psychiatric educational experience with electronic teaching and administrative tools, presentation software, teleconferencing, specialized task-oriented software, digital video, and other forms of multimedia. Digital information is quickly and conveniently accessible on demand around the clock; is compact, portable, flexible, and transmissible via wireless technology; and can contain embedded cross-references. Disadvantages of these sorts of technologies may include cost and, in some instances, lack of available support staff.

In this chapter we discuss these issues, as well as barriers to implementation, the impact of the Health Insurance Portability and Accountability Act of 1996 (P.L. 104–191; HIPAA), and the importance of security regarding patient care issues. Exciting frontiers at the interface of psychiatry and technology are also discussed.

We hope that readers will be inspired by the tools presented and will harness their teaching creativity and learning abilities in new and useful ways. Balance is certainly required between the utilization of these tools and maintenance of an environment conducive to learning. We hope that our material is presented and described in a language suitable for beginners in information technology. Special technical skills are not a prerequisite to understanding or utilizing this information.

For the sake of simplicity, our discussion presents software available for the Windows operating system and makes notation when and if a corresponding software version for the Macintosh (Mac) operating system is available. The reader should be aware that because Web page addresses change frequently, there may be invalid uniform resource locators (URLs) listed in the following pages. In such cases, the desired page is usually easily found by using an Internet search engine such as Google (http://www.google.com). All URLs were accessed as recently as May 26, 2005. It should be noted that no endorsement of the described hardware or software is either intended or implied and that any lists of products are representative and not necessarily comprehensive.

PERSONAL DIGITAL ASSISTANTS

PDAs have emerged as indispensable tools for education, training, and patient care. Students and residents use these units to track and document their patient care experiences (by maintaining case logs), to access digital texts and pharmaceutical databases for diagnosis and treatment, to prepare consultation and evaluative reports, to document coding and billing, to use study aids, and even to access electronic medical records and laboratory results wirelessly.

The two principal types of PDAs vary by their operating systems (OSs): Palm OS and Windows Mobile 2003 OS for Pocket PCs (formerly Windows CE; for the sake of simplicity we refer to this OS as Pocket PC). The general advantages and disadvantages of each OS are discussed elsewhere (Table 7–1). Our focus is on the applicability of these devices to medicine and psychiatry. The Palm OS has been available for a longer time, and currently there are many more compatible medical software programs for it than for the Pocket PC OS. The Pocket PC OS is a version of the Microsoft

TABLE 7–1.   Internet resources for general computer information

Primers on personal digital assistant (PDA) usage, reviews of current products, and purchasing guidelines can be found on these Web sites:

PC Magazine	http://www.pcmag.com
Consumer Reports	http://www.consumerreports.org
PDA Buyers Guide	http://www.pdabuyersguide.com
ZDNet	http://www.zdnet.com
Handheld Computing Magazine	http://www.hhcmag.com
Pocket PC Magazine	http://www.pocketpcmagazine.com

Windows OS for personal computers (PCs). Palm OS and Pocket PC OS are not compatible with each other, although both will currently work with Windows-based PCs and Apple Macintosh computers. However, third-party software permitting either OS to connect with a Mac may cost $30–$70 extra in some cases.

Simple, inexpensive units store thousands of addresses, appointments, memos, to-do lists, programs, and data. However, some entry-level units have only 2 megabytes (MB) of internal memory—not enough to accommodate most reference texts, which are often several megabytes in size each. Higher-priced units generally have color screens, faster processors, more memory for storage, and rechargeable batteries. They also usually have more bells and whistles, such as a built-in voice recorder, digital camera, digital music player, Global Positioning System, built-in thumb keyboard, wireless capability, and software that permits the PDA to act as a universal remote control device for televisions, videocassette recorders, and DVD players. Prices of PDAs range from $79 to $800.

Wireless connectivity (Wi-Fi and Bluetooth) allows one's PDA to log on to wireless networks and exchange information with other wireless devices like a desktop PC, printer, camera, or cellular phone. Many PDAs allow e-mail exchange. However, there is usually an associated service cost. Many units will allow exchange of Microsoft Office documents (native for Pocket PC; third-party software is required for some Palm units). There has also been a convergence of technologies, because some models of PDAs are also cellular phones. See Table 7–2 for a list of PDA manufacturers and their Web sites.

Ultimately, users must choose a PDA with features that meet the needs of their daily practice. One of the most useful PDA capacities is the ability to access digital textbook and reference information on demand. It bears repeating that this type of software resource consumes relatively large

TABLE 7–2.   Personal digital assistant (PDA) manufacturers and their Web sites

Palm OS (merged with Handspring)

palmOne	http://www.palmone.com/us
Sony	http://www.sonystyle.com
Garmin	http://www.garmin.com

Pocket PC OS

Casio	http://www.casio.com/index.cfm
Dell	http://www.dell.com
Hewlett-Packard iPAQ	http://welcome.hp.com/country/us/en/ prodserv/handheld.html
Toshiba	http://www.toshibadirect.com/td/b2c/ toshibapda.to
Viewsonic	http://www.viewsonic.com

Combination cellular phone/PDA (Smartphones)

Samsung	http://www.samsung.com/Products/index.htm
palmOne (merged with Handspring)	http://www.palmone.com/us
Kyocera	http://tools.kyocera-wireless.com/ phoneshowcase.do
Hitachi	http://www.hitachi.com

Note.   OS=operating system.

amounts of internal memory (e.g., mobilePDR takes up more than 5 MB). Some digital texts will run only in the PDA's fixed internal memory, not on external memory cards. Therefore, it is recommended that users consider purchasing a device with ample internal memory (16 MB minimum). However, as the technology matures, an increasing number of manufacturers will probably produce digital texts that will also run on external memory cards. In anticipation of this possibility, users may wish to consider devices with expansion slots for external memory so that they can increase their memory capacity as their needs grow. Digital media, such as audio or video files, and some applications also typically consume large amounts of memory, and external memory cards are useful to accommodate these applications. Rechargeable batteries are also a benefit because they cost less than disposables in the long run. However, higher-end units with faster processors consume battery power more quickly. Users with this type of unit may have to recharge daily to prevent data loss that occurs if the battery drains to 0%.

One should not consider a PDA as a replacement for a laptop—for one thing, typing extensively on Chiclet-size keys is rather tricky, although normal-size plug-in keyboard attachments are commercially available from third parties. Viewing a PowerPoint presentation on the small screens also leaves something to be desired. However, hardware and software additions such as Margi (http://www.margi.com) allow one to load and present PowerPoint slides on an LCD projector directly from a PDA. Demonstrations of and teaching about PDAs can be facilitated by using software such as Handshare (http://www.mobilityware.com/HandShare/HandShareProduct.htm), which allows the projection and control of a PDA on a computer or LCD screen. Finally, regarding limitations, one should not expect seamless wireless connectivity; users can expect disruptions in their connections. Although wireless coverage has improved, good coverage is not yet ubiquitous. PDA software for psychiatry is discussed later in this chapter.

ONLINE TEACHING TOOLS

The Internet provides a vehicle to conduct classes at any time of day. Web-based instructional software allows faculty members to construct a course online. Teaching materials—including lectures, notes, photos, and videos—can all be accessed in sequential or nonsequential fashion. References may be linked to full-text journals or textbooks. Exam questions are answered online, with test results immediately available. These tools are summarized in Table 7–3. A review of these programs and more can be found at the EduTools Web site (http://www.edutools.info/index.jsp).

TABLE 7–3.   Online teaching tools

ANGEL	http://www.cyberlearninglabs.com
Desire2Learn	http://desire2learn.com/welcome.html
Gradepoint	http://www.gradepoint.net
WebCT	http://www.WebCT.com
Blackboard	http://www.blackboard.com
Centra	http://www.centra.com/solutions/training.asp
ToolBook Instructor	http://www.sumtotalsystems.com
Educator	http://www.ucompass.com
FirstClass	http://www.softarc.com
KEWL	http://kewl.uwc.ac.za
KnowEdge eLearning Suite	http://www.internetion.net/lms.asp
My Course	http://mycourse.thomsonlearning.com

Communicating with students outside of class time can take place face-to-face during office hours or virtually via the Internet through a chat room at a designated time period. Asynchronous communication can occur through other Internet mediums. E-mail can provide both individual communication and group communication. An e-mail list (Listserv) permits group notices and discussions, with the communication delivered to the student's or resident's e-mail address. Newsgroups and bulletin boards can provide opportunities for group discussions, with the latter allowing for threaded discussions (whereby discussion topics are labeled). Many pagers now have the capacity to receive e-mail text messages consisting of up to 150 (or in some cases 250) characters. It is now easy to contact a group of residents or students and e-mail "blast" a brief message to announce, for example, a last-minute lecture cancellation or to remind a group to obtain their annual tuberculosis test.

LEARNING TO USE POWERPOINT

There are many presentation creation software products available from which to choose. To name a few, Microsoft PowerPoint, Apple Keynote, and CRE:8 Multimedia are all worthy tools. One of the most commonly used programs in the medical environment today is PowerPoint. Due to space limitations, we have placed our tutorial, "PowerPoint for Beginners," online (http://www.admsep.org/tc.html).

DIGITAL, WIRELESS, AND NONLINEAR TOOLS

Digital cameras and camcorders now allow the direct transfer of images to media such as CD-ROM and DVD as well as to the Internet, making it easier to create multimedia teaching tools. Programs such as Easy Media Creator (http://www.roxio.com), DVD MovieFactory (http://www.ulead.com), and Studio Video Solutions (http://www.pinnaclesys.com) facilitate such productions. PowerPoint even allows the incorporation of digital video clips.

Wireless capability, in addition to increasing mobility, enables new opportunities for information exchange. Wireless-equipped classrooms permit instantaneous download of speakers' PowerPoint presentations to students' notebook computers, the delivery of spot quizzes with answers beamed backed to a central computer for real-time tabulation, and—to the possible detriment of the speaker—real-time critiques communicated among students using instant messaging.

Hypertext linkage permits the development of nonlinear forms of teaching exercises. *Nonlinear* refers to the capacity to move from one area of a document to another and back in a nonsequential fashion. This is analogous to the difference between watching a videotape and a DVD, where in the latter instance one can move freely from one part of the story to another without the need for rewinding. Using hypertext linkages and Web authoring software (without necessarily going to the Internet), one colleague created a computer version of *Jeopardy* to teach a complicated treatment protocol.

TEST-WRITING SOFTWARE

Writing exams for psychiatry residents or medical students can prove to be both time-consuming and difficult. However, several test-writing software products currently on the market can assist with this task. The products discussed do not contain prefabricated psychiatry test questions, nor do they contain any psychiatric reference text. They do, however, help users write and organize test questions in a way that speeds final test assembly and enables significantly greater test security, as explained below.

Typically, on opening the software the user creates test questions in one of several available formats. The program then assists the user in building test question databanks (collections of questions grouped by category). Most programs have a test-writing wizard, which walks beginners through the test construction process. And most have word processing capabilities.

Later, when an exam is needed, the test author then specifies a certain number of questions to be taken from one or more databanks (e.g., five questions from Bank A, four from Bank B, eight from Bank C, and so on). The software then randomly picks the specified number of questions from each databank and randomly orders the entire final collection. The exam is then ready for printing or online administration (on the Internet or local network). A corresponding bubble-sheet answer key may be created and can be printed to match each exam. If this cycle is repeated, a different exam will be created, also with random question ordering, and as the size of the databanks increases, the number of duplicate questions between exams will decrease. Potentially, with extremely large databanks, one could create a totally unique exam for each student, although this is unnecessary, because the construction of just a few different test versions per exam sitting is probably adequate to foil any unethical test-taking behaviors.

The examinations created can be printed or administered online (on the Internet or local network) so that it can be taken on a PC. If the exams are taken using a computer, the software will automatically grade the test. Also, the software will automatically perform varying degrees of test-item analysis as students make their answer choices. One can include images and other

TABLE 7–4.   Test-writing software products

Product	Web address	Web-based course management system interface?	Price
Random Test Generator	http://www.hirtlesoftware.com	No	$99
Diploma 6	http://www.brownstone.net	Yes	$49
Respondus	http://www.respondus.com	Yes	3 tiers: free, $79, and $139
ExamView Test Generator	http://www.examview.com	Yes	$99
Question Tools Exam 2	http://www.questiontools.com	No	3 tiers: free, $736, and $3,689

multimedia files with individual questions, such as radiographic data, photographs, video, or audio. And one can import test data from other sources—for example, a test previously written in Microsoft Word. These programs allow the instructor to manually review students' tests and compare student answer selections against the true answers. They have built-in software that allows one to upload Internet tests to a Web server. Tests administered in "Practice" test mode through a Web browser permit students to review and see detailed answer explanations once their tests are complete in any test format (screen, paper, and Internet). The products usually provide the ability to password-protect access to the test bank files. They permit sharing of question banks with other instructors. Finally, they usually allow inclusion of reference (source) information for every test item created.

These test-writing software products are summarized in Table 7–4.

ADMINISTRATIVE TOOLS

Several residency management software programs are now commercially available. These programs provide various tools that are useful in the daily administration of residency programs:

- *Resident evaluations:* This tool permits each program to place its own resident and faculty program evaluation forms on the Internet. These forms are then filled out online and tabulated externally. Summary reports are

TABLE 7–5. Residency management software products

New Innovations	http://www.new-innov.com\residency.asp
Advanced Informatics	http://www.advancedinformatics.com
Residency Partner	http://www.residencypartner.com/products/ rp_product_overview.asp
thinresidency	https://www.thinresidency.com
MedHub	http://www.medhub.com/?mhp=2
eResidency	http://www.eresidency.net/rms/index.cfm

thus available to the program director. Delinquent evaluations are tracked, and automated e-mail reminders are sent out. Faculty members and residents may view their own evaluations in summary form. Evaluations by individual residents are never viewed, thus maintaining anonymity.

- *Procedure logs:* Procedures performed by residents may be tabulated and confirmed by supervising faculty members. These procedure logs could also be patient logs to document the diversity of clinical experience. The logs can be maintained on PDAs and the data transmitted during synchronization via secure Internet lines to the host company, where the data are collected and analyzed. Summary reports are provided to the program director and are available to the resident.
- *Demographic database:* Demographic information on residents can be exported from the Electronic Residency Application Service application materials directly to these management software systems.
- *Resident scheduling:* This tool enables scheduling of residents for the entire residency period. Rotation schedules can be viewed and/or printed by postgraduate year or rotation; in addition, allows planning of on-call schedules, rounds, conferences, etc.
- *Resident and/or attending attendance:* Attendance of residents at lectures, meetings, or conferences can be documented.
- *Graduate Medical Education readiness preparation:* This tool permits tracking of issues of importance.

More specific details on these programs can be found on the Web sites listed in Table 7–5.

Residency programs requiring simply a patient log tracking system can utilize software such as Pendragon Forms (http://www.pendragon-software. com), Intellisync Mobile Suite (http://www.intellisync.com/pages/Products/ Intellisync-Mobile-Suite), or WiFile Pro (http://www.handshigh.com/html/

wifile.html) to create log forms for PDAs. After data are entered on the PDA, they can be synchronized onto a single desktop computer or through a channel on the Internet. Both programs require some additional programming time to set up.

Traditional software suites such as Microsoft Office are generally packaged with at least a word processor, database program, and spreadsheet application and sometimes presentation and desktop publishing software. Spreadsheet software (e.g., Microsoft Excel) provides an inexpensive means of tracking stipend utilization as well as providing an easy way to shuffle potential rotation assignments when making out a schedule.

Spreadsheets provide a matrix of cells, each of which may be identified by row and column. Each cell may contain a label, a numerical value, or the result of a mathematical formula or equation. Each spreadsheet or page can also be linked with other pages. In the case of a residency program divided among, for example, four sites with four concomitant sources of funding, each resident in the program may have an individual spreadsheet page with stipend assignments for each academic year. All the individual spreadsheet pages may be linked to a summary page. Thus, whenever a resident's rotation and stipend assignment is changed, the summary page will be updated automatically and will reflect that change. An easy-to-follow guide on using spreadsheets is *Excel 2003 for Dummies* (Harvey 2003).

Desktop publishing software can assist in the production of recruitment brochures, newsletters, and flyers. The costs become minimal after the initial software purchase, and the resulting pieces can be quite professional in appearance through the easy incorporation of color photographs.

Many institutions also provide intranet capability. Intranets are private networks, with access limited to members of a particular institution, that can be linked to the Internet. Call schedules, pager numbers, departmental policies and announcements, and online teaching modules can be posted on an intranet with the knowledge that the information will not be accessible by the general public. Portions of the intranet can have further password protection—for example, to limit the viewing of faculty members' home telephone numbers to department members.

SPEECH RECOGNITION SOFTWARE

In the clinical setting there are occasions when the time spent completing patient-related paperwork exceeds expectations and impinges on the time allotted for teaching and learning. Some of this lost education time can be recovered through the use of speech recognition software (SRS), which can increase the rate and ease of completing medical record notes. SRS can also benefit educators and trainees because it can decrease the time required for authoring scientific articles or presentations. In the future it may be important for attending physicians, residents, and students to become familiar with this type of technology because it may gain an increasing foothold in academic settings over the slower conventional typing and dictation mechanisms.

With today's SRS a user speaks continuously and naturally into a headset microphone connected to a computer, and the software captures and translates this audio signal into digital text in real time. That is, the SRS "types" what is spoken into the microphone. The ability to dictate information directly into a computer without touching the keyboard has several advantages over writing or manually typing documents or using conventional dictation transcription services:

- People can speak far more quickly than they can type, and with the speed of today's computer processors, the SRS can "type" almost as fast as the speaker can talk. SRS frees users from using a pen or keyboard, allowing them to hold papers, graphs, or books, or just to relax.
- Persons who are susceptible to carpal tunnel syndrome or repetitive strain injuries will experience little if any injury while speaking instead of typing.
- An instant voice-to-print product eliminates delays incurred through conventional voice dictation (i.e., transcriptionist turnaround time). The product is complete as soon as the speaker finishes speaking and editing, unlike with a dictated note, which first goes to a transcription service for processing and is returned to the author for editing and completion.
- The text is always legible and spelled correctly, unlike handwritten notes.

Other positive attributes include the fact that although SRS is not perfect, its accuracy rate has greatly improved over the past few years. According to a testing conducted by *PC Magazine*, the accuracy rate of several voice recognition products is 96%–98% "after only a couple hours of use" (Alwang 2002, 2003). These products are more affordable than they once were, with entry-level products starting at about $50 (including headset microphone), and they reduce or eliminate transcription processing costs. Last, users can personalize and build the program's vocabulary recognition through ongoing usage.

Disadvantages of this technology include the fact that noisy environments can affect accuracy rates. Users must be able to depend on the availability of quiet surroundings. Older computers may lack adequate computer processor speed or memory capacity to provide accurate results. And users with accents may experience more initial accuracy problems.

One of our favorite programs is Dragon NaturallySpeaking 8 ($59 and up). It makes dictation, correction, and voice control of one's PC surprisingly fast and easy. Initial training of the program—done by reading a passage from a prepared text—requires little time. Included package literature states this training can be done in "about 5 minutes," but our experience was that training took a little longer, perhaps 20 minutes. If the program misrecognizes a word, one can use voice commands to correct the misrecognition in a way that further refines the program's understanding of the user's pronunciation of specific words or phrases. Accuracy rates are quite high after initial training and improve as the program learns from the user's corrections. Users may add words to the program's vocabulary either on the fly or with the program's vocabulary optimizer. This tool analyzes one of the user's previously written documents for vocabulary and writing style. And one may also dictate into any program that accepts text, such as word processors like Corel WordPerfect, Microsoft Word, WordPad, and other supported programs. The user-friendly interface makes mastery of the program rather straightforward. Step-by-step wizards also guide beginners through the set-up process. Dragon NaturallySpeaking Version 9 now supports certified Pocket PC devices as well as additional digital handheld recorders, array microphones, and cordless microphones (support for Pocket PC and handheld recorders is available for Preferred and Professional Editions only). A medical professional version is available; however, it is considerably more expensive than the Essentials version, but it reportedly utilizes a more advanced speech recognition engine. Advanced voice scripts, like those found in the IBM Speech Recognition product ViaVoice Pro, come only with Dragon NaturallySpeaking 8 Professional ($700 street).

A number of other similar continuous SRS products are on the market; another highly rated program is IBM's ViaVoice. A nice review article from *PC Magazine* (Alwang 2002, 2003) can be read on the Internet (http://www.pcmag.com/category2/0,4148,4830,00.asp). Table 7–6 summarizes the available speech recognition products.

TELECONFERENCING

The same equipment for telemedicine can be applied to teleconferencing. High-resolution cameras transmit visual images and sound along special telephone lines (integrated services digital network [ISDN]) or via Internet

TABLE 7–6. Speech recognition product summary

Product	Manufacturer's Web site	Price
Dragon NaturallySpeaking 8	http://www.scansoft.com	$59 and up
IBM ViaVoice	http://www-306.ibm.com/software/ voice/viavoice	$49 and up
IBM ViaVoice, Mac OS X Edition	http://www.scansoft.com/viavoice/ osx	$59 and up
Pro-Med Medical Solutions	http://www.speechtechnology.com/ dragon/promed.html	$729
Voice Studio 1.4	http://www.voicestudio.us	$99

Note. OS=operating system.

protocols, permitting two-way audio and visual communication between remote physical sites. The standard for good video quality is a minimum refresh rate of 30 frames per second with a 4-kHz frequency for telephone-quality audio. Such systems require at least two units (one at each site) and can cost $20,000–$30,000 each. "Plain old telephone service" (POTS) lines are not sufficiently reliable for clinical work but might suffice for remote clinical supervision that requires only head shots, as might Web camcorders over the Internet. With the use of such devices, supervision, case conferences, administrative meetings, and educational programs can take place in real time with full participation from multiple locations. Any transmission of clinical data requires HIPAA compliance.

ONLINE CONTINUING MEDICAL EDUCATION

Many practitioners and educators find valuable continuing medical education (CME) and other professional development content online. The advantages of online psychiatry CME material are its intrinsic multimedia capacities, its on-demand availability, its always-on nature, the ability of users to self-pace, the presence of hyperlink referencing, and the capacity for online quizzes and interactive testing (with immediate performance assessment). Most sites refresh their CME topics regularly. The formats of these psychiatry CME sites vary—for example, they may include simple Web pages, PowerPoint presentations, webcasts, and streaming video presentations. Some previously recorded lectures and Grand Rounds presentations are available. The online CME activities can be divided into two camps: regular subscription basis and à la carte. Several of the à la carte CME sites are free. Although there are myriads of psychiatry CME activities online, we have attempted to filter out what we feel are, to the best of our knowledge, reliable, established authoring entities. These are summarized in Table 7–7. In addition to music, iPods and other MP3 players can be used to capture digitally recorded lectures to play back at a later time (Google "pod casting" for more information).

ELECTRONIC REFERENCE SOURCES

Electronic media have some advantages over traditional textbooks. One is the speed with which one can retrieve information during a search—that is, after entering a search term in an electronic media product, it usually takes only a few minutes to retrieve the desired information. Second, electronic media can be easily updated over the Internet, so that the latest advances in scientific knowledge are accessible on demand. Third, electronic media are more compact than conventional textbooks. For example, the entire *Encyclopædia Britannica* (a 32-volume set in hardcover) fits on a CD-ROM 2-disk set. This compactness means enhanced portability, permitting use at the point of care. For example, a clinician-educator can simply power on his or her PDA and within a few moments display the possible side effects of a new medication for discussion with patients and trainees. Finally, in some cases electronic media are more adaptive to users with disabilities. The disadvantages include the fact that a PC is required to view the information and that technical glitches may interfere with usage. Electronic-based texts are not for everyone. Although notebook computers and PDAs provide advantages, many individuals prefer reading text on paper rather than on a computer screen.

Ironically, few psychiatric textbooks are currently available in optical media formats (e.g., CD-ROM or DVD). However, perhaps for the sake of user convenience and to curtail unauthorized replication, the large majority of portable electronic psychiatric titles have shifted from optical media formats to the PDA format and subscription-based online content. Nonetheless, one CD-ROM–based reference deserves mention—the *PDR Electronic Library* ($99, Thomson Healthcare, http://www.pdrbookstore.com). This useful source of drug information and prescribing information can be accessed in several different ways. For example, in addition to product lookup, one can access drugs by category, manufacturer, indication, and contraindications. And one can enter several medications to determine whether there are drug interactions.

In regard to psychiatric reference software for the PC, several valuable drug reference programs are available. These programs can be updated on demand by the end user via the Internet, and some are free. For example,

TABLE 7–7. Online continuing medical education

Regular, monthly CME based on annual subscription

Oakstone Medical Publishing	http://www.cmeonly.com
Audio-Digest Foundation	http://www.audio-digest.org

À la carte CME (from trusted sponsors)

American Psychiatric Association	http://www.psych.org/members/grandrounds
Cleveland Clinic	http://www.clevelandclinicmeded.com/online/psychiatry.htm
Harvard Medical School	http://cmeonline.med.harvard.edu
Duke University	http://www.healthstream.com/physician/promos/duke.asp?PID=56&SID
George Washington University Medical Center	http://66.40.168.196/index.htm
Johns Hopkins University	http://www.hopkins-advantage.com
Columbia University	http://cpmcnet.columbia.edu/dept/video/frametpcs.html
New York University	http://www.med.nyu.edu/Psych/itp.html
University of Pittsburgh	http://www.cmeinfo.com/472.html
Journal of Clinical Psychiatry	http://www.psychiatrist.com/cmehome
eMedguides	http://www.emedguides.com
Journal Watch Psychiatry	http://psychiatry.jwatch.org/misc/about_jwpsy_cme.shtml
eMedicine	http://www.emedicine.com/med/psychiatry.htm
Medscape	http://www.medscape.com/psychiatryhome
CME, Inc.	http://www.medinfosource.com/online/index.html

Online journals

	The sheer number of online journals precludes full listing here. A more extensive list is available at: http://www.admsep.org/links.html#journals

Free miscellaneous CME

Lectures in psychiatry, various topics	http://www.emedicine.com/med/contents.htm
	http://www.medscape.com/viewprogram/2675
Interactive Testing Modules in psychiatry, various topics	http://www.med.nyu.edu/psych/psychiatrist/itp.html

TABLE 7–7. Online continuing medical education *(continued)*

Psychiatry Slide Lecture/ Slide Library, various topics	http://www.cene.com/Psychiatry/SlideLibrary/ SlideLibrary.asp
Past Grand Rounds Series, various topics	http://www.medicalrounds.com/index.php3?page=inc/ list&category=psychiatry http://www.mentalhealth.ucla.edu/opce/gr0001.html
Webcasts regarding psychiatry topics	http://psychiatry.uchicago.edu/grounds http://www.xpertcme.org/live http://www.cene.com/Psychiatry/Webcast/ Webcast.asp http://cpmcnet.columbia.edu/dept/video/topics.html
Interesting sites	
Digital slice of brain	http://medstat.med.utah.edu/eccles/slice/brain.html
Virtual Naval Hospital Online	http://www.vnh.org/Providers.html
National Library of Medicine Collaboratory for High Performance Computing and Communications	http://collab.nlm.nih.gov
Psychiacomp (for residents in training)	http://psychiacomp.com

many users rely on ePocrates (free, ePocrates Inc., http://www2.epocrates. com), and the print version of the *Physicians' Desk Reference* (PDR) has been converted to a PDA format called mobilePDR (free, Thomson Healthcare, http://www.pdr.net). MobileMICROMEDEX is yet another free PDA drug reference program (free, Thomson Healthcare, http://www.micromedex. net). For a small monthly fee, Tarascon Publishing offers Pocket Pharmacopoeia Deluxe ($2.29/month, Tarascon Publishing, http://www.tarascon. com). Finally, Johns Hopkins University offers a free antibiotics reference program (free, Johns Hopkins Point of Care IT, http://hopkins-abxguide. org).

Other important PDA psychiatric reference texts can be downloaded from the Internet. For example, American Psychiatric Publishing offers *Quick Reference to the DSM-IV-TR® Diagnostic Criteria*, *DSM-IV-TR® Handbook of Differential Diagnosis*, and *Quick Reference to the APA Practice Guidelines for the Treatment of Psychiatric Disorders* (all of these can be purchased at http:// www.psychiatryonline.com/eBooks.aspx). Skyscape's Web site (http://www.

skyscape.com) offers more than a dozen reference texts (e.g., *The Washington Manual® Psychiatry Survival Guide* [$29.95], *Griffith's 5-Minute Clinical Consult 2005* [$64.00], *Psychiatry Recall* [$32.95], *Manual of Psychiatric Therapeutics* [$49.95]). Medspda (http://www.medspda.com) is another vendor that offers psychiatry titles (e.g., *eMedicine Psychiatry* [$49.00], *Clinical Psychiatry 2006* [$9.95], *The Massachusetts General Hospital Handbook of Neurology* [$39.95]).

Numerous other reference programs can be found on the Internet. Although an exhaustive cataloging of these resources is beyond the scope of this chapter, some of the principal sites that provide freeware, shareware, and commercial PDA software are Handango (http://www.handango.com), Download.com (http://www.download.com), PDA.com (http://www.pda.com), pdaMD.com (http://www.pdaMD.com), PalmGear.com (http://www.palmgear.com), FreewarePalm (http://www.freewarepalm.com), PocketPC Freewares (http://www.pocketpcfreewares.com/en/index.php), MemoWare (http://www.memoware.com), Eurocool (http://www.eurocool.com), and PocketPC Software (http://www. ipaqsoft.net/php/freeresults.php?type=emul).

Psychiatric information is available in several other media formats, such as electronic journals, databases, and other Web-based content. These sources can be located through an Internet search engine such as Google (for more information on using Internet search engines, see "Finding Medical Information on the Internet," below).

COMPUTER-ASSISTED PSYCHOTHERAPY

PC-based software for psychiatry is largely focused on practice management for large systems (e.g., patient scheduling, electronic medical records, and billing). These are certainly important tasks in everyday practice; however, decisions regarding these types of tools are more likely to be made for administrative reasons rather than for their value in psychiatric education. These software tools can be reviewed elsewhere in the literature. Excluding these topics, currently there are some rather fascinating commercially available programs for psychiatrists. For example, computer-assisted psychotherapy (CAP) offers the potential advantages of decreased cost of treatment, improved access to psychotherapy, high levels of patient satisfaction, reliability and consistency of function, reduction of burden on the therapist for repetitive tasks, unique (patient) learning experiences, and promotion of the self-help component of therapy (Wright 2004).

Currently the clinical applications for CAP include cognitive-behavioral therapy (CBT) and virtual-reality therapy (VRT). According to Wright (2004), although there are admitted limitations, 9 of 10 controlled trials found efficacy for computer-assisted CBT. VRT is grounded in the exposure-based therapies for phobias and posttraumatic stress disorder. VRT usually involves the use of a collection of technological devices:

> A computer capable of interactive 3-D visualization, a head-mounted display, and data gloves equipped with one or more position trackers. The trackers sense the position and orientation of the user and report that information to the computer that updates (in real time) images for display. (Riva 2003)

More information on CAP and the available products can be obtained by following the URLs in Table 7–8. Most mental health professionals advise the use of digital therapies only by those trained to use them, in combination with traditional treatments.

VIDEO MEDIA FOR BOARD PREPARATION

There are many ways users may enhance their skills in preparation for the American Board of Psychiatry and Neurology (ABPN) board exam Parts I and II. Although it is not new, the video format is still quite useful in this regard. Table 7–9 lists video-based resources that are available for home study. We do not presume to include all the resources available in this area.

HIPAA AND SECURITY

The Health Insurance Portability and Accountability Act of 1996 (HIPAA) provides standards for ensuring patient confidentiality as well as penalties for failures to comply. Hence, precautions must be taken to secure patient information, because HIPAA rules provide for substantial penalties for violations. Although their small size helps make PDAs convenient to use, the same feature makes PDAs easy to lose or to steal. The same holds true for notebook computers and peripherals.

Password protection inhibits physical access to a machine by requiring that a code be typed before the computer or PDA is usable. However, the password program on many PDAs is easily defeated, requiring more powerful add-on password programs. In the event that the password is compromised, encryption scrambles data to render it unreadable without the proper decoding information. There are several different types of encryption algorithms, some more sophisticated than others. Encryption capability is available on some of the newer high-end devices. Third-party encryption software for the PDA is listed in Table 7–10.

TABLE 7–8. A sample of computer-assisted psychotherapy resources

Topic	Web address	Information
Wright JH, Wright AS, Beck AT: *Good Days Ahead: The Interactive Program for Depression and Anxiety.* A PC-based CBT program	http://www.mindstreet.com	Mindstreet; Single-User Self-Help Edition DVD, $99; Professional Edition, 10-User Package, $595.
Beating the Blues	http://www.ultrasis.com/products/btb/btb.html	A CBT-based multimedia program. See Web site for cost.
Immersive Virtual Telepresence in Health Care, Rehabilitation, and Neuroscience	http://www.cybertherapy.info/pages/main.htm	A reference page with free articles on the technique, the technology involved, studies conducted, and virtual-reality software development tools.

Note. CBT=cognitive-behavioral therapy.

TABLE 7–9. Video media for Board preparation

Item	Web site	Description	Cost
Pass the Boards	http://www.psychboards.org/chou.shtml	Several videotapes for Part II board review; author also offers private tutoring and live courses	10-tape set, $1,200; individual tapes, $150; phone: 914–591–4868
The Boards Videotape II	http://www.columbia.edu/~seh5/video.html	Two sets of videotapes for Part II board review	Institutions/libraries, $195; individuals, $125
Strategies for Passing the Oral Boards	http://www.psychboardprep.com/video.html	Three different videotapes for Part II board review; author also offers private tutoring	$95 per tape
A Comprehensive Review of Psychiatry	http://www.cmeinfo.com/psychiatry.html	Part I board review; 40 AMA-PRA category 1 credit hours; videotape, DVD, audiotape, CD	$995
Intensive Psychiatric Board Review Course	http://www.mhsource.com/boardreview/index.html	Part I board review; 50 hours CME credit; CD-ROM, audio CD, audiotape, video	40 audio CDs, 4 CD-ROMs, or 26 DVDs, $1,199

TABLE 7–10. Third-party encryption software for the PDA

MovianCrypt	http://www.moviansecurity.com
SureWave Mobile Defense (formerly PDA Defense)	http://www.jpmobile.com
PDA Secure	http://www.trustdigital.com
Pointsec	http://www.pointsec.com
Teal Lock	http://www.tealpoint.com/softlock.htm

Note. PDA=personal digital assistant.

PDAs should utilize one of any number of security programs that not only provide password protection but also encrypt specific data files. These programs can be set to automatically activate after a certain period of time.

Antivirus software isolates and eliminates the entry of malicious computer code before it can do damage. However, new viruses and worms are created daily, and antiviral programs must be regularly updated. Firewalls, both hardware and software, provide a barrier between one's computer and anyone on the Internet who wants to access the computer while it is logged on. Computers that are constantly logged on to the Internet are especially vulnerable.

Notebook computers are similarly vulnerable to theft. Drive encryption software can protect these data as well. Available products include DriveCrypt (http://www.securstar.com) and Pointsec for PC (http://www. pointsec.com/solutions/solutions_pointsec.asp). In addition to software solutions, there are some basic precautions to be taken. Notebook computers should never be left unattended, even for a few moments, in an empty classroom or even in a hotel room. They are easily placed into a briefcase or duffel bag and quickly removed. Wire security cables can provide a initial deterrent to thieves and can be attached to special security slots on almost every modern notebook or glued to smaller desktop PCs and peripheral equipment.

FINDING MEDICAL INFORMATION ON THE INTERNET

There is no master filing system on the Internet and no single, established reference desk from which to seek trained assistance. There are basically two ways of finding information, including medical information, on the Internet. These methods are the direct method and using an Internet search engine.

If one already knows the exact Web page address, one can, using the direct method, enter it into the browser and go straight to the Web site. However, Web addresses are often unintuitive, long, and not amenable to memorization. Therefore, the direct route to a Web page is clearly used the minority of the time.

Many Internet users instead rely on Internet search engines to find their information. In fact, there are 550 million search requests made each day worldwide (Roush 2004). And the Internet's content is growing by some 60 terabytes a day (Roush 2004). This gives the expression "finding a needle in a haystack" an altogether new meaning. Needless to say, use of the Internet without search engines would prove exceedingly difficult.

Just as most people learn to play baseball most expediently by actually engaging in the sport, one can learn to use Internet search engines most effectively by using a hands-on approach. To facilitate this type of experience for the reader, the remainder of this guide is situated on the Internet (http://www.admsep.org/tc.html). In this manner the reader can not only become acquainted with the five different types of Internet search engines, their applications, and their strengths and weaknesses, but the user will gain actual experience through this immersion.

BARRIERS TO IMPLEMENTATION: LEARNING CURVES AND FISCAL REALITIES

Fiscal costs are only the first expense in setting up new technology. There are very few software or hardware packages that are truly turnkey solutions (i.e., applications that can be used right out of the box). Most involve some set-up/installation time and a learning curve. Instruction books or classes can help, so one should plan to spend several hours to learn the nuances of the items that have just been purchased. More complicated software may even require some programming skills, and this may require the assistance of the information technology department, a knowledgeable colleague, resident or student, or a paid consultant or technician. One also must budget annually for maintenance, equipment replacement, and software upgrades. Systems stop working or begin making errors, hardware breaks down or becomes obsolete, and new versions of software may provide useful features that were absent from the earlier version.

There is seldom a good time to purchase new technology. The longer one waits, the more likely it is that the price will come down and more features will become available. Yet it will be that much longer before the new investment can be put to use. The price of acquisition, maintenance and replacement expenses, and the cost of time spent by people learning and installing new technology are all part of that investment.

Implementation of new technology may meet with resistance from faculty, residents, students, and staff, although each new class of medical students and residents bring with them increased levels of computer competence. One should be prepared to encounter pockets of opposition to change in general and to new methods of operation (e.g., faculty members filling out evaluation forms on the Internet). Patience and persistence—and adequate training programs—will go a long way toward countering the opposition.

SUMMARY

The role of technology in the educational process is not to replace the educator but to provide tools to assist the teacher and to augment the learning process. Technology provides additional means to convey new information and to assess the assimilation of that information. It also provides access to learning unencumbered by conventional workday hours, because online learning is available 24 hours a day, 7 days a week. However, some data are being accumulated that suggest that learning is best accomplished earlier in the day and not in the wee hours of the morning. Finally, like most tools, technology has its costs as well as its benefits.

REFERENCES

Alwang G: Better (but still not perfect) speech recognition. PC Magazine 21(21):46, 2002

Alwang G: From your lips to the PC's ears. PC Magazine 22(8):52, 2003

Harvey G: Excel 2003 for Dummies. Hoboken, NJ, Wiley, 2003

Health Insurance Portability and Accountability Act of 1996, Pub. L. No 104-191

Riva G: Applications of virtual environments in medicine. Methods Inf Med 5:524–534, 2003

Roush W: Search beyond Google. Technol Rev 107(2):25–32, 2004

Wright J: Computer-assisted cognitive-behavior therapy, in Cognitive-Behavior Therapy (Review of Psychiatry Series, Oldham JM and Riba MB, series eds). Edited by Wright JH. Arlington, VA, American Psychiatric Publishing, 2004, pp 55–82

CHAPTER 8

TEACHING PSYCHIATRY RESIDENTS TO BECOME EFFECTIVE EDUCATORS

Brock P. Nolan, M.D.

Brenda Roman, M.D.

David Bienenfeld, M.D.

The American Medical Association (2003) notes in its *Graduate Medical Education Directory* that "residents must be instructed in appropriate methods of teaching and have ample opportunity to teach students in the health professions." This short statement appears understandable on the surface, yet its implementation has led to a degree of confusion among directors of medical student education and residency training across the country. Although the American Psychiatric Association (2001) has released a brief practical manual on the subject, recent literature searches and communications with those who hold the above positions reveal a lack of any codified, formal model for carrying out the American Medical Association directive. A global medical education model for instructing residents to become effective educators will follow a discussion regarding the importance of such an endeavor.

IMPORTANCE OF TRAINING RESIDENTS TO TEACH EFFECTIVELY

CONSOLIDATING ONE'S OWN KNOWLEDGE

It is an accepted principle of education that by teaching a topic to another individual, the teacher's own mastery of the subject improves. The review and preparation necessary before presentation of material, combined with the actual teaching session, serve a cementing role in the educator's own understanding of a given issue. When a resident is tasked with providing a brief overview of second-generation antipsychotics for a group of medical students on an inpatient service, for example, that resident must first examine his or her own understanding of the topic. This process is ideal for the identification of deficits in one's knowledge base. Furthermore, as a result of the process of organizing such a presentation, the resident may formulate or group the agents in ways not done when he or she confined consideration of the topic to its clinical utility only. Finally, the actual process of standing before a group of students, fielding questions, and providing answers can strengthen the house officer's sense of competence by reinforcing the mastery developed in the few years since medical school. Thus, by teaching residents to be effective teachers and requiring them to use these skills, the overall learning experience of the residency is improved.

A STRONG BASIS FOR RECRUITMENT

Feifel et al. (1999) explored the precipitous decline over the past 25 years in the number of medical student graduates who choose careers in psychiatry. Unfortunately, their conclusions indicate that many students' negative opinions regarding the consideration of a psychiatric career are formed prior to medical school matriculation. Given this finding, our field must concentrate its efforts on providing positive experiences for students during their preclinical years and especially during their junior clerkships. Strong, demonstrably competent psychiatric resident role models are critical to this process.

Students need to envision themselves as capable members of the larger medical community before they can comfortably choose to enter a given field. It seems obvious that placing skillful resident clinician–educators in front of students will only improve their opinion of psychiatry, and medical literature supports this. Lee et al. (1995) surveyed students who did and did not pursue psychiatry residency training and found that positive experiences with psychiatric faculty and residents correlated with choosing to enter the field, whereas a "poor psychiatric clerkship" was more commonly reported by those who did not choose the field. The authors also found that "psychiatric residents' satisfaction with their careers" and "the amount of intellectual challenge" available in psychiatry were of major importance to students who entered psychiatry. With improvement in psychiatry residents' abilities to interact with, educate, and intellectually stimulate the medical students with whom they work, the field's ability to recruit talented postgraduates should improve.

IMPROVING PATIENT CARE BY EDUCATING NONPSYCHIATRIC PROVIDERS

A large degree of the treatment and "face time" given to patients with emotional illnesses is delivered by nonpsychiatric providers. Clinical psychologists, social workers, nurses/ancillary staff, and nonpsychiatric physicians all have a substantial role in the treatment responses our patients will exhibit. Particularly on inpatient wards, but in other treatment environments as well, the resident (far more than the attending physician) is the psychiatric provider with whom treatment team members from the above disciplines have the most contact.

Whereas the exchange of information and experience flows in a complex fashion among members of all these disciplines, the discipline of psychiatry allows its members an opportunity to educate members of each of these disciplines in important ways. Training in psychopharmacology, psychotherapy, social skills considerations, and disease etiology allows the psychiatrist a unique perspective on emotional disorders which (when effectively communicated among disciplines) can improve patient outcomes. Thus, the development of effective teaching skills in the psychiatric resident is important to the patients he or she serves.

IMPROVING PATIENT CARE BY EDUCATING PATIENTS THEMSELVES

The word *doctor* derives from the Latin word *docere*, meaning "to teach." In its more paternalistic days, medicine deviated from this origin, but due to the enlightened practice styles of William Osler and those like him, modern medicine has regained its sense of partnering with the patient to improve outcomes. Far from simply wanting ailments cured, today's patients desire education from their physicians. They expect explanations regarding etiology, prognosis, treatment options, and prevention much more at present than in decades past. This concept is critical in psychiatry as emotional illness remains largely stigmatized and poorly understood by the lay public and requires an even deeper commitment to patient education than may be true for other fields of medicine.

As mentioned previously, most formal medical education focuses on mastery of disease and treatment concepts with very little attention given to developing or improving the ability to communicate this tremendous body of knowledge effectively to patients. As noted by one author, "While subject expertise is important, it is not sufficient" (Spencer 2003, p. 592). By endeavoring to develop and institute formal "teaching skills" programs in residency training curricula, we are ultimately improving care for patients and fulfilling the commitment to patient beneficence.

PROPOSED MODEL FOR TEACHING PSYCHIATRIC RESIDENTS TO TEACH

EXPANSION OF ALTERNATIVE LEARNING MODELS IN THE MEDICAL SCHOOL CURRICULUM

A certain degree of the success a residency program will have in instructing its house officers to become effective educators is dependent on skills and learning methods developed during the undergraduate training years. Problem-based learning and, more recently, team-based learning are two examples of alternative teaching strategies that foster skills crucial in would-be residents. Learning from other team members' successes and mistakes prepares a student to participate in a more collaborative fashion as a resident later. This focus on group learning rather than individual study promotes a team-oriented concept, fosters a sense of responsibility in participants for others' learning, and reinforces principles of education that are helpful for future resident–teachers. (The reader is directed to the literature devoted to these learning models for details.) Continued emphasis on various medical school teaching models will ultimately result in residency graduates who are more effective teachers.

TARGETED RECRUITMENT

As a result of personal areas of focus in medicine (e.g., research interests), some medical professionals are simply less interested in the importance of developing teaching and preceptor skills. In such cases, no amount of teaching in instructional methods is likely to result in the candidate's becoming an accomplished teacher. For this reason, residency selection committees need to incorporate consideration of a candidate's interest in and commitment to developing teaching skills into the committees' overall recruitment, evaluation, and selection processes. Beyond this, actually targeting medical students who have teaching experience or who take positions of leadership and explaining the importance of these backgrounds to the field of psychiatry may lead to increased numbers of residents with an interest in developing teaching skills.

The importance of these qualities in a potential psychiatric resident is not usually evident to senior medical students. In the first author's recruitment to psychiatric residency, the impact of a training director commenting on his multiple prior teaching positions and explaining the benefits they would provide in the field was instrumental in his choosing not only the field of psychiatry but also the specific program. Actively recruiting and selecting for residency candidates with interest or past experience in teaching will facilitate the process of their developing further teaching skills.

OBJECTIVES FOR TRAINING

Before designing any curriculum, educators would be well advised to consider the results for which they are aiming. These objectives should match the general philosophy and goals of the entire residency training program. For example, a program that emphasizes community psychiatry would likely include psychoeducation and public education as training objectives. A program that emphasizes empirical research would put greater weight on objectives such as scientific presentation skills.

A proven method for choosing objectives begins with brainstorming: the responsible group simply lists possible ideas for objectives, going "around the table" without regard to rank or seniority, without questions or revisions. The process continues until all ideas are in front of the group. Participants can then revise, reword, and combine items to narrow the list. To reduce it further to a manageable size, members may rank-order the items according to perceived importance or send them to a group of content experts, such as acknowledged excellent teachers, for feedback on the relevance of the objectives to the final achievement of the desired skills.

Table 8–1 lists some representative objectives for resident training.

POSTGRADUATE YEAR 1

Because new interns come to programs with varying degrees of psychiatric expertise, many programs begin with basic psychiatric didactic topics such as the psychiatric interview, the mental status examination, and so forth. Nonetheless, some formal didactic time must be set aside early in the academic year to begin residents' instruction in appropriate methods of educa-

TABLE 8–1.   Representative objectives for residents as teachers

Formats

Formal lecture

Small-group leadership

Bedside teaching

Team learning

Individual supervision

Liaison with other medical professionals

Public education

Psychoeducation

Knowledge and skills

Assessment of learners

Provision of feedback to learners

Principles of evidence-based medicine

Use of presentation software

Creation of handouts

tion. One excellent source for beginning this process, *Residents as Teachers: A Guide to Educational Practice* (Schwenk and Whitman 1993), was originally written for a family practice audience but is easily adaptable to the needs of psychiatric education. This work describes in detail concepts such as active versus passive styles of teaching and learning and the benefits and drawbacks of various teaching styles (e.g., group discussions, lectures, tutorials, preceptorships) and covers strategies for effective teaching in specific situations (e.g., lectures, grand rounds, morning reports, journal clubs, bedside teaching). A copy of this work could be given to all incoming psychiatric residents early in the intern year and should be discussed with a faculty member skilled in educational methods. Where schedules do not allow formal didactic time to be devoted to such an introductory course, residents could discuss relevant issues in a journal club format.

Another source of effective teaching methods appropriate for introduction in the intern year is a review article that surveys the effectiveness of various teaching methods in family practice, internal medicine, and pediatrics (Heidenreich et al. 2000). Despite not specifically focusing on the field of psychiatry, this article describes common medical teaching methods used for clinical instruction. Such methods include orienting the learner, prioritizing learning needs, priming, pattern recognition, effective questioning, and the provision of feedback. (The reader is referred to this article for a discussion of formal methods of education.) The acquisition of skills such as these early in residency is important for the resident as teacher.

It may be worthwhile to explore additional resources outside the psychiatry department or the school of medicine as a whole. Most departments exist as part of a larger university and should fully tap these resources, if available. Faculty members in the department of education (or medical education), for example, may be willing to host a two- or three-session seminar for interns covering basic methods of instruction and feedback. These ancillary resources combined with the department's formal teaching curriculum can provide junior psychiatry residents with a good foundation on which to develop teaching skills throughout their residency.

Senior resident–to–junior resident mentorship in a training program is a crucial component of the model for teaching house officers to teach. Most psychiatry programs staff their inpatient wards with a combination of interns and more-experienced residents. Also, a large portion of the intern year is spent rotating through internal medicine, emergency medicine, and neurological services, on which more-senior nonpsychiatric residents perform many teaching duties both for the psychiatric intern and for any medical students who may be rotating on the service. These encounters with more-seasoned residents and the observation of the seniors' teaching methods constitute an invaluable "shadow curriculum" experience on which new house officers can draw. Allowing time in the postgraduate year 1 didactic curriculum for interns, in the presence of a faculty facilitator, to discuss the teaching they have observed during their time on the wards, the techniques that seemed effective, and what they found less useful can help interns to begin the process of evaluating teaching methods and molding them into their own style of teaching.

Finally, residents should receive written evaluations of their teaching skills from the students they supervise. With thoughtful consideration of student criticism, teaching skills can be enhanced. Consistent areas of concern, as well as high praise, can be noted in the resident's file for review by the residency training director.

POSTGRADUATE YEAR 2

After completing an internship, the second-year psychiatric resident has developed a degree of competence in psychiatric matters and educational techniques sufficient to allow the assignment of official teaching duties. This is not to imply that first-year residents are unable to teach students with whom they work, but rather that as the trainee moves further into residency, he or she becomes better equipped to handle formal teaching responsibilities. Although some residencies staff their inpatient wards with residents from all postgraduate classes, for most programs the bulk of day-to-day ward coverage is still by second-year residents. Also, given that medical students are generally assigned to inpatient wards for their psychiatric clerkships, it is at this level of training that most residents will experience their greatest opportunities for formal clinical instruction.

A standard medical school psychiatry clerkship consists of 6 weeks at a university or community hospital's inpatient ward. Allowing half of 1 week at the beginning and the end of the rotation for orientation and to wrap up affairs leaves approximately 5 weeks for clinical instruction of students by on-service residents. This allows three-times-weekly sessions of 30–60 minutes' duration each during which on-service residents must cover a topic in suitable depth for the third-year students. If we assume that the average service has three residents assigned at any given time, each resident could be responsible for one session weekly, which should leave ample time to meet clinical obligations on even the busiest inpatient services.

Although each department can emphasize topics of its choosing, the following 15 topics (3 topics weekly for 5 weeks) are proposed as an example:

- The psychiatric interview/mental status exam
- Substance abuse
- Suicide/homicide/safety considerations
- Psychotic disorders
- Mood disorders
- Anxiety disorders
- Personality disorders
- Eating disorders
- Delirium/dementia
- Psychotherapies
- Antidepressants
- Antipsychotics
- Mood stabilizers
- Anxiolytics
- Electroconvulsive therapy

This list can easily be modified for a given department's purposes, but as written it provides a broad overview of psychopathology and therapeutics. Importantly, the resident is encouraged to make links between lecture content and currently treated patients to bridge the gap between academic information and real-world applications. This is a crucial issue, because whereas students frequently receive lectures on these topics over the course of their preclinical years and clerkship, the psychiatry clerkship may be the only setting in which they receive clinical examples of the principles being taught.

At Wright State University, many residents on the inpatient wards find it most convenient to meet with students over lunch in a small office or conference room away from the distractions of the service. During the discussion, residents not presenting on a given day cover responsibilities for the presenter and assigned students, to limit interruptions and maximize the value of the time spent. When possible, interns attend the sessions as well. Through careful note taking, the intern can build up his or her own library of presentations for use later. Interestingly, many find the sessions more productive if other residents do not attend. It is important for the students to know who is teaching and for the developing resident–teacher to have the authority and attention requisite to teach well. Some find this approach to education counterintuitive. Given that issues such as learning from co-residents' teaching endeavors and supervisory concerns are real, this topic will be addressed later in "The Teaching Case Conference" section.

The mechanism of developing a library of such mini-lectures is left to each individual department and, in some respects, to the individual resident. At Wright State University, some faculty members have well-worn, scripted presentations that are easily adaptable to this purpose. Other possibilities include "translating" from various review manuals a presentation to address a given topic. Still other residents (particularly as they gain experience) prefer to give presentations off the cuff, with less predetermined structure. The Wright State University department is in the process of developing a resident teaching manual that will contain outlines of each topic for use during student mini-lectures. It is hoped that this manual will increase the standardization of teaching across residents' and students' rotation sites.

Beyond the development of "lecturer role" skills, it is appropriate for residents in the second postgraduate year to begin learning to handle supervisory issues as well. Day-to-day supervisory skills in a resident ideally develop as the result of receiving excellent attending supervision throughout training. Nonetheless, specific skills need to be identified for development in the resident as supervisor. Involving the student as an active member of the treatment team (as opposed to enabling passive observation) is an important skill. This includes assigning students to collect patient information from collateral sources, which teaches them about the kinds of questions to ask as well as how to ask. Additionally, students can be coached to research patient education materials and even take the lead in providing this valuable service to patients and families. Identifying questions during patient rounds in which the principles of evidence-based medicine can be utilized by the student to prepare a brief report to the team can be invaluable in helping all educators move away from the historical models of "in my experience" and "see one, learn one, teach one." Finally, residents should be actively involved with attending physicians in assessing student performance and in submitting constructive comments to be used in evaluations.

POSTGRADUATE YEAR 3

In many psychiatry residencies, a resident's time working in the presence of medical students is at its lowest during the third postgraduate year. At times, medical students may rotate through an outpatient clinic where a third-year resident is assigned, but more often than not, the teaching opportunities for a postgraduate year 3 resident center on ancillary staff and patients themselves. Nonetheless, these are important population targets for educational activities and should be covered in a residency's teaching plan.

Ancillary staff members such as nurses, clinical psychologists, social workers, and office technicians often interface with a psychiatrist's patients, and for this reason, the psychiatrist has a vested interest in their competence. The physician is ultimately responsible for the education and care his or her staff delivers; the time to develop these supervisory skills is during residency, rather than waiting until one is out on one's own. In some cases, the level of experience of some ancillary personnel will be greater than that of even a senior resident; thus, "political care" is necessary when structuring teaching opportunities, to avoid awkward situations. The structure of a given teaching encounter should vary according to the nature of the audience targeted. For the most part, several of the mini-lectures described in the "Postgraduate Year 2" section are appropriate for use with ancillary staff. Modifying certain presentations (e.g., focusing more on the long-term clinical considerations of dementia and less on delirium in a presentation to social workers) may be necessary. Also, the fact that most staff members encountered by the third-year resident serve outpatients rather than inpatients must be considered. Overall, three to four supervised presentations to ancillary personnel over the course of one's residency (most likely accomplished in the third postgraduate year) should be attempted.

Educating patients goes to the heart of what it means to be a physician. It is disappointing, then, that so few residency programs require from their residents any demonstrated mastery of the ability to educate patients and families. Although this skill is developed at all points during a resident's training, the third postgraduate year offers the most seamless opportunity for a trainee to demonstrate this critical ability, because of the longer-term nature of the resident's relationship with outpatients during the third year, the (presumed) larger amount of time allowed for patient encounters, and the more structured, steady nature of the third-year workday. Whereas supervisory considerations will be deferred to "The Teaching Case Conference" section, residents should document at least three cases of comprehensive patient education during the third year. Topical content of these cases should include an explanation of the diagnosis and prognosis, a recommended course of treatment, alternatives to this recommendation, risks and benefits of all possible courses of action, and responses to any questions from the patient and/or the patient's family.

POSTGRADUATE YEAR 4

The final year of psychiatric residency has historically been a time for knowledge consolidation and exploration of elective areas of topical interest. Nonetheless, there are important teaching skills to be acquired during the final year of training. Two specific skill areas proposed here are junior–resident mentorship and attending physician skills.

A fourth-year psychiatric resident can offer a wealth of experience and knowledge to junior residents in the department. As alluded to earlier, these skills can be developed and tapped by requiring senior residents to engage in formal mentorship duties with younger trainees. Such duties can take a number of forms, from chief-resident responsibilities to the development of resident-driven board preparation courses to the facilitation of a resident psychotherapy process group. The actual activities chosen are less important than the overall experience in mentorship activities and time spent in appropriate reflection and supervision by appropriate faculty.

Attending physician skills encompass a vast array of qualities, which are difficult to define and even more difficult to establish guidelines for competency demonstration. As used here, however, such skills refer to a finite set of duties typically required of an attending physician who leads an inpatient psychiatric service. Sometimes referred to as "sub-attendingships" or "senior resident internships," these rotations serve as the final opportunity for a resident to attain and demonstrate the skills necessary to manage, teach, and evaluate a team of residents and students. Although only a small percentage of psychiatrists will go on to practice in an inpatient capacity, those who do may find their work to be much different (relative to their inpatient residency experiences) than the work of their outpatient-practicing counterparts. For this reason, fourth-year residents could be strongly encouraged (if not required) to spend several weeks back on the inpatient wards running the service in a sub-attending capacity.

SUPERVISORY ISSUES

FORMAL, VIDEO-BASED SUPERVISION

Without sufficient quality supervision, no quantity of instruction or required teaching experiences will make residents effective educators. For this reason, any medical education model should include the assignment of a "teaching supervisor" to each house officer, whose responsibility it is to meet regularly with the assigned resident to discuss teaching experiences. The interaction can be patterned after the traditional psychotherapy trainee–supervisor relationship; depending on the amount of teaching being performed by a trainee at a given time, meetings with the supervisor can occur weekly, biweekly, or monthly.

The resident is expected to come to supervision on each occasion with a teaching case for discussion. Background information such as location, targeted audience, topical content, and methods of presentation should be quickly reviewed with the supervisor, followed by a more in-depth examination of the resident's effectiveness. The supervisor should review the factual basis of a resident's teaching, but more worthwhile will be the exploration of what worked well and what did not as the trainee's delivery rather than content is critiqued. In-person observation of the resident's teaching may at times be beneficial, but as with the practice of psychotherapy, the extra person in the room may alter the encounter and prevent a true rendering of the resident's work. For this reason, frequent videotaping of a resident's teaching encounters for supervisory review is helpful. Taping can be easily done in a variety of formats, and nearly all of the teaching formats outlined in previous sections can be recorded with minimal interruption of the teaching session. The one exception may be the patient-education sessions in the third postgraduate year, because of confidentiality concerns with the patient. With appropriate explanation and documentation of informed consent, however, this exercise should also be able to be incorporated into the videotaping experience.

Taping serves multiple ends. It provides the supervisor and resident with a true representation of a resident's teaching and offers far more opportunity for improvement than a simple narrative account by the trainee. Furthermore, it allows the resident to build a library of teaching experiences for reflection and review as he or she progresses in training. Finally, it enhances group learning when reviewed, as covered in the next section, with a group of co-residents.

THE TEACHING CASE CONFERENCE

A central activity for teaching residents to be effective teachers is the teaching case conference. This format offers a training program the opportunity to develop and refine its residents' teaching skills in a team-based, collaborative fashion. Although a given program may modify the parameters to suit its needs, the basic structure of this conference should imitate the psychotherapy case conferences now in place at many programs around the country.

Residents are assigned in groups of 8–10 to a senior faculty member with experience, interest, and skill in medical education. Frequency of meetings may vary in response to other demands within a program, but sessions occurring at least monthly are desired. At each session, one resident is responsible for writing up a brief description of a recently completed teaching session. Several minutes are spent discussing the unique objectives of the assignment, followed by a review of the resident's videotape from the session. The tape is periodically stopped and the resident's teaching style critiqued by members of the group. Alternative ways of presenting the material are discussed, and the targeted audience's reception of the material is explored. Ideally, a resident will have tapes of multiple sessions in which he or she taught the same material (e.g., a presentation on antidepressants given early in the second year and one given at the end of the second year). This will allow for comparison and contrast between sessions and will provide the occasion to evaluate improvement in a resident's skills over time.

The value of the teaching case conference is clear. It affords junior residents the opportunity to observe the teaching of certain concepts before they themselves are required to do so. Senior residents receive yet another opportunity for mentorship and consolidation of teaching skills. Departmental faculty members can see firsthand the teaching their residents do and can potentially document competencies. Finally, the conference provides the opportunity for collegial group learning and experience sharing, which is more morale-building and efficient than other learning styles.

OBSERVED STRUCTURED TEACHING EXAMINATIONS

Like observed structured clinical examinations (OSCEs), observed structured teaching examinations (OSTEs) provide an opportunity to standardize situations in which the examinee (i.e., preceptor) interacts with a standardized student (i.e., medical student or resident). OSTEs have been utilized in recent years as tools in faculty development to evaluate teaching skills and identify areas of strengths and weaknesses (Gelula 1998; Lesky and Wilkerson 1994). Theoretically, direct measures of teaching performance could be assessed and even used as part of teaching portfolios, but in most instances, OSTEs are used solely as formative exercises.

Because today's residents have experience with OSCEs during medical school, it seems a natural progression to use OSTEs as part of their development as educators. A variety of standardized clinical scenarios are possible. For instance, a "standardized third-year student" (who has been appropriately trained in a rigorous fashion) presents a clinical case to a resident examinee, who listens, offers formative feedback, and provides clinical teaching. In another scenario, a resident examinee may need to address professional lapses in the standardized student. After the exercise, the standardized learner provides feedback to the resident about how effectively the resident utilized clinical teaching skills. Videotapes of these encounters can be viewed later by the group of residents who have gone through the OSTE. These reviews (facilitated by faculty members) can provide constructive suggestions for change by examining the residents' teaching skills. Areas of evaluation should include appearing interested, listening appropriately, being open to concerns, using a collaborative approach, encouraging questions, and checking the student's understanding of the concepts. Additionally, the provision of effective feedback that encourages rather than discourages the student should be assessed during the video review.

Although OSTEs may not be ideal tools for specific teaching evaluation, they do provide an opportunity to examine behaviors in action, to practice teaching skills, and to allow immediate feedback to the teacher. Dunnington and DaRosa (1998) found that residents self-assessed great improvement in their teaching through the use of OSTEs. Indeed, the ultimate goal should be teaching improvement.

FORMAL INSTRUCTION

A formal curriculum should exist for residents being asked to become more reflective and self-critical of teaching skills. This curriculum should include current educational theories and techniques in medical student education, a working knowledge of evidence-based medicine concepts, provision of effective feedback to students, and concepts of learner-centered learning, with more-active "learner contracts" established whenever possible. Instruction in effective PowerPoint presentations, note development, and evaluation tools can also be included.

At Wright State University, senior residents have been trained as examiners for a required observed and evaluated student interview of a live patient. As residents evaluate the interviewing skills of medical students, they are also reassessing their own skills. Residents find that by being examiners in this process, they are more confident and comfortable participating in their own oral examinations. Having residents assist in question development for medical students' exams and quizzes can also be invaluable. Residents develop first-line experience with the challenge of writing good United States Medical Licensing Examination–style exam questions, and when students express frustration, the residents may defend the exam rather than collude with the student criticism. Through this process, residents read and learn material at a depth that is not otherwise obtained.

FEEDBACK

Of paramount importance is the provision of worthwhile feedback to trainees regarding their teaching endeavors. Such feedback forms the basis of professional reflection, which, "in the context of professional practice….is the key to learning from experience" (Heidenreich et al. 2000, p. 236). Other authors note that "teachers must reflect on their teaching if they are to identify ways to improve it" (Skeff et al. 1997, p. 696). By providing timely, appropriate, constructive feedback, a psychiatry department can guide residents to reflect on their teaching practices in an effort to improve them.

The first piece of formal feedback to consider is a year-end award within the residency for excellence in teaching. This can be voted on and bestowed by medical students, ancillary staff, the residents themselves, or faculty members with special knowledge of the residents' teaching activities. In some cases, a combination of the above groups may be best suited to determine the recipient of the award—or, alternatively, multiple awards can be given. Where possible, a financial stipend should be given in conjunction with the award, and naming the honor after a respected department figure (perhaps a past chairperson with special interest in teaching) can provide additional incentive for residents to strive for excellence in teaching.

Another important item of feedback for residents can be the comments solicited from populations the residents are assigned to teach. Although the bulk of these comments will be from medical students on their junior clerkships, other populations mentioned above offer a source of 360-degree feedback that is important to draw on in evaluating residents. There are at least two methods for using these comments. First, at the end of each academic year, each resident can be given all comments submitted regarding his or her performance in teaching activities. This distribution should occur yearly, with submitters' names deleted to protect the anonymity of the evaluators. This anonymity is critical to guarantee the evaluators' candor. The resident can then reflect with a supervisor on the reviews received and contemplate possible improvements in technique, and so forth. Second, various anonymous evaluations of residents can be read by the faculty discussant and responses to the evaluations explored. This allows all residents to contemplate and reflect on teaching strengths and shortcomings (regardless of whether each individual resident possesses any given one) and improve the group's overall grasp of educational concepts.

FINAL THOUGHTS: IMPLEMENTATION CONCERNS

In the arena of psychiatric training coordination, no new entity can be integrated into an existing residency model without encountering resistance or without displacing other important activities already in place within the department. The zero-sum nature of time within our programs makes the implementation of this model quite challenging for psychiatry residencies, where demands on faculty members' and residents' time are already great. However, many aspects of this model could be integrated through avenues already in place within most departments. There will certainly be bumps in the road and further demands on the time of all involved if a model such as this is undertaken. If "teaching takes time" (Heidenreich et al. 2000), then we can expect teaching "how to teach" to take even more time. Nonetheless, there are rich potential rewards for the successful implementation of such an endeavor throughout our field for our faculty, our residents, our students, and, ultimately, our patients.

REFERENCES

American Medical Association: Graduate Medical Education Directory. Chicago, IL, American Medical Association, 2003

American Psychiatric Association: Psychiatric Residents as Teachers: A Practical Guide. 2001 (Revised from Psychiatric residents as teachers, prepared by APA Committee on Medical Student Education, American Psychiatric Association, 1988)

Dunnington GL, DaRosa D: A prospective randomized trial of a residents-as-teachers training program. Acad Med 73:696–700, 1998

Feifel D, Moutier CY, Swerdlow NR: Attitudes toward psychiatry as a prospective career among students entering medical school. Am J Psychiatry 156:1397–1402, 1999

Gelula MH: Using standardized medical students to improve junior faculty teaching. Acad Med 73:611–612, 1998

Lesky LG, Wilkerson L: Using "standardized students" to teach a learner-centered approach to ambulatory precepting. Acad Med 69:955–957, 1994

Heidenreich C, Lye P, Simpson D, et al: The search for effective and efficient ambulatory teaching methods through the literature. Pediatrics 105:231–237, 2000

Lee EK, Kaltreider N, Crouch J: Pilot study of current factors influencing the choice of psychiatry as a specialty. Am J Psychiatry 152:1066–1069, 1995

Schwenk TL, Whitman NA: Residents as Teachers: A Guide to Educational Practice. Salt Lake City, University of Utah School of Medicine, 1993

Skeff KM, Bowen JL, Irby DM: Protecting time for teaching in the ambulatory care setting. Acad Med 72:694–697, 1997

Spencer J: Learning and teaching in the clinical environment. BMJ 326:591–594, 2003

CHAPTER 9

THE ACCREDITATION PROCESS

Challenges and Benefits

Jerald Kay, M.D.

Nothing strikes more fear in the heart of a young training director than the accreditation process. Moreover, seasoned program directors, residency staff, and faculty are not immune to the trials and tribulations of preparing for an accreditation visit. I have been a training director and a site visitor and am currently a department chair serving on the Residency Review Committee (RRC) for Psychiatry. Based on these experiences, in this chapter I hope to provide a relevant, multidimensional view of the accreditation of a psychiatry residency. Because of the rapidity in turnover among training directors these days, it will be necessary to review the organization, policy procedures, and responsibilities of the RRC for Psychiatry as well as those of training directors and their faculty. Some of the more common problems in preparing for an accreditation visit are also presented.

WHY HAVE AN ACCREDITATION PROCESS?

Unlike some other countries, the United States has separate and autonomous agencies that are responsible for assessing and maintaining the quality of undergraduate medical education and graduate medical education (GME), as well as licensure and specialty certification. The fundamental reason for accreditation is to improve the quality of health care in this country by ensuring and improving the quality of physicians in training. This goal is accomplished through the creation of national standards for all specialties and subspecialties and the performance of regular valid, fair, open, and ethical assessment of all programs. National standards for GME are developed with extensive input of all specialties and are therefore responsive to change and innovation in education and current practice. The accreditation process emphasizes effective measurement tools to evaluate residents' competence and due process. It is free from political or economic influences and is carried out by individuals who are expert in their disciplines and trained in the work of accreditation. In this age of increasing physician accountability, the accreditation of programs should provide the highest form of professional self-evaluation. Moreover, it should serve as a critical forum for program self-study.

WHO IS RESPONSIBLE FOR ACCREDITATION?

The Accreditation Council for Graduate Medical Education (ACGME) has two functions. It is responsible for establishing the "Essentials of Accredited Residencies in Graduate Medical Education" (Accreditation Council for Graduate Medical Education 1998) and for conducting evaluations of residency programs. The "Essentials" consist of program requirements, which mandate program obligations for each specialty and subspecialty, and institutional requirements, which define the responsibilities of the educational institution such as a university medical school and affiliated teaching hospitals (American Medical Association 2003, pp. 13–16). The authority for the accreditation process resides in each specialty or subspecialty RRC, and the ACGME monitors the activities of each RRC to ensure compliance with policies and procedures.

The ACGME has broad representation and is composed of members from the American Board of Medical Specialties (ABMS), the American Hospital Association (AHA), the Association of American Medical Colleges (AAMC), the American Medical Association (AMA), and the Council of Medical Specialty Societies (CMSS). It also includes representation from specialty organizations such as the American Psychiatric Association (APA).

WHAT IS THE RRC FOR PSYCHIATRY, AND WHAT DOES IT DO?

The RRC for Psychiatry consists of members sponsored by the APA, the American Board of Psychiatry and Neurology (ABPN), and the AMA. It also has a resident member and is staffed by the ACGME. The RRC has the following responsibilities:

- To propose program requirements (the Essentials) and to revise these requirements on a regular basis, thereby improving both the accreditation process and the quality of training
- To determine whether residency training programs (RTPs) are following both the program specialty requirements and the institutional requirements
- To recommend to the ACGME improvements in accreditation policies and procedures.
- To communicate effectively with the APA, the American Association of Directors of Psychiatric Residency Training (AADPRT), the ABPN, and the subspecialty societies

It is important that each training director of the general residency, child and adolescent residency, and all the fellowship programs (forensic, addictions, geriatrics, psychosomatic medicine, and soon to be pain management) be very familiar with the Essentials. The Essentials detail the administrative, clinical, and didactic obligations to trainees. They are contained in the annual *Graduate Medical Education Directory* (American Medical Association 2003, pp. 324–332, the "green book") and can be found on the ACGME Web site (http://www.acgme.org). The form required from all training directors for accreditation purposes attempts to validate whether a program is in compliance with the Essentials. Last, it is important to note that training directors and specialty societies have great influence on the development and revision of the Essentials. When the call goes out to the field for suggestions about new essentials or the modification of existing ones, psychiatric educators must provide input.

There is a tendency for some program directors to view the RRC as adversarial or contentious. Nothing could be further from the truth, and the significance of feedback from the field can never be overemphasized. It is also helpful to keep in mind that members of the RRC are training directors, chairs of departments of psychiatry, and ABPN directors and are all active teachers in their respective training programs.

WHAT IS A SITE VISIT, AND HOW DOES A PROGRAM PREPARE FOR IT?

To begin on a positive note, the findings of a site visit can be a remarkable asset to the residency program and its department of psychiatry. Deficiencies in institutional support, facilities, clinical experiences, and supervision can provide a mechanism for remedying problem areas. As examples, inadequate space for residents' offices, poor on-call facilities, lack of safety in clinical sites, poor library or informatics resources, and inadequate diversity of clinical experiences for residents prompt action from the department, sponsoring academic institution, and teaching hospitals. No dean, chair of psychiatry, or hospital chief executive officer relishes the uncovering of shortcomings in a graduate program. Frequently, the findings of a disappointing accreditation decision provide the residency training director (RTD) with leverage for securing additional resources. Second, if properly prepared for, a site visit prompts intense departmental self-study. It can identify deteriorating morale among residents and faculty, poorly run courses, unnecessary repetition or absence of required topics and areas in the curriculum, and inadequate clinical and didactic evaluation procedures, to name but a few possibilities. If approached properly, the accreditation process offers the opportunity to redesign or strengthen a residency. Third, for a recently appointed RTD, the accreditation visit can be a reason for networking with more experienced program directors through the AADPRT or through the hiring of an experienced outside consultant.

The timing of a site visit is determined by the RRC. For most programs with minor deficiencies, this may occur every 4 or 5 years. Other programs with significant problems can anticipate less time between visits. This could be as frequent as even 1 or 2 years. In every instance, the notification of an accreditation visit should mobilize the RTD to undertake a program review through the department's residency training committee, which includes key teaching faculty and adequate resident representation. Even for the most experienced of RTDs the required documentation for a site visit is challenging.

It is the responsibility of the program director to coordinate the accurate completion of the Program Information Form (PIF). This lengthy and detailed document provides the site visitor with a view of the program's administrative and educational characteristics and is used by the site visitor to evaluate the program's compliance with the Essentials. It is also closely scrutinized by the RRC at the time of accreditation decisions. It is available online from the ACGME Web site (http://www.acgme.org).

CHRONOLOGY OF A SITE VISIT

1. The RTD is notified by the ACGME that a site visit is required. Ample time is provided to prepare. It is the responsibility of the RTD to **contact the site visitor to schedule the visit.** Either a field sur-

veyor or a specialist site visitor (SSV) is assigned to review the program. The former are physicians and nonphysicians who perform
more routine surveys of training programs in good standing and often
review a number of specialty programs in a single institution during
one visit. An SSV is always a psychiatrist and is assigned to programs
with significant deficiencies, including those on probation. Application for a new program is always conducted by an SSV. The RTD
should never establish a site visit date when the department chair or
key teaching faculty will be unavailable, because they must meet with
the field surveyor or SSV.

2. Key faculty and all residents must be informed immediately of the date
   of the visit and that they are required to participate by meeting with the
   site visitor. As is true in the residency selection process, the **administrative assistant** of the training program plays a crucial part in preparation for the site visit.

3. Ideally, **preparation for a site visit** should begin with an intensive review of the program approximately 1 year before the scheduled date.
   This self-study provides an opportunity for faculty and trainees to suggest new ideas about the training program and to note components that
   are going poorly. It should be remembered that there is nothing like the
   eventuality of a site visit to motivate the examination of a curriculum
   and to establish a more cohesive teaching faculty. However, the better
   programs in the country have a continuing curriculum review process
   on a yearly basis.

4. Particularly in the case of a new program director, one should never
   underestimate the time that is required to **complete the PIF accurately,** because faculty members must assist the RTD in this task. Like
   many aspects of a program, such as evaluations of residents, the RTD
   will have to remind and push faculty members to complete the parts
   of the PIF that describe the teaching and clinical services for which
   they are responsible. **Goals and objectives** for clinical experiences
   and years of the curriculum are required on the PIF. Recently appointed RTDs should carefully examine the Essentials and become
   very familiar with them to ensure that all areas are being covered in
   the training program.

5. The RTD and administrative program assistant begin a review of all
   resident records to ensure that selection materials, residents' logs,
   evaluation of residents, evaluation by residents of their instructors,
   and minutes of training committee meetings are up to date. Inadequate **selection files** of residents transferring to the program are easily noted when there is no letter from the applicant's previous program

stipulating his or her educational experience. **Documentation for international medical graduates** must also be complete. RTDs must include in each graduated resident's file a **letter testifying to the resident's ability to practice in an ethical and competent fashion.** Files for residents who have struggled during their training and required probation or remediation must contain adequate documentation about the nature of the **deficiencies and a plan to assist the resident** in overcoming problems. This plan should contain an objective method of ascertaining the resident's progress and how it will be measured. Files of residents who have **prematurely terminated** their training through either dismissal or transfer to another program or specialty should also contain adequate documentation. In the case of dismissal, there must be thorough documentation of **due process.** Residents' files should contain evidence that each trainee has taken a **written examination** (most often the Psychiatry Resident In-Training Examination) as well as **clinical examinations** at regularly scheduled times. Brief **curricula vitae of teachers** central to the educational mission should be updated. Because all programs are required to have a faculty committed to scholarship, recent publications and other scholarly activities should be added and any publications by residents should be appropriately noted.

6. All **letters of institutional affiliation** must be current. New institutions that have been added to the RTP since the last site visit should have formal affiliation letters.

7. The RTD should ensure that the program has completed **internal reviews** conducted by the graduate education committee of the school or hospital. The RRC frowns on a last-minute internal review that merely attempts to follow the letter of the law but not the spirit.

8. It is imperative to conduct a **mock site visit** before the site visitor's arrival. This reduces anxiety for faculty members and residents who have never participated in a site visit. It often identifies missing information or confusion about the curriculum.

9. The RTD should be prepared to show the site visitor residents' **offices and classrooms,** and in the case of an SSV, there may be a request to **examine clinical charts** to ascertain that clinical care is responsibly documented. If there has been a particular problem with inadequate facilities or supervision—for example, in the psychiatry emergency service—the site visitor may wish to observe that location. Programs often utilize more than one site for resident rotations, but it is up to the site visitor to indicate that he or she wishes to see them. Because of time limitations, this may not always be possible.

10. The RTD should arrange for **residents to meet with the field surveyor or SSV.** Larger programs may wish to select a representative number of residents from each year of the program. Smaller residencies often have all residents meet with the site visitor. The purpose of this meeting is to verify that educational and clinical experiences as described in the PIF are in fact offered and current. It also provides an opportunity to gauge the morale of a program and to identify administrative and supervisory deficiencies.

11. Some site visitors also request a meeting with a **dean or director of GME** at an institution. This interview is especially helpful when it is clear that proper institutional support is not being provided.

12. As mentioned, site visitors always wish to interview the **chair of a department of psychiatry.** The purpose of this meeting is to assess that the chair is providing solid departmental and personal resources to the training program and RTD. Site visitors are attentive to the success or problems in this relationship.

13. All site visitors insist on meeting with **faculty who are centrally involved** in the RTP. This includes, for example, directors of inpatient, outpatient, consultation-liaison, child and adolescent, and emergency psychiatry. If a program designates associate RTDs in each of its affiliated institutions, then these faculty members should also be available to the site visitor.

HOW DOES THE RRC REVIEW SITE PROGRAMS, AND WHAT IS THE NOTIFICATION PROCESS?

The RRC meets twice yearly, once in the fall and once in the spring. The ACGME staff of the RRC for Psychiatry assigns each RRC member programs to review. Each program is evaluated by two people. Programs in child and adolescent psychiatry are generally reviewed by RRC members who are child psychiatrists. Other postresidency programs such as addiction and forensic psychiatry may not be reviewed by psychiatrists with subspecialty training.

Reviewers carefully study both the PIF and the site visitor's report to assess concordance between the two. The site visitor's report will also address issues that cannot be identified through the PIF. These include resident and faculty morale and issues of evaluation and administration, facilities, due process, selection, duty hours, supervision, and adequacy of resident files, to name but a few. Each site visitor's report notes specific deficiencies or inadequacies in the requirements. Site visitors also examine very closely whether the program has adequately dealt with all previous deficiencies and whether progress notes requested by the RRC are in fact accurate and reflect careful intervention.

Each RRC reviewer assigned to a program must prepare a written report, which is also distributed to other members of the RRC with the exception of those with a potential conflict of interest. The two program reviewers present their reports to the entire RRC and recommend an action. After deliberation, the RRC makes an accreditation recommendation, which may or may not agree with the recommendation of the two reviewers. The ACGME then prepares a written report on all actions taken by the RRC at a meeting, and this must be signed off on by the chair of the RRC. Finally, the staff sends a letter to the RTD advising the program of the RRC's action.

The RRC is governed by strict impartiality and careful attention to due process. Reviewers with any conflict of interest—such as those who belong to a department in the same state as the program being reviewed—are neither permitted to participate in reviewing a program nor allowed to be present when accreditation decisions are formulated. All decisions are based only on written records from the PIF, the site visitor report, and the reports of the two reviewers on the RRC. Recommendations about accreditation status never come from personal opinion.

There are three basic accreditation categories and two nonaccreditation categories:

1. **Provisional accreditation** is granted for new programs or programs that had ceased functioning but are once again wishing to train residents. Programs with provisional accreditation generally receive a site visit and are reviewed within 2 years.
2. **Withhold accreditation** is a decision based on a new program's inability to comply with the Essentials. As is the case with all written reports from the RRC to the RTD, areas that are not in compliance with the Essentials are noted, and the program must reapply for approval to begin or restart training.
3. **Full accreditation** reflects the finding that a program is in substantial compliance with the Essentials. Such a program may have minor deficiencies, about which the RRC requests a **progress report** from the RTP describing actions taken to rectify them. The maximum interval between program reviews is 5 years, although shorter cycles can be recommended by the RRC.
4. **Probationary accreditation** status is given to a program that is fully accredited but is no longer in substantial compliance with the essentials

of training. Programs that receive this type of accreditation are almost always reviewed again within 2 years, but the RRC can decide that the problems are such that the program should be reviewed in only 1 year.

A program is not permitted to have probationary accreditation for more than 4 years, after which time it must be given full accreditation or the program must withdraw from training. Continued probation is therefore a possible option, but only for two review cycles.

5. **Withdrawal of accreditation** of a training program can occur if a program with either provisional or probationary accreditation is not in compliance with special essentials. When a program receives this type of decision it can complete training of residents only until the end of the academic year; future classes cannot be accepted, and residents who are not graduating must find new training opportunities.

Adverse actions such as probation and withdrawal can be appealed to an ACGME appeals panel, which is composed of experienced psychiatrists who are not on the RRC. This panel can either sustain or rescind the decision of the RRC. If the former occurs, then no additional appeal action is permitted. Figure 9–1 summarizes all of the possible accreditation possibilities.

WHAT ARE SOME COMMON MISTAKES MADE IN THE ACCREDITATION PROCESS?

Although it is by no means comprehensive, Table 9–1 addresses problems that I have experienced over the last 20 years as a site visitor and RRC member. Other actions that reflect poorly on the program and its faculty and staff at the time of the site visit are noted in Table 9–2.

HOW ARE SUBSPECIALTY PROGRAMS ACCREDITED?

The RRC for Psychiatry is responsible for the accreditation of all 1-year specialty residencies whose successful trainees are then eligible to sit for the ABPN exams that confer added qualifications in geriatric, forensic, addiction, and psychosomatic psychiatry. The ability to initiate and continue such a 1-year program is dependent on its related general psychiatry program being satisfactorily accredited. If the parent program is on probation or its accreditation is withdrawn, then the subspecialty residency cannot continue. There are specific essentials developed in conjunction with the

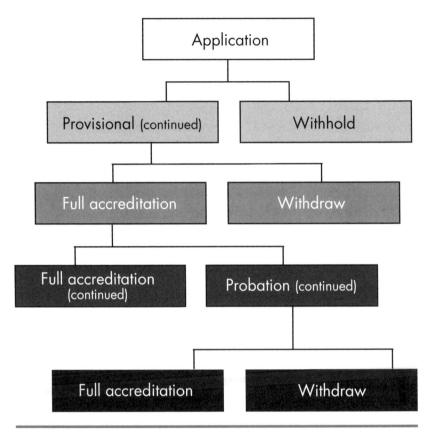

FIGURE 9–1. Categories of accreditation.

subspecialty societies, the APA, the RRC, and the ABPN for each of the subspecialty residencies. Like the general psychiatry and child and adolescent essentials, those for the subspecialty programs mandate clinical, curricular, supervisory, evaluative, and scholarly activities and administrative responsibilities. The accreditation categories differ slightly from those of general and child and adolescent psychiatry because the subspecialty residencies are dependent on the status of their parent programs. Even though the subspecialty training program meets all requirements, it may be placed on accreditation with warning (administrative) or withdrawal of accreditation (administrative) when the parent general residency program is doing poorly. The other categories of accreditation are identical to those in general and child and adolescent psychiatry (accreditation, withhold accreditation, accreditation with warning, and withdrawal).

TABLE 9–1. Common mistakes in completing the Program
Information Form (PIF)

---

1. There is a discrepancy between the **block diagram** (section 7 of the PIF) that illustrates resident rotations and other material contained in the PIF. A careless completion of the block diagram may also demonstrate the program's noncompliance with mandated duration of experiences.

2. The program has failed to notify the Residency Review Committee (RRC) when it has **changed department or program leadership** or has added or deleted **positions and affiliated institutions.**

3. The program has not implemented all the changes to **correct deficiencies** as requested by the RRC or as promised in the progress note if required.

4. The program claims that certain **subjects are taught,** but the "Scheduled Seminars and Conferences" section (section 8.0 of the PIF) contains no mention of teaching activities about these topics.

5. The PIF does not include **up-to-date affiliation agreements** between institutions used for resident rotations.

6. The PIF stipulates that residents **have specific clinical responsibilities** with selected treatments and patients, but the reviewer ascertains during the meeting with residents that in fact few if any trainees can attest to these experiences.

7. The residency training director (RTD) does not place in a graduating resident's file a letter attesting that there was no evidence of unethical or unprofessional behavior and serious questions of clinical competence.

8. The file of a resident departing from a program does not contain a letter from the program director describing the type and length of rotations for which credit was granted. If full credit is not given to a departing resident, this letter must also indicate why.

9. The RTD does not provide all entering residents with a copy of the **"Essentials** of Accredited Residencies in Graduate Medical Education" or the **"American Medical Association Principles of Ethics** With Special Annotations for Psychiatry."

10. The program has no record of the systematic evaluation of faculty teaching by its trainees.

ADVERSE ACTIONS AND THE RIGHT TO APPEAL

When the RRC votes to take an adverse action, the program receives a letter explaining the intent to take the proposed action. The program then has the opportunity to rebut by letter the findings of the RRC. At the very next meeting, the RRC will then reconsider the specific concerns and the evidence from the program that contests the findings. The committee then has the option to either sustain or rescind each specific deficiency or inade-

TABLE 9–2.   Mistakes to avoid during the site visit

1. Numerous **corrections and additions to the Program Information Form (PIF)** are given to the site visitor when he or she arrives at the department. Site visitors prepare for each accreditation visit by thoroughly reviewing past Residency Review Committee (RRC) actions and the PIF. They are not prepared to address large amounts of new data on the spot.

2. The **PIF is received** by the site visitor **much later than agreed on** because the program waited until the last moment.

3. **Residents' records** are not easily available for inspection.

4. **Key faculty members or administrative personnel** are unable to meet with the site visitor.

5. A program's **required internal review** by its institution's graduate medical education body was conducted immediately before the accreditation visit.

6. The **program director misleads** the site visitor about components of the training program, which is readily discovered in speaking with other faculty members and residents.

7. The program director instructs faculty members and residents who are scheduled to meet with the site visitor to provide an **inaccurate description** of the administration, evaluation, and curriculum of the program.

8. Residents are instructed to mention nothing about important **morale problems** or inadequate supervision of clinical experiences.

9. The residency training director and/or faculty members **argue with the surveyor** about findings or the value of certain essentials. Any disagreements or concerns about the evaluation process should be addressed to the RRC and not to the site visitor.

10. The program director and/or faculty members press the **site visitor for feedback.** Surveyors are prohibited from providing such information.

quacy. Once again, this step of the accreditation process consists of a thorough re-review of the history of the program, the surveyor's report, the PIF, and the program's rebuttal information before the decision to rescind or sustain is made.

If the program is dissatisfied with the final RRC decision it has the right to ask for a formal appeal, which is considered by an ACGME appeals panel and not the RRC. As noted above (under "How Does the RRC Review Site Programs, and What Is the Notification Process?"), this panel is composed of leaders in psychiatric education who are not currently members of the RRC. If the result of the appeals hearing upholds the RRC's adverse decision, this decision is final.

SOME FINAL THOUGHTS ABOUT THE ACCREDITATION PROCESS

There resides among new RTDs a significant mythology about the RRC. The most helpful method to counter misunderstanding of the accreditation process is to consult with senior educators and attend the RRC updates given at the annual AADPRT meeting. Each year the ACGME holds its annual educational conference in Chicago. This 3-day meeting has a number of sessions that may be of use to the new RTD and his or her administrative assistant. Typical presentation topics include the following:

- What to expect when anticipating a site visit
- The program's administrator's/coordinator's role in the accreditation process
- Administrator's/coordinator's sessions in which best practices are described that are helpful in site visit preparation as well as individual program approaches addressing compliance with the Essentials
- How to teach and assess the general competencies
- Latest research on outcomes measurement in the RTP and new tools for assessment of residents
- How to implement the common duty hours standards and establish ways of ensuring a program's continued compliance

Another approach is to become an SSV. Because SSVs retire from education or move on to different aspects of psychiatry, there is a need to recruit new psychiatrists who have a commitment to improving the quality of residency training. Training sessions for becoming a site visitor are often held during the AADPRT annual meeting in late winter. Another way of making one's interest known is to speak directly with a current member of the RRC.

Last, the most important function of accreditation is the establishment of methods to improve the quality of care in this country. The future of accreditation will be characterized by the increasing focus on clinical care outcomes and the development of new methodologies of assessing these outcomes. This process requires constant input from RTDs regarding the practicality of proposals and the revision of the psychiatry essentials.

REFERENCES

Accreditation Council for Graduate Medical Education: Essentials of Accredited Residencies in Graduate Medical Education. Chicago, IL, Accreditation Council for Graduate Medical Education, 1998. Available at: http://www.acgme.org/GmeDir/Sect2.asp. Accessed July 1, 2004.

American Medical Association: Graduate Medical Education Directory 2003–2004. Chicago, IL, American Medical Association, 2003

CHAPTER 10

EVALUATION OF RESIDENTS

Carl Greiner, M.D.

Jerald Kay, M.D.

GOALS AND PRINCIPLES OF EVALUATION

Educational assessment and appropriate communication of those assessments are at the core of the activities of the residency training director (RTD). The RTD plays a substantial role with residents and faculty in setting a credible atmosphere for legitimate evaluations. Developing valid evaluations and sharing a thoughtful review to a resident is generally a rewarding experience; it is exciting for the resident to appreciate the milestones reached in professional development and to move toward competency. The Accreditation Council for Graduate Medical Education (ACGME) guidelines on the six competencies provide a structured and outcome-based approach for the resident (Accreditation Council for Graduate Medical Education 2004, Section III.E.1). Developing the necessary competencies during the course of the residency provides clarity to the resident and the program about essential work. In mentoring residents, the RTD makes contributions based on his or her role as educator, psychiatrist, and administrator.

As an educator, the RTD needs to be aware of fundamental teaching techniques and the tools of evaluation. The resident's clinical performance

I would like to thank Amy Longo, J.D., for her commentary; Vicki Hamm, graduate medical education coordinator at the University of Nebraska Medical Center, for her updates on the Accreditation Council for Graduate Medical Education; and Betsy Porter for her comments.

should be benchmarked with those of similar experience. The RTD can be particularly helpful in assisting the resident to acquire an improved understanding of his or her learning style. Appreciating the resident's learning style is important in working with the resident's strengths and weaknesses.

The art of synthesizing assessments from faculty, staff, and students is one of the most important tasks. Becoming familiar with Bloom's (1956) *Taxonomy of Educational Objectives* can provide a rational platform to discuss the status of the resident's psychiatric sophistication. Being able to highlight the resident's abilities in degrees of sophistication is important; the scale ranges from the ability to recall factual issues in diagnosis to synthesizing complex cases. Using standard literature from education will allow the RTD to be a better moderator of discussions about the resident's strengths and liabilities.

The value of educating through intensive dialogue was demonstrated as early as Plato's (1944) *Republic*. Discussing future career planning and aspirations can be one of the most valuable experiences for a resident during the training period. Assisting the resident in the development of complicated skills and comprehension of psychiatric concepts is accomplished through supervisory dialogue. If there is a need to address a resident's attitudinal problems, a focused dialogue on the specific issue is conducted.

As a psychiatrist, the RTD is alert to the vagaries of evaluation. Interpersonal jealousies, rivalries, and issues of transference and countertransference can complicate the achievement of adequate assessments. Bringing potential inconsistencies (e.g., a faculty member who gives all residents high grades but complains about the quality of residents) to the forefront can improve the quality of faculty assessments. The role of the RTD is not to provide psychotherapy to the relevant parties but to alert the evaluating individuals that significant discrepancies are present in the assessments.

As an administrator, the RTD uses the evaluations for two central reasons: 1) it is an opportunity to determine whether the training program is meeting its clinical and educational goals, and 2) it provides required documentation for site reviews. The evaluation process plays an integral role in the development of residents and the ongoing revision of a residency training program. Developing an evaluation style that anticipates fine performance yet acknowledges genuine deficiencies when necessary is an essential task of the RTD.

The RTD in psychiatry also needs to master the new requirements in the general and specific competencies. The American Association of Directors of Psychiatric Residency Training (AADPRT) provides ongoing recommendations, and other medical specialty RTDs in one's institution are other potential sources of assistance. The psychiatric RTD faces the additional challenge of the different models of conceptualizing psychiatric disorders—biological and psychodynamic—and relevant practice arising from each. Luhrmann's (2000) book *Of Two Minds* provides a useful review for the RTD.

The RTD needs to maintain the attitude of "honest appraisal." The ongoing credibility of the RTD in eliciting change in residents' behavior is strongly influenced by the trustworthiness of the assessments. The RTD's opportunity to provide honest appraisals is enhanced or limited by the standard culture of the department and home institution.

ORGANIZING THE EVALUATION

The primary goal of evaluation is to assess the resident's competency. The RTD should consider the elements of who, what, when, why, and how in the evaluation process.

"WHO" COMPONENT

The RTD reviews the residents in PGY-1 through PGY-4 unless they are child psychiatry residents. Typically, the subspecialty residents are evaluated by the fellowship director. If residents are on off-site rotations, it is important that they be in regular communication with the RTD and receive their evaluations. If the resident is on a leave of absence or on maternity or paternity leave, the RTD should note that the regular evaluation will be done on the resident's return.

The RTD needs to clearly define the relationships for evaluation of general residents, child psychiatry residents, and fellows. Although the fellowship director has overall authority for the assessment of fellows and child psychiatry residents, the assessment from the general residency is important. The fellows interact with residents and other fellows; the quality of that interaction should be assessed and shared.

"WHAT" COMPONENT

The ACGME offers a specific outline for the requirements of evaluation in the "New Special Requirements" (Accreditation Council for Graduate Medical Education 2004). Sections III.A–D and VI.A provide the guidelines for the RTD. The word *must* is included in describing the evaluation requirements; this is a significantly stronger expectation than *should*. The guidelines provide a template to which the RTD can refer in discussions with the department chair, faculty members, and residents.

The RTD has responsibility for evaluating the residents in both the general competencies for all residents and the specific requirements for psychiatry. The general guidelines for competency have provided a sea change in the approach to residency training. As Dr. David C. Leach (2003) noted, "Competent is different than 'qualified,' the latter documents that a physician has achieved certain educational milestones that are associated with the potential to be competent; whereas competence is a demonstrated habit that expresses itself in the physician's everyday practice" (p. 3).

The ACGME has devoted considerable talent and energy to the discussion and references for the six basic competencies. Each training program needs to develop a clear listing of expectations for the residents in the respective areas. The expectations provide a platform for the resident to measure his or her progress in the residency. According to the ACGME "Common Program Requirements" (Accreditation Council for Graduate Medical Education 2004, Section V.B, p. 19), residents must demonstrate the following:

- "**Patient care** that is compassionate, appropriate, and effective for the treatment of health problems and the promotion of health." Examples include conducting a comprehensive examination of a patient, garnering a complete psychiatric history, and providing a comprehensive biopsychosocial treatment plan. Learning the techniques of brief, intensive, and group therapies is essential. Assisting residents in developing a psychodynamic understanding of patients has been a prevalent weakness in many residency programs.
- "**Medical knowledge** about established and evolving biomedical, clinical, and cognate (e.g., epidemiological and social–behavioral) sciences and the application of this knowledge to patient care." Examples include knowing the side effects of common psychopharmacological agents and pertinent drug interactions and assessing risks to self and others (Teich 1998). Understanding the theoretical contributions of dynamic, behavioral, and cognitive approaches is a core issue in the development of psychiatric residents.
- "**Practice-based learning and improvement** that involves investigation and evaluation of their own patient care, appraisal and assimilation of scientific evidence, and improvement in patient care." Examples include reading the scientific literature in a critical fashion, assimilating best-practice guidelines, and recognizing the need for lifelong learning. Comparing the resident's self-assessment of practice ability and the relevant faculty assessment is an additional technique in assisting the resident to make an accurate acknowledgment of his or her clinical abilities and learning.

- **"Interpersonal and communication skills** that result in effective information exchange and collaboration with patients, their families, and other health professionals." Much of these interpersonal skills are provided in the psychotherapy training. Additional skills include maintaining an effective communication in a timely completion of the medical record. An appreciation of using the Internet and e-mail in ways that are compliant with the Health Insurance Portability and Accountability Act of 1996 (P.L. 104-191) should be encouraged.
- **"Professionalism,** as manifested through a commitment to carrying out professional responsibilities, adherence to ethical principles and sensitivity to a diverse patient population." Examples include developing an awareness of the major tenets of medical ethics promulgated by the American Psychiatric Association (APA), adhering to institutional by-laws on medical records, and providing medical coverage as requested. This particular area has often been seen as the "gray zone" of residency. Clearer definitions of expectations may reduce problematic behavior.
- **"Systems-based practice,** as manifested by actions that demonstrate an awareness of and responsiveness to the larger context and system of health care and the ability to effectively call on system resources to provide care that is of optimal value." Examples include referring patients to advocacy groups, working with third-party payers, and referring to an appropriate level of care in the community. An appreciation of risk management activities in psychiatry would be helpful.

These competencies are addressed in depth on the ACGME Web site (http://www.acgme.org). Reviewing the checklists of common competencies for other medical departments can be helpful. Dr. Leach (2003) advocated conversation with other educators to develop local guidelines.

The special requirement for psychiatry taps into a broad range of competencies in the biopsychosocial model. Psychiatry has placed particular emphasis on developing cultural competency. Donini-Lenhoff (1999) noted that the American Medical Association (AMA; 1999) has published the *Cultural Competence Compendium*, and *Academic Psychiatry* has published journal issues on specialized curricula for special health care needs of minority groups.

Another more recently approved competency in 2001 addressed the resident's learning of psychotherapy skills. This inclusion in the special requirements was the result of more than a decade of study by the AADPRT and other educational groups and was undertaken as a response to a perceived lapse in education and training in this area as well as a persistent concern that the biopsychosocial training model was slipping back into a narrower biomedical one. As a result, new competencies were adopted in five different therapies: psychodynamic, brief, supportive, cognitive-behavioral, and combined treatment. Although it is highly likely that the psychotherapy competencies will be consolidated in the next revision of the specific requirements, evaluation of these treatments will nonetheless remain relevant.

Assessing psychotherapy competence is challenging and resource intensive (Yager and Bienenfeld 2003; Yager and Kay 2003). Although no generally accepted method exists for addressing all five psychotherapy competencies, the Columbia Psychodynamic Psychotherapy Competency Test (Mullen et al. 2002) is a very helpful tool for assessing dynamic psychotherapy that is being used by a growing number of training programs. Currently, many programs supplement supervision by faculty with the requirement that residents tape sessions with their patients. Most educators believe that exclusive reliance on psychotherapy process notes may be a disservice to the resident, because it misses important teaching opportunities. (At Wright State University, all resident offices are equipped with inexpensive wall-mounted cameras, videocassette recorders, and small monitors, permitting residents to tape as many sessions as they desire beyond the required yearly number for presentation in psychotherapy case conferences.) Although there has been a great deal of resistance over the years centering on the potentially intrusive nature of taping, most educators feel that this threat has been exaggerated and that the resistance may be more reflective of clinicians' discomfort with having their work exposed than of their concern for patients' privacy.

The process-folio method is one comprehensive approach to evaluating psychotherapy competency. It consists of the following information, which is reviewed by supervisors:

- **Initial case write-up and formulation,** including consideration of the indications for the recommended type of therapy, the goals of treatment, and the problems likely to be encountered in the treatment of the particular patient
- **Follow-up summaries of the treatment,** completed on a regularly scheduled basis (at least every 3–6 months), that describe major themes and problems and how they were handled
- **Indication that reading was done** on the conduct of psychotherapy for the treatment of the particular patient and demonstration of how that reading influenced or deepened the resident's knowledge
- **Termination summary,** addressing the process of termination, goals met and unmet, and plans for treatment should additional problems arise or the patient desire further treatment

(Refer to Appendix 10–A for general psychotherapy competencies and to Appendix 10–B for sample psychotherapy-specific competency evaluation forms.)

"WHEN" COMPONENT

The general requirements mandate a resident review twice each year. The evaluation should occur in such a way that the resident has the opportunity to remediate deficiencies or consider fellowships or local and national awards. The RRC requires semiannual reviews; a set schedule such as October–November and April–May allows the resident to plan for the event. In addition, such scheduling avoids other busy times such as recruiting season and the beginning of the academic year. The resident can anticipate and prepare personal goals and objectives, and faculty members can finish late paperwork.

Increased frequency of evaluations may be used for those who are transferring into the program or are beginning their first postgraduate year. Helping the new resident with establishing goals and reviewing progress can be useful.

If issues of performance such as risk management problems (e.g., poor documentation, ill-considered medication usage, conflicts with patients) emerge, an early appointment should be set to review the resident's performance. Quickly addressing patient dissatisfaction or injury is an important aspect of practice and an important experience for the residents in dealing with untoward events (Teich 1998).

"WHY" COMPONENT

Assisting residents to appreciate their specific strengths and weaknesses is the most important reason for performing the evaluation reviews. Formative evaluations provide the equivalents of "course correction" in navigation (Angelo and Cross 1993). The practice of psychiatry is easy to do poorly and difficult to do well. The RTD and other faculty members are in an important position to assist the resident in thinking critically and meaningfully about the presentation of psychiatric illness. Dr. Edward Silberman (personal communication, January 2004) warned about "plausible psychiatry," by which he meant that residents could develop an uncritical approach to psychosis, anxiety, and depression. Identifying symptoms without placing them in a larger diagnostic context is a temptation. The competent resident needs to be able to distinguish significant nuances and differential points in determining accurate diagnoses and management plans.

Reliable formative evaluations will also prepare the resident for summative evaluations in going from the second to the third year of residency. An absence of reliable formative evaluations leaves the resident in poor shape for taking Parts I and II of the American Board of Psychiatry and Neurology (ABPN) exam.

"HOW" COMPONENT

The "how" components of a complete evaluation include thoroughness, appropriate process, and the usage of appropriate tools. For the new director, the demand for evaluations can be bewildering. Maintaining contact with a senior colleague at another institution or asking for a basic review by the graduate medical education committee in one's home institution will greatly aid the first series of evaluations.

- **Thoroughness.** A review of all of the relevant experiences since the previous review is necessary. Some attending physicians do not complete the reviews in a timely way, and it may be necessary to make telephone calls or write letters to obtain the relevant information. Describing a resident's strength is not difficult; the challenge comes in describing areas of weakness. Typical areas may include difficulty with angry or seductive patients or with particular age groups. Ongoing areas of weakness can plague residents when they take Parts I and II of the ABPN exam.
- **Appropriate process.** The RTD should follow contractual and institutional guidelines if there are deficiencies, potential probationary status, or suspension. The wise RTD must be aware of the possibilities of litigation if there is a negative assessment. Communication dictates that residents be fully aware of the implications of a negative evaluation and what avenues they have to remediate the problem.
- **Tools.** The RTD has a range of choices, which can include resident self-assessment, faculty supervisor rotational review, and scores on the Psychiatry Resident In-Training Examination (PRITE). Recommended additional reviews include assessment by the chief resident, live performance assessments such as objective structured clinical examinations (OSCEs) and mock boards, and 360-degree reviews.

The semiannual review provides an ideal opportunity to synthesize the different sources of the resident's evaluation. The self-evaluation can be one of the most valuable insights into the resident's development. Providing written personal goals allows residents to put their best foot forward and provides a background for ongoing review. Knowledge of these personal goals enables the RTD to recommend appropriate mentors who could facilitate the resident's growth. This recommendation is particularly important for the junior residents, who may not have a clear idea about the range and depth of the faculty.

A well-constructed faculty review is one of the most important assessments. The faculty member can comment on each of the six competencies and provide specific examples of attitude, skills, and knowledge. The overall assessment of the resident's developing judgment is essential. Every educator has had experiences with residents who have "book knowledge" but who experience significant difficulty translating that knowledge in urgent and emergent situations. The daily observations of patient care, interaction with staff, and professionalism are major resources for the RTD in giving a balanced review.

The PRITE, a 300-item exam, provides an important quantitative measure of performance that compares the resident to all general residents as well as to residents at his or her own level of training. The PRITE helps to identify strengths and weaknesses in performance and is a useful tool for providing specific feedback. The PRITE scores allow the RTD to address current performance and to review possible areas for improvement before residents take the ABPN exams.

The chief resident's insights can be invaluable and are often distinctive evaluations of attitude and willingness to work with others (Reuben and Noble 1990). The critical material that is often absent from faculty evaluations may be present with a near-peer review. In addition, reviews from "on call" can be an early warning for residents who have challenges in clinical capability. The chief resident can have a particularly strong sense of how the resident compares with others in his or her class. The chief resident may have a greater opportunity to know the resident over time and to provide relevant insight into a resident's strengths, weaknesses, and possible problematic performance.

Loschen (1993) provided an excellent description of OSCEs. He noted that mock boards have the usual limitation of examining only one or two patients. In distinction, Loschen described the OSCE as using examination stations to test discrete clinical skills in short sessions (5–15 minutes). For practical considerations, a group of six stations has typically been used. A variety of materials could be used such as clinical data, an emergency scenario, or standardized patients. Residents could receive feedback from the standardized patients. Faculty members are discouraged from using rare or unusual case material, and standards for performance are specified before the exam. The virtue of this type of exam is its comprehensiveness, fairness, and objectivity, which may be lacking in a supervisory commentary. As residency programs face increasing demands to certify residents' competence, performance-based exams will become more important.

The mock boards are informative about how the resident actually interviews patients unknown to him or her. Unfortunately, as the clinical world becomes busier, there are fewer opportunities for the faculty to participate in a resident's complete interview of a patient. The mock board provides an important glimpse on the establishment of rapport, capacity for empathy, and ability to do a focused interview. The real-time assessment of a resident's competency in understanding a patient and providing a reasonable diagnosis and plan is invaluable. The RTD should strongly encourage his or her faculty to provide yearly examinations.

The 360-degree review, which garners information from staff members, students, and patients, is a powerful tool in reviewing residents' performance. Although there are concerns about the time and potential expense of this approach, it speaks to the competency of professionalism. How a resident relates to an attending physician may not be indicative of the relationship with nurses or staff members. Although supervisor assessments are the core of our system, a 360-degree review offers a valuable added perspective.

If the RTD reviews this range of material before the semiannual review, he or she will have the opportunity to provide succinct and reasoned assessments of the resident's strengths and weaknesses. Common patterns will appear, such as the resident with strong descriptive skills but with a great hesitancy to examine intrapersonal and interpersonal issues. Other patterns include the bright resident with limited confidence, the relationally skilled resident with a minimal knowledge base, and the resident who has excellent skills in one domain but has limited ability to connect with patients of other groups. The RTD can make specific recommendations about ways to broaden and deepen the resident's capacity to work with a wide variety of patients.

An important educational development is the incorporation of performance-based examination, which can aid the RTD in evaluating how the resident handles complex problem solving. Swanson and colleagues (1995) reviewed four important performance-based assessments: patient management problems, computer-based clinical simulations, oral examinations, and standardized patients. These newer techniques are to be used in combination with multiple-choice tests.

RECORD KEEPING

It is difficult to imagine the range of paperwork, scheduling, and assessments that need to be processed by a new RTD. Necessary tasks include maintaining an organized record of residents' reviews, recording which faculty evaluations have been turned in and which need to be solicited, and arranging applicant interviews.

"The devil is in the details" is a widely quoted aphorism. New RTDs will quickly confront the reality that they have inherited the job of being a record keeper. They face the same range of challenges as the medical records department and must employ their ingenuity in trying to keep records up to date. How one maintains sanity during these experiences is an early test of the RTD's adaptive capacity. Some thoughts on surviving this task follow:

- Hiring or developing a responsible executive secretary who has a strong sense of joint ownership in the residency will greatly ease the burden of maintaining program records. The RTD must actively participate in the record keeping. This participation will usually require that the RTD have institutional authority to encourage wayward faculty members to provide required documentation. The executive secretary *can* provide a list of delinquent evaluations, missing residents' patient lists, and up-to-date management of correspondence; what the secretary *cannot* do is generate a departmental atmosphere for the importance of records. This is a task for the RTD and department chair. An ongoing negotiation for the RTD is to acquire adequate space and resources to maintain the residency program.

- Giving regular attention to records gives the RTD the advantage of access to a full range of materials for the semiannual reviews. It is in the RTD's best interest to have a system that functions effectively.

- Establishing sensible guidelines for releasing information on residents who completed their training in the distant past is highly recommended. Health maintenance organizations and hospital medical staff services ask for detailed training assessments to use for credentialing. Providing such assessments for a resident who graduated a decade or more ago can be a challenge. Older files prepared with different expectations are often inadequate. One can do very little about the content of old records. However, the RTD can improve his or her life and that of a successor if a final, summary assessment of each resident is made. This approach avoids the problem of commenting on a former resident's probation when there is no clear record about the specific issue or its resolution. Without further information, the RTD is left with the unpleasant task of simply noting that the resident had been subject to disciplinary action.

- Developing a computer-based record-keeping system will minimize the paper avalanche. E-mail simplifies communication regarding management issues. Some evaluations, such as the semiannual review, should be kept on paper unless there is a foolproof backup system; keeping residents' patient logs on computer disks permits them to be stored at an off-site location. Maintaining patient logs on a computer system allows a better assessment of the range of patient contacts and categories of treatment as well as a more rational review of what types of training experiences need to be improved.

OBSTACLES TO EVALUATION

Many obstacles may impede the giving and receiving of a comprehensive evaluation. Some of these obstacles are attitudinal. Rosenthal (1995) noted overarching themes such as "permanent uncertainty" and the "necessary fallibility" that accompany clinical work. The faculty may be hesitant to identify and assess errors because of the knowledge that everyone makes errors. However, failing to identify and discuss errors places the resident, faculty, and institution at risk.

Although these elements may play a role, there are other more common concerns: sometimes faculty members do not make evaluation a priority. Some faculty members feel uncomfortable giving negative reviews, fearing that the resident may decrease his or her evaluation of the attending physician's service. Some members of the faculty fear that any negative comment has a potential to result in litigation. If the faculty member has a well-founded and well-documented approach to a resident's deficiencies, the fear of litigation is excessive. Inviting the hospital attorney to a faculty meeting for a question-and-answer period may assist in establishing more comfortable guidelines for assessments.

Although the faculty may be well trained regarding collusion in psychotherapy, less attention may be paid to this factor when reviewing one's residents. Avoiding the identification of a deficiency is an easy shortcut. The RTD may face the serious challenge that a poorly performing resident may have no reliable, written assessments of deficiencies until a crisis occurs. In an age of due process, the RTD is placed in a difficult position of identifying appropriate steps. The RTD is forced to assume a greater degree of personal risk than an educational community would warrant; that is, the RTD is assuming an unnecessary level of corporate responsibility for the management of the resident's deficiencies.

Time limitations present further obstacles. In a busy clinical setting, evaluation may appear to be a peripheral and unwanted exercise. A thorough evaluation requires a commitment of time. Thoughtful consideration must be given to place the resident's performance in a context of relative experience (e.g., being in the first year of residency), difficulty of assignment (e.g., a hectic consultation-liaison service), and training contingencies (e.g., the death of a beloved teacher). With increased clinical demands on faculty, one is more likely to hear faculty members claim to be too busy to provide a thorough evaluation. Faculty members who are too busy must understand that unless they participate fully in the evaluation process, further assignment of residents to their service may not be possible.

Organizational obstacles exist as well. The RTD must ensure adequate department financial support for staffing the residency training office. In addition, a close working alliance with the department chair is critical to the RTD's success. The emerging new patterns in psychiatric practice make it a confusing time for clearly articulating a model (or models) of the excellent psychiatrist. The department chair and RTD can help define and model the expectations for competency in their particular program.

If the institution does not have a tradition of honest evaluation of faculty and students, the RTD's challenges will be greatly increased. A lack of accountability among the faculty will easily translate into lack of accountability for residents' behavior. Assessment committees often avoid this difficult connection. The wise RTD will try to maximize the evaluation of residents in the context of departmental and institutional traditions.

Finally, the lack of a consensus on the moral and professional issues that are part of the evaluation process presents a unique obstacle. Wagner (1993) highlighted this issue in his discussion of medical students' cheating and the controversy concerning what the outcomes should be. Although lack of consensus can provide the springboard for a more comprehensive understanding, the RTD and training committees have a more complex task in formulating and presenting a credible evaluation process. One potential way to address this problem would be establishment of a departmental committee for evaluation of misconduct that focuses on whether the administrative action is consistent with published professional codes (such as the ethics guidelines of the AMA and the APA) or mission statements of the home institution.

Some residents provoke polarized reactions from faculty, students, and staff. An important role for the RTD is to mediate between varied evaluations to arrive at an honest appraisal. It is one of the more stressful experiences for an RTD to sort through the starkly different assessments by various attending physicians. Simply identifying the polarity of evaluations may assist the promotions committee to recognize that a fundamental problem with the resident may exist. An important differential evaluation would include whether the resident has simply had varying performance throughout the academic year, has uncovered an ideological split in the department, or has a capacity to polarize affect. More of this discussion is presented below under "Due Process Procedures and the Problem Resident."

RESIDENTS WITH DISABILITIES

The RTD is expected to provide training to residents within a broad spectrum of ages and physical health statuses. For example, a beginning resident may have completed a successful career in another area of medicine and be starting a new career in her 50s. A resident may have a chronic illness that might require absence from the residency.

The Americans With Disabilities Act of 1990 (P.L. 101-336) provides that "no qualified individual with a disability shall, by reason of such disability, be excluded from participation in or be denied the benefits of the services, programs, or activities of a public entity, or be subjected to discrimination by any such entity" (42 USC §2132). The booklet *The Disabled Student in Medical School* is essential reading (Association of American Medical Colleges 1993). An abbreviated list of the summary recommendations follows:

- Schools should judge persons based on their ability to complete the educational program rather than on their status as disabled persons.
- "Reasonable accommodations" or "modifications" may be needed and, if so, must be provided.
- Each school must determine the "essential functions" or "essential eligibility" requirements of its program.

Amy Longo, R.N., J.D., an Omaha hospital attorney, provided an important insight when she noted that the essential functions remain constant, but the way they are accomplished may be flexible. The institution must demonstrate that reasonable attempts have been made to accommodate the resident's needs. The potential resident has the responsibility to describe what needs are to be addressed. For example, a potential resident may request a limited call schedule due to auditory impairments and vertigo. It is important to remember that special needs are usually a *prospective* matter of identifying an issue and working toward an accommodation; a resident's claiming of special needs *after* academic failure should be viewed with caution.

The hospital attorney can be helpful in reviewing recent case law on what types of conditions have been considered disabilities. The RTD should request legal assistance in providing a legitimate review of a potential resident's requests.

DUE PROCESS PROCEDURES AND THE PROBLEM RESIDENT

It is important for the RTD to be thoroughly familiar with both the departmental and institutional requirements for a resident who is facing academic sanctions. Not surprisingly, most litigation occurs when dismissal from medical school becomes necessary (Helms and Helms 1991). Discussions with the associate dean for graduate medical education at one's institution will be informative about recent institutional experiences.

A developing body of literature on disruptive physicians is available and is worth reviewing. Gawande's (2002) reflections on "when doctors go bad" from a surgical resident's point of view are informative. He concluded that colleagues "tend to be entirely unequipped to do anything about them."

The RTD is responsible for advising the resident in a timely fashion about the action being contemplated and avenues for redress, and for notifying the appropriate institutional committee. The RTD needs to be aware that departmental and institutional guidelines must be followed. The specific requirements may include identification of the problem, a recommended solution, and the organized supervision that will monitor compliance. Many issues overlap with the problem resident; however, most of these residents find themselves facing warnings or sanctions due to being disorganized or unskilled rather than because they have a major illness or personality disorder.

In many ways, the problem resident has been a continuing theme in the discussion of the arduous aspects of evaluation. It is helpful to consider the duration, intensity, and gravity of impairment. Since the early 1970s, the AMA has provided important readings on physician impairment. The assessment of resident vulnerability by Tokarz and colleagues (1979) is an impressive work; they noted that 9% of physician addicts die by suicide. The American Medical Association's 1995 report on substance abuse among physicians provided a critical review of the literature and offered an international perspective on drug and alcohol abuse and dependence; the claims of drug dependence 30- to 100-fold greater than the national average are not supported by data. However, several thought-provoking articles have come from the United Kingdom. Brooke et al. (1991) clearly identified a central problem in effectively evaluating the substance-impaired physician:

> Awkward moral overtones intrude; we are embarrassed to confront a colleague and uncertain what course to follow. The afflicted doctor continues in misery while colleagues turn away, having furtive meetings, but failing to get to grips with the problem. (p. 1011)

Firth-Cozens (1987) reported that residents experience a higher level of emotional distress than other occupational groups, with 50% reporting emotional distress, 28% having evidence of depression, and approximately 20% having frequent bouts of heavy drinking. Although RTDs need to be familiar with common illnesses among trainees, they should focus their concerns in terms of competency to do the work.

A helpful checklist for more common problems could include the following items:

- Is the resident frequently listed for late dictations and mismanaged discharges? New compliance reviews are more active in identifying residents who do not follow up on paperwork.
- Is the resident experiencing an unusual number of conflicts with students, fellow staff members, and faculty? An unwillingness among other residents to trade call with a particular resident is an important marker.
- Are there indications of gradually increasing absenteeism and declining job performance? The RTD needs to maintain an index of concern for drug and alcohol abuse. Unfortunately, it may require an extended period before residents or faculty members identify the issues, usually after the forgiveness of residents and faculty members has been exhausted.
- Is the resident withdrawing from usual activities and failing to participate in social events? The resident's decreased availability may come as a delayed report to the RTD from other residents or faculty members.
- Is the resident having repeated difficulty with diagnosing and treating patients while on call? The challenge of call reveals confidence, base of knowledge, and ability to manage a wide range of disorders. Problems on call should be reviewed quickly by the RTD.
- Are there indications of a resident's having problems with maintaining appropriate boundaries with patients? Defining the issues for the resident in a straightforward and useful manner is perhaps the single most complex challenge to the RTD.

The RTD should maintain an attitude of trying to find an appropriate intervention that could allow the resident to continue in the program. Drug and alcohol treatment, leave of absence, and anger management programs can all be considerations.

THE DANGEROUS RESIDENT

Although it is not a common issue, the RTD needs to be alert to the possibilities of severe misconduct. It is sobering that a physician who was later convicted of murdering patients had a brief experience as a psychiatric resident. He was hired despite having informed the program that he had been in jail (Stewart 1999). The program had not done an adequate background check regarding the imprisonment or prior dismissals from other residencies. The RTD needs to maintain an index of suspicion if there is a pattern of boundary violations (Gutheil and Gabbard 1993), aggressiveness, or deception. The RTD should have the opportunity to discuss these concerns with other senior RTDs, the department chair, or administrative officials at the institution. The state board of medical examiners has investigatory capability beyond the scope of the training program.

SUMMARY

For both newer and more seasoned RTDs, the new competency guidelines are creating exciting challenges in assessment. At its best, the development of departmental specifics to meet the six competencies can be a "norming" experience for the resident and faculty. There can be a clearer sense of what it means to accomplish the goals of the residency. The RTD needs the cooperation of the faculty to address the increased level of expectation in meeting the six educational goals. Maintaining a clear sense of the RTD's role as an educator provides for a more rewarding experience.

Keeping records that are accurate, timely, and comprehensive is an RTD's best policy. Then, if litigation occurs, the necessary documentation is available. The alert RTD will keep abreast of changes in the legal arenas of disability and common law for misconduct. A good relationship with the university or hospital attorney is helpful. Similarly, thorough familiarity with the due process requirements of one's institution will encourage a reasonable and uniform approach to dealing with misconduct. RTDs need to assist residents in developing their maximum level of skill. By including aspects of faculty evaluation and self-evaluation in the process, the experience of evaluation becomes more of a bilateral experience than a unilateral one. Such a format will best express regard for the colleague in training.

The institutional requirement for the RTD is to monitor whether or not the program itself is a persistent factor in a resident's diminished performance. Overwork can be one of the major stresses in residents' lives. If the evaluation process reveals that some services are "outliers" in the expectation of residents and results in a high rate of poor performance, the RTD needs to work with the service chief to modify the experience. The RTD is in a special position to recommend changes in the training that will allow a successful educational experience.

RESOURCES

Local resources include the director of graduate medical education, the hospital attorney, Alcoholics Anonymous (particularly if there are Caduceus Groups), the state board, and the state resources for impaired physicians. At a national level, there are supports through the AMA Wellness Office, the ACGME, and senior RTDs in AADPRT.

REFERENCES

Accreditation Council for Graduate Medical Education: Graduate Medical Education Directory 2004–2005. Chicago, IL, American Medical Association, 2004

American Medical Association: Substance Abuse Among Physicians. Report 1 of the Council on Scientific Affairs (Report A-95). Chicago, IL, American Medical Association, 1995. Available at: http://www.ama-assn.org/ama/pub/article/2036-2538.html. Accessed July 3, 2004.

American Medical Association: Cultural Competence Compendium. Chicago, IL, American Medical Association, 1999

Americans With Disabilities Act of 1990, Pub. L. No. 101-336

Angelo TA, Cross KP: Classroom Assessment Techniques: A Handbook for College Teachers, 2nd Edition. San Francisco, CA, Jossey-Bass, 1993

Association of American Medical Colleges: The Disabled Student in Medical School: An Overview of Legal Requirements. Washington, DC, Association of American Medical Colleges, 1993

Bloom BS: Taxonomy of Educational Objectives: The Classification of Educational Goals: Handbook I: Cognitive Domain. New York, Longmans, Green, 1956

Brooke D, Edwards G, Taylor C: Addiction as an occupational hazard: 144 doctors with drug and alcohol problems. Br J Addict 86:1011–1016, 1991

Donini-Lenhoff F: Cultural competence requirements in GME. ACGME Bulletin, October 1999, p 9

Firth-Cozens J: Emotional distress in junior house officers. Br Med J (Clin Res Ed) 295:533–536, 1987

Gawande A: Complications: A Surgeon's Notes on an Imperfect Science. New York, Metropolitan, 2002

Gutheil TG, Gabbard GO: The concept of boundaries in clinical practice: theoretical and risk-management dimensions. Am J Psychiatry 150:188–196, 1993

Health Insurance Portability and Accountability Act of 1996, Pub. L. No 104-191

Helms LB, Helms CM: Forty years of litigation involving students and their education, I: general educational issues. Acad Med 66:1–7, 1991

Leach DC: From qualified to competent: on the way and oriented toward fulfillment. ACGME Bulletin, August 2003, pp 1–3

Loschen EL: Using the objective structured clinical examination in a psychiatric residency. Acad Psychiatry 17:95–104, 1993

Luhrmann TM: Of Two Minds: The Growing Disorder in American Psychiatry. New York, Knopf, 2000

Plato: The Republic. New York, Heritage Press, 1944

Mullen LS, Rieder RO, Glick RA: The Psychodynamic Psychotherapy Competency Test. New York, Columbia University Medical Center, 2002

Reuben DB, Noble S: House officer responses to impaired physicians. JAMA 263:958–960, 1990

Rosenthal MM: The Incompetent Doctor: Behind Closed Doors. Philadelphia, PA, Open University Press, 1995

Stewart J: Blind Eye: How the Medical Establishment Let a Doctor Get Away With Murder. New York, Simon & Schuster, 1999

Swanson DB, Norman GR, Linn RL: Performance-based assessment: lessons from the health professions. Educational Researcher 24:5–11, 35, 1995

Teich C: Risk management in the psychiatric setting, in The Risk Manager's Desk Reference, 2nd Edition. Edited by Youngberg BJ. Gaithersburg, MD, Aspen, 1998, pp 328–341

Tokarz JP, Bremer W, Peters K: Beyond Survival: A Book Prepared by and for Resident Physicians to Meet the Challenge of the Impaired Physician and to Promote Well-Being Through Medical Education. Chicago, IL, American Medical Association, 1979

Wagner RF: Medical student academic misconduct: implications of recent case law and possible institutional responses. Acad Med 12:887–889, 1993

Yager J, Bienenfeld D: How competent are we to assess psychotherapeutic competence in psychiatric residents? Acad Psychiatry 27:174–181, 2003

Yager J, Kay J: Assessing psychotherapy competence in psychiatric residents: getting real. Harv Rev Psychiatry 11:1–4, 2003

APPENDIX 10–A

GENERAL PSYCHOTHERAPY COMPETENCIES

- Obtain and present information clearly and in detail.
- Establish initial rapport and maintain therapeutic alliance.
- Develop and articulate appropriate treatment goals.
- Use supervision.
- Formulate a case using each of the five specific psychotherapies.
- Articulate indications for each of the five forms of psychotherapy.
- Obtain informed consent.

From the Wright State University Department of Psychiatry Residency Training Program, David Bienenfeld, M.D., Director of Residency Training.

APPENDIX 10–B

SAMPLE PSYCHOTHERAPY COMPETENCY EVALUATION FORMS

From the Wright State University Department of Psychiatry Residency Training Program, David Bienenfeld, M.D., Director of Residency Training.

PSYCHODYNAMIC PSYCHOTHERAPY

Resident: _____   Date: _____

Supervisor: _____

Number of cases supporting this evaluation:_____

Number of cases observed directly or on tape:_____

1. Does not meet reasonable standards for the level of training
2. Sometimes adequate but often falls short of expectations
3. Usually meets expectations, but rarely exceeds them
4. Consistently meets and often exceeds expectations
5. Usually exceeds expectations, often by a substantial margin

Rate resident's ability to:	Superior				Poor	N/A
	5	4	3	2	1	0
1. Obtain and present information clearly and in detail.	❏	❏	❏	❏	❏	❏
2. Establish initial rapport and maintain a therapeutic alliance.	❏	❏	❏	❏	❏	❏
3. Develop and articulate appropriate treatment goals.	❏	❏	❏	❏	❏	❏
4. Use supervision.	❏	❏	❏	❏	❏	❏
5. Articulate indications for psychodynamic psychotherapy in each particular case.	❏	❏	❏	❏	❏	❏
6. Obtain informed consent.	❏	❏	❏	❏	❏	❏
7. Formulate a case using a genetic-dynamic framework.	❏	❏	❏	❏	❏	❏
8. Recognize and describe defenses and resistances.	❏	❏	❏	❏	❏	❏
9. Interpret and manage transference.	❏	❏	❏	❏	❏	❏
10. Use a variety of interventions, including facilitation and clarification.	❏	❏	❏	❏	❏	❏
11. Make plausible, clear, timely, tactful, evocative interpretations.	❏	❏	❏	❏	❏	❏
12. Pace frequency and length of sessions.	❏	❏	❏	❏	❏	❏
13. Manage termination.	❏	❏	❏	❏	❏	❏
14. Handle fees.	❏	❏	❏	❏	❏	❏
15. Establish, communicate, and maintain appropriate therapeutic boundaries and maintain confidentiality.	❏	❏	❏	❏	❏	❏
16. Recognize and manage countertransference.	❏	❏	❏	❏	❏	❏
17. Use literature as an aid to understanding treatment.	❏	❏	❏	❏	❏	❏

SUPPORTIVE THERAPY

Resident: _____ Date: _____

Supervisor: _____

Number of cases supporting this evaluation:_____

Number of cases observed directly or on tape:_____

  1 Does not meet reasonable standards for the level of training
  2 Sometimes adequate but often falls short of expectations
  3 Usually meets expectations, but rarely exceeds them
  4 Consistently meets and often exceeds expectations
  5 Usually exceeds expectations, often by a substantial margin

Rate resident's ability to:	Superior				Poor	N/A
	5	4	3	2	1	0
1. Obtain and present information clearly and in detail.	❏	❏	❏	❏	❏	❏
2. Establish initial rapport and maintain a therapeutic alliance.	❏	❏	❏	❏	❏	❏
3. Develop and articulate appropriate treatment goals.	❏	❏	❏	❏	❏	❏
4. Use supervision.	❏	❏	❏	❏	❏	❏
5. Articulate indications for supportive therapy in each particular case.	❏	❏	❏	❏	❏	❏
6. Obtain informed consent.	❏	❏	❏	❏	❏	❏
7. Formulate a case using a biopsychosocial approach.	❏	❏	❏	❏	❏	❏
8. Balance protection, containment, and limit-setting with promotion of autonomy and independence.	❏	❏	❏	❏	❏	❏
9. Assess and enhance strengths, coping skills, and ability to use environmental supports.	❏	❏	❏	❏	❏	❏
10. Assess and maximize healthy defenses.	❏	❏	❏	❏	❏	❏
11. Generate and convey empathy.	❏	❏	❏	❏	❏	❏
12. Understand and enhance treatment compliance.	❏	❏	❏	❏	❏	❏
13. Focus on the here and now and encourage patient activity.	❏	❏	❏	❏	❏	❏
14. Provide a role model for identification.	❏	❏	❏	❏	❏	❏
15. Use interventions including clarification, explanation, and confrontation appropriately.	❏	❏	❏	❏	❏	❏
16. Provide psychoeducation to patients and families.	❏	❏	❏	❏	❏	❏

COMBINED PSYCHOTHERAPY AND PSYCHOPHARMACOLOGY

Resident: _____ Date: _____

Supervisor: _____

Number of cases supporting this evaluation:_____

Number of cases observed directly or on tape:_____

    1   Does not meet reasonable standards for the level of training

    2   Sometimes adequate but often falls short of expectations

    3   Usually meets expectations, but rarely exceeds them

    4   Consistently meets and often exceeds expectations

    5   Usually exceeds expectations, often by a substantial margin

Rate resident's ability to:	Superior				Poor	N/A
	5	4	3	2	1	0
1. Obtain and present information clearly and in detail.	❏	❏	❏	❏	❏	❏
2. Establish initial rapport and maintain a therapeutic alliance.	❏	❏	❏	❏	❏	❏
3. Develop and articulate appropriate treatment goals.	❏	❏	❏	❏	❏	❏
4. Use supervision.	❏	❏	❏	❏	❏	❏
5. Articulate indications for combined therapy in each particular case.	❏	❏	❏	❏	❏	❏
6. Obtain informed consent.	❏	❏	❏	❏	❏	❏
7. Formulate a case using a biopsychosocial framework.	❏	❏	❏	❏	❏	❏
8. Describe effects of medication and psychodynamics upon each other.	❏	❏	❏	❏	❏	❏
9. Identify symbolic significance of medication (e.g., transitional object, placebo).	❏	❏	❏	❏	❏	❏
10. Manage medications based on psychosocial stressors.	❏	❏	❏	❏	❏	❏
11. Understand and manage dynamically and personality-based resistance to medication effects.	❏	❏	❏	❏	❏	❏
12. Address practical issues of treatment compliance (e.g., scheduling, cost, cognitive capacity).	❏	❏	❏	❏	❏	❏
13. Develop initiation and/or discontinuation plan for medication.	❏	❏	❏	❏	❏	❏
14. Understand and address abuse/misuse of medications.	❏	❏	❏	❏	❏	❏
15. Deal with medical and psychological consequences of adverse effects.	❏	❏	❏	❏	❏	❏

BRIEF PSYCHOTHERAPY

Resident: _____ Date: _____

Supervisor: _____

Number of cases supporting this evaluation:_____

Number of cases observed directly or on tape:_____

1 Does not meet reasonable standards for the level of training
2 Sometimes adequate but often falls short of expectations
3 Usually meets expectations, but rarely exceeds them
4 Consistently meets and often exceeds expectations
5 Usually exceeds expectations, often by a substantial margin

Rate resident's ability to:	Superior				Poor	N/A
	5	4	3	2	1	0
1. Obtain and present information clearly and in detail.	❏	❏	❏	❏	❏	❏
2. Establish initial rapport and maintain a therapeutic alliance.	❏	❏	❏	❏	❏	❏
3. Identify a therapeutic focus and develop reasonable goals by the end of session #2.	❏	❏	❏	❏	❏	❏
4. Use supervision.	❏	❏	❏	❏	❏	❏
5. Articulate indications and contraindications for brief psychotherapy in each particular case.	❏	❏	❏	❏	❏	❏
6. Obtain informed consent.	❏	❏	❏	❏	❏	❏
7. Formulate a case using a biopsychosocial framework.	❏	❏	❏	❏	❏	❏
8. Set and adhere to a termination date.	❏	❏	❏	❏	❏	❏
9. Develop appropriate disposition plans with the patient by the end of therapy.	❏	❏	❏	❏	❏	❏
10. Demonstrate an appropriate level of therapist activity within the therapy.	❏	❏	❏	❏	❏	❏
11. Employ one of the established brief therapy models.	❏	❏	❏	❏	❏	❏

COGNITIVE THERAPY

Resident: _____　　Date: _____

Supervisor: _____

Number of cases supporting this evaluation:_____

Number of cases observed directly or on tape:_____

1　Does not meet reasonable standards for the level of training
2　Sometimes adequate but often falls short of expectations
3　Usually meets expectations, but rarely exceeds them
4　Consistently meets and often exceeds expectations
5　Usually exceeds expectations, often by a substantial margin

Rate resident's ability to:	Superior				Poor	N/A
	5	4	3	2	1	0
1. Obtain and present information clearly and in detail.	❑	❑	❑	❑	❑	❑
2. Establish initial rapport and maintain a therapeutic alliance.	❑	❑	❑	❑	❑	❑
3. Develop and articulate appropriate treatment goals.	❑	❑	❑	❑	❑	❑
4. Use supervision.	❑	❑	❑	❑	❑	❑
5. Articulate indications for cognitive therapy in each particular case.	❑	❑	❑	❑	❑	❑
6. Obtain informed consent.	❑	❑	❑	❑	❑	❑
7. Formulate a case using a case conceptualization diagram.	❑	❑	❑	❑	❑	❑
8. Use collaboration during therapy.	❑	❑	❑	❑	❑	❑
9. Demonstrate an appropriate level of therapist activity.	❑	❑	❑	❑	❑	❑
10. Identify and elicit automatic thoughts.	❑	❑	❑	❑	❑	❑
11. Identify and elicit core beliefs.	❑	❑	❑	❑	❑	❑
12. Use guided discovery as a tool.	❑	❑	❑	❑	❑	❑
13. Use the structured session model, including:						
a. mood check	❑	❑	❑	❑	❑	❑
b. bridging from prior session	❑	❑	❑	❑	❑	❑
c. agenda setting	❑	❑	❑	❑	❑	❑
d. review of homework	❑	❑	❑	❑	❑	❑
e. capsule summaries	❑	❑	❑	❑	❑	❑
f. feedback	❑	❑	❑	❑	❑	❑
14. Use dysfunctional-thought records.	❑	❑	❑	❑	❑	❑
15. Use activity scheduling.	❑	❑	❑	❑	❑	❑
16. Use behavioral techniques.	❑	❑	❑	❑	❑	❑
17. Devise appropriate homework assignments.	❑	❑	❑	❑	❑	❑

(BACK OF EACH EVALUATION)

Summary/narrative comments (REQUIRED). Please include particular strengths and areas for improvement. Please make note of quality and timeliness of documentation, ability to conduct "split therapy," where resident is managing either psychotherapy or pharmacological management while someone else is managing the other, and ability to manage financial considerations (e.g., setting and collecting fees).

_____   _____
Supervisor   Resident

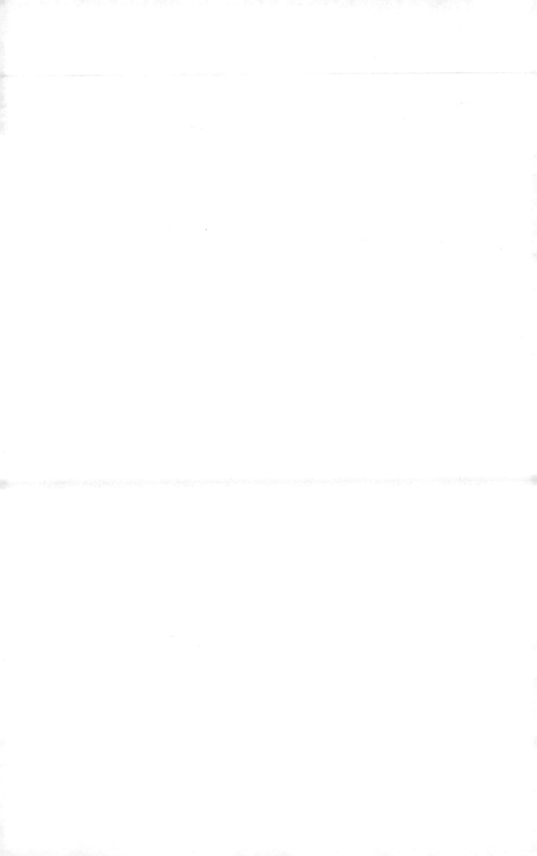

CHAPTER 11

SPECIAL PROBLEMS AND CHALLENGES IN THE RESIDENCY PROGRAM

Paul C. Mohl, M.D.

Most residency training directors (RTDs) seek their jobs out of an interest in education, supporting residents, and developing curricula. However, their success will be judged primarily by how they perform at two other functions: recruitment and handling of problems and problem residents. This chapter addresses the latter of these two functions. Effective handling of special problems will be almost invisible to both residents and faculty, garnering little praise. Ineffective handling will be noticed by all, provoke intense criticism, erode morale among both faculty and residents, and compromise efforts in other areas.

In considering various special problems it is useful to keep in mind the numerous roles of the RTD: personnel officer, mediator, evaluator, icon and caricature, role model, parent (as seen by the faculty), and curriculum developer. Difficulties encountered handling the problems enumerated in this chapter can be understood as arising from inherent conflicts in these roles. Most problems require some form of personnel officer management, something very few RTDs are prepared for. Yet the personnel officer decisions (enforcing institutional or departmental procedures, protecting the program from legal liability) must be modulated by the impact on the training of the particular resident involved and on the curriculum as a whole.

TABLE 11–1.   Roles of the residency training director

Systems engineer
Expert in psychiatric education
Personnel officer
Public relations agent
Caricature and icon
Parent surrogate
Mediator
Role model
Evaluator
Curriculum developer

Although the service impact of a particular decision is not the immediate concern of the RTD, a significant change in the service load must be seen as affecting the training of other residents and thus the clinical curriculum (Table 11–1).

Another important dimension is the true source and nature of the RTD's power and authority to solve problems. Ultimately, the RTD has only one concrete weapon vis-à-vis the faculty: the power to assign or not assign residents to a particular site. This is a truly blunt instrument, one that will be wielded rarely if at all. All faculty members have been through residency—often having rather different experiences from one another—and have opinions about what a program should look like (usually with their particular site or area of interest being more prominent than it currently is). To them the RTD is in some ways just another faculty colleague; in others, an authority with the power to dole out a highly valued resource.

Among the residents the RTD's power emerges from being seen as the person who gave them a place. The RTD is a transference object: the good parent, the principal, the withholder of support in conflicts with faculty, the enforcer, the rescuer, and so forth.

In fact, the RTD's real authority is moral and is rooted in knowledge, especially knowledge about the field of psychiatric *education:* that is, where the field is moving, what the new accreditation requirements are, what teaching goes on at site A versus site B, how the didactics are structured, what the most recent relevant legal rulings about sick or unprofessional residents are, how the overall structure of the program accomplishes various educational objectives, and so forth. None of the special problems enumerated in this chapter can be solved effectively by an RTD who has lost his or her moral authority or who is unable to articulate clear commitment to an educational vision and knowledge of the vast range of opinion and policy regarding residencies. Regular demonstration to the faculty that the RTD possesses extensive information that they do not have, and to the residents of the RTD's commitment to their education, maintains the necessary moral authority to solve problems.

In general, there are two basic models for training directors: the *charismatic* type and the *honest broker* type. Charismatic types take advantage of all the projections coming their way to make decisions and make them stick. Honest broker types see themselves as *systems engineers*, whose job is to use their knowledge of psychiatric education and their moral authority to make a program composed of complex pieces function smoothly and effectively to train and educate the residents optimally. Honest brokers are more concerned with how fair the system is—and is *perceived* to be—than with how good they are seen to be.

My opinion is that the honest broker type is far superior to the charismatic type, and the solutions to problems suggested in this chapter reflect that belief. Faculty members and residents will accept many disappointments if they believe that the system of decision making is fair and has considered their points of view. The key word here is *believe*. It is important that the system not only be fair, but that it *be perceived as fair*. Much of what I advocate relates to this important distinction. This means constant ongoing consultation and keeping important people informed well in advance as things develop. Often the direction of a decision may be obvious, but the process of informing people and soliciting their input is crucial to the *perception* of fairness.

> *Residents and faculty members, if they believe themselves to be part of a fair and honest system knowledgeably committed to legitimate educational goals, will work hard to solve problems that arise. This means that RTDs must know not just what to do, but whether to do anything, when to do it, when not to step in (to avoid possibly interfering with others' attempts to solve a problem), and how to appear to be doing something when in fact they are temporizing.*

In the discussion of specific problems to follow, I may not always refer back to these principles, but they are the basis for the solutions suggested.

ILLNESS OR INJURY IN A RESIDENT

Many of the problems described in this chapter fall under the general category of a resident's not being available to a clinical service that was expecting the resident and depending on the presence of that resident to assist in the care of patients. Not only does this threatened absence tap into the faculty's perception that they "need" the resident and cannot function without him or her, it raises the specter, if the site functions effectively without a resident for a period of time, that the RTD might conclude that the site can do without a resident during future shortages. Furthermore, sites and faculty are often in a complicated competitive position with each other about which one is the better rotation. All of this conspires to create a "give us our body" message from the faculty. They will watch the RTD's response carefully to try to gauge to what extent the RTD understands the needs of the site, how the role of the service is perceived, and how valued the faculty's educational efforts are.

Residents are exquisitely sensitive to schedule changes. Their fundamental issue in almost any conflict is the feeling of not being in control of their lives. Nothing reinforces this feeling more than an abrupt, unexpected shifting of the schedule, even if only one resident is involved only for a brief time. At the same time, the other residents assigned to the same service as the ill or injured resident fear that they will have to carry an extra service load. This subgroup of residents becomes a group pressuring to change the schedule and a source of anger, ambivalence, and guilt among the rest of their class. Compounding this sentiment is the general reaction among the residents of wondering "Could this happen to me?" How such a situation is handled becomes a test case in the residents' eyes for the compassion with which they will be dealt should something untoward occur to them, how they are truly viewed by the faculty, and whose side the RTD is on.

Thus, even a routine event of life raises fundamental questions in the minds of both faculty members and residents. The RTD must keep all this in mind.

If the resident's illness occurs in connection with the residency (e.g., as a result of a violent act by a patient), then the issues are compounded further. The faculty experience some sense of guilt, and the residents see before them the lifelong risks of their chosen profession and the human limitations of the faculty to provide for their security, welfare, and well-being. In the past 10–20 years, medical education has become increasingly paternalistic in its stance toward students; my perception is that as a result of this stance medical school graduates arrive at their internships still seeing themselves as students, dependent on the faculty. They are still in the very early stages of development of a fully autonomous, professional identity. They look to the faculty as protectors, as still being the ultimately responsible physicians, and many faculty members accept that role.

A number of principles should guide the handling of these situations. First, as an RTD I want the staff at every site to believe that it is the best, most important site in the program. Any site director who does not believe this is willingly accepting a second-rate position. Similarly, I also want the residents to have difficulty deciding which service is the most educational. Second, I want the residents to feel and behave, both individually and as a group, like professionals. I want them to feel professional ownership of the sites and to feel responsible for assisting sites, fellow residents, and faculty members who are faced with some difficulty. If these values are in place, the RTD has much more latitude to respond to any problem. Instilling these values requires the systems engineer role to be implemented in a variety of verbal and nonverbal ways over a period of time.

If there is a reasonable sense of the two values listed in the preceding paragraph, *the first thing the RTD should do is…nothing.* This will give everyone a chance to see the problem, digest it, think about it, and conduct dialogue on-site about it. In my experience, the residents and faculty will solve it 90% of the time. Either the faculty will say, "We can survive for this brief time with one less resident" or the residents will say, "We need to help out." Commonly, both residents and faculty will put pressure on the RTD to make the decision quickly, to avoid processing the complicated feelings that are stimulated. The RTD should say something like "Why don't we see how things go for a couple of days first?" or "Get together with the faculty up there and see what you come up with."

If it becomes clear after a few days that the problem is not moving toward a solution, the RTD's first action should be to set up meetings with everyone involved. These days, such meetings often consist of group e-mail strings. A secondary issue is being able to determine when the e-mail string needs to be replaced by more personal contact, by phone or in person. When a problem such as this cannot be solved on-site between the residents and faculty, there is often something else going on. Through such situations I have discovered important issues at sites—such as changes in the service demands, structure, personnel interactions, and so on—of which I was unaware. Once these issues are clarified and addressed, the residents and faculty will often proceed to solve the issue.

If it becomes clear—either through the failure of residents and faculty to find a site-based solution or through consensus of both sides—that a schedule change is necessary, the implementation must be handled carefully. Within a year or two after I became an RTD, I identified in my own mind which sites could not tolerate the loss of a resident without serious damage to their educational programs, and which sites were much less resident dependent, able to function effectively in a shortage situation. Such assessments are open knowledge, with the rationale being clearly explained to all attending physicians. This openness creates a sense of security among the sites and prevents a sense of surprise when a resident has to be pulled. At times I have met with an entire resident class, explained why I thought a schedule change was necessary, and asked for volunteers. Other times I have called two or three residents and asked them to make the change. I always select the resident whose education will be most enhanced (or least damaged) by the change, and I always apologize for asking and appeal to the resident's sense of helping out both his or her fellow residents and the faculty (I have yet to be turned down). When informing a service director that a resident will be pulled, I express appreciation for the service director's contribution to the overall functioning and quality maintenance of the program, and I suggest to the faculty members who will get the resident that they call to express their gratitude to the site that is losing the resident.

The principle is to continually reinforce to all parties that we are in the situation together, trying to maintain the best possible educational program in an unfortunate circumstance. It is "their" program, not mine, and we are all trying to keep it going as best we can.

In many programs it is the PGY-2 class where the most pressure is experienced if a resident becomes unavailable. In our program, the psychiatric emergency service (PES) is extremely resident dependent. Some programs have, at all times, a designated resident on a particular rotation who is to cover for any other resident who misses more than a day or two for any reason. Recently, our PGY-2 class, on its own, brought a plan to me for what to do if the PES needed coverage. We see here an RTD-generated plan in the former case and a resident-generated plan in the latter. The former situation creates certainty and a sense of support from the administration among the residents. The latter represents the class working together as professionals to anticipate and solve a problem.

The worst situation of this sort that I have encountered was when a patient struck a resident who was pregnant, precipitating premature labor in the resident and necessitating bed rest for 4 months. Because I had established the modus operandi described in the preceding paragraphs, the site director called me to let me know what had happened and then said, "Let us handle this." Another inpatient unit director at the same hospital volunteered to rotate his residents into the empty slot, wisely asking his residents to help out first, then assigning them the task of setting up the schedule. The faculty at the site organized a resident/faculty review committee that met at the injured resident's home for a "psychological postmortem" to assist the resident in processing her experience and to review how preventable the incident was. They tried but failed to get the patient, when he improved, to send a note to the resident.

PSYCHIATRIC ILLNESS, SUICIDE ATTEMPT, OR SUICIDE COMPLETION IN A RESIDENT

The most extreme and disturbing variation on the issue of illness in a resident is when a resident attempts or completes suicide. I am not aware of any data on the topic, but because psychiatrists are generally more sympathetic toward applicants who have histories of psychiatric illness, the psychiatric residency may have an increased risk for such occurrences. In such an event, the loss of function is overwhelmed by everyone's emotional reaction to the nature of the event. Perhaps most prominent is guilt, which may be dealt with by projection of responsibility onto the RTD ("Why didn't she/he see it coming and prevent it?"). But the fundamental issue is that although psychiatrists have no doctor–patient relationship with residents, suicide prevention is such a fundamental part of their professional roles and identities that when a colleague or trainee makes or completes an attempt, they are hit hard by it and do much soul-searching.

I have not had a resident attempt or complete suicide during my tenure as an RTD, nor even during my entire career. I have heard of such events and have known students who entered psychiatry in another program and eventually committed suicide. Therefore, I cannot speak from my own experience. But I would imagine that this kind of event calls for vigorous, collective intervention. Multiple meetings with residents individually and in groups, between faculty members and residents, and with faculty members individually and in groups are all indicated. This is a traumatic loss for all, in which help is needed to sort through the complicated professional roles, identity issues, responsibility issues, guilt, fear, and more. Perhaps even a retreat with facilitation by a suicidologist or a series of educational events about suicide risk in the profession and suicide prevention as friends and coworkers might be indicated. Above all, efforts to promote a shared grieving and processing must be prominent. The community of residents and faculty must be helped to come together in dealing with the event, and not to split apart.

When residents become psychiatrically ill, both faculty members and residents tend to be very sympathetic and solicitous, making the issues discussed above under "Dealing With Illness or Injury in a Resident" often easier to work through. More complicated issues arise when a resident has a substance abuse problem. In some ways, the now-long history and application of impaired physicians committees facilitates the making and implementing of decisions. However, the special confidentiality provisions, some of which are enacted in various state laws or regulations, create an aura of secrecy that goes against much of what I have advocated. Because the resident becomes administratively under the purview of the impaired physicians committee, I have found it easy to simply say that the committee is currently responsible for decisions related to the resident's return to clinical responsibility. Both faculty and residents understand what this means and have always responded very professionally. We are fortunate that in our system the impaired physicians committee defines its purview to include any impairment in clinical functioning due to any medical condition. This has enabled me to activate it rather than administrative disciplinary actions in rare situations when the resident is impaired psychiatrically but is resistant to entering treatment.

PREGNANCY IN RESIDENTS

Of all the special situations in residency training, the issue of pregnant residents has probably received the most attention in the literature. Until around 1980, when there was a dramatic increase in enrollment of women in medical schools (with a substantial proportion choosing psychiatry), a pregnant resident was a relatively rare occurrence. Now it is routine. Most residency programs consist of more than 40% women, and it is a virtual certainty that sometime during any 1- to 2-year period, at least one of these women residents will become pregnant.

The issues here are the same as those involved in illness and injury, with two important complicating factors. First, pregnancy is viewed by many residents and faculty members as a resident's choice. Second, feelings arise about special treatment that is made available to some residents but not to all. In terms of the shortage resulting from the pregnancy leave, compared with injury and illness, one has lead time in preparing for the absence. This is a mixed blessing. On the one hand, there is plenty of time to prepare; on the other, there is plenty of time for individuals to become very upset about the situation. In addition, the absence of the sense of crisis that accompanies an unexpected injury or illness reduces the shared need to find a solution.

The residents' reaction to the news that one of their peers is pregnant is usually mixed. There is delight and excitement, and there is resentment and envy. Interestingly, the split is rarely along gender lines. Men tend to split, with some being very supportive, even overly solicitous, of the pregnant resident. Other men can be very resentful, feeling as if the resident is "getting away with something" and taking advantage of her position to dump work on the rest of the resident group. Some women, especially those who are married, who have children, or who may be contemplating pregnancy, are also very supportive, even militantly so, demanding special privileges and consideration. Ironically, the most venomously resentful residents I have encountered are other women, commonly unmarried, who see any special considerations as undermining of their roles and position among their peers. Whereas men recognize the unique biological function of childbearing—although they may resent the timing—some single women may see marriage and motherhood as a choice or happenstance that excludes them.

The faculty is usually, these days, very supportive of pregnant residents and are concerned simply with site coverage. However, there are still a few old-guard types (which can include some senior women faculty members who delayed their childbearing until after residency), who deeply resent the resident's choice to become pregnant. This small but vocal group can effectively stir up everyone, resulting in a totally unnecessary uproar. I have had faculty members literally say to me, "Why did you let this happen?"—leaving me with the feeling that I should have been standing at the exits each night passing out birth control pills.

The stance of the pregnant resident herself becomes crucial in this situation. Some take an "I'm tough!" stance, planning to work full-time, taking their full measure of call right up to the moment of delivery, and determined to return to work 2 weeks afterward. Others engage in special pleading, demanding relief from call as soon as they learn they are pregnant, requesting easier rotations, resenting that they may have to make up some educational time if they take 6 months off before returning, and generally acting entitled. One year I had two pregnant residents in the same class, which was already slightly smaller than most classes, who were going to deliver at approximately the same time. One was at the tougher end of the continuum, negotiating with her classmates to take extra call during her second trimester so that she could take less during the third, if necessary. The other acted much more entitled and spoke openly about the special status of pregnant women. The resident group practically fell over themselves helping out the first resident while being very resistant and resentful toward the second.

The single most important aspect of keeping this now-routine part of residency training from becoming a special problem is to have a written policy in place. The RTD should ensure that the policy is well known and well disseminated and should promote residents' and faculty members' acceptance of the policy as fair and humane. Such a policy is best proposed by a committee of residents and faculty, representing all subgroups and factions. In my opinion the committee is best chaired by a woman. A way of keeping the committee from getting bogged down by the emotional reactions raised by this issue is to charge it with harmonizing program policy with affiliated institutions' policies, with reviewing the program's obligations under the Family and Medical Leave Act of 1993 (P.L. 103-3), and with distinguishing between the program's educational obligations and those resulting from its role as employer of the residents. Other important issues that such a committee must wrestle with are whether residents may use sick leave for their time off, how much unpaid leave can be taken without requiring an extension of the resident's time in the program, whether new adoptive mothers should be treated any differently from biological mothers, and at what point the resident is obligated to inform the training director of her pregnancy. Once the committee comes up with a policy, it should be widely circulated, reviewed, and voted on by the residency training committee (RTC). It should then be included in every new resident's orientation packet.

The presence of this policy will reduce conflict over the issue. In our program, we require notification of the RTD at least 6 months before the expected delivery date. This maximizes the opportunity to negotiate any necessary schedule changes. In fact, it will usually enable the schedule for the year to be made out with the anticipated absence in mind. In addition, I have found it very helpful to counsel pregnant residents at the time they notify me of their pregnancy. This counseling includes three major elements: informing residents of what they can do to maximize the support available to them from both peers and faculty members, explaining anticipated patient responses, and preparing them for how difficult it will be to return to work. Professionally oriented women, in my opinion, seem to be particularly unprepared for the emotional changes that occur within them in the presence of their first infant. For that reason, I discourage them from making any final commitment to how long they plan to be out until late in their middle trimester.

If handled well, the issue of pregnant residents can be a problem the entire department takes great pride and pleasure in. In our program, we post announcements of the birth throughout the department, announce it at various meetings, and send flowers.

PATERNITY LEAVE

The issue of paternity leave is similar to that of maternity leave, with the additional component that it has far less acceptance in society. Therefore, the reactions of both residents and faculty tend to be much more along the lines of "Why does he need it?" and "He's getting away with something."

The solution is essentially the same as for maternity leave: have a written policy. It is probably best to have the same committee that proposes a policy on maternity leave propose one for expectant fathers as well. This ensures a coherent proposal that, more than anything else, defines the program's attitude toward gender issues. In addition, it is amazing how many of the "old boys" who resist the importance of maternity leave—no matter how much they believe in the crucial role of early attachment—will mellow in their opposition when confronted with a parallel benefit for male residents.

The parental leave policy of the Department of Psychiatry at the University of Texas Southwestern Medical Center is presented in Appendix 11–A.

RESIDENTS WHO CHOOSE TO LEAVE THE PROGRAM

Apart from the scheduling difficulties posed by the situation when a resident chooses to leave the program, the primary problem—regardless of the reason—is morale among both faculty and residents. Reasons for leaving vary: a decision to change specialties or transfer to another psychiatry program, financial issues, spouse or significant other being employed elsewhere, other personal reasons (e.g., to seek treatment for substance abuse), or being one step ahead of dismissal. The reasons for the resident's decision may be well known to fellow residents, known only to a few, known only to the RTD and a few trusted faculty members, or known only to the resident. A reason may be promulgated that is not the full rationale, and this may or may not be obvious to the other residents and the faculty. The RTD may know why the resident is leaving but not feel at liberty to convey it, which can cause tension.

Regardless of the specifics, the reaction of both the residents and faculty is most likely to be "Is there something wrong with us?" These days, this question can include "What's wrong with our field?" If the reason for the departure needs to be kept confidential, this stirs fantasies about what may have been going on and represents a challenge to the trust between the RTD and both residents and faculty. A further complication is that every so often a class experiences far more than its fair share of comings and goings. Such a class often becomes a wounded group that fails to develop class cohesion or loses what cohesion it did have. It is hard enough on residents that they know that as with college and medical school, they are in a situation that will entail a parting in 4 years, so unexpected and multiple partings can become anticipatory traumas.

When a resident informs the RTD that he or she will be leaving and the reasons for it, an important part of the discussion becomes who knows, what they know, and what the resident's preferences are about what may be said about the decision. Unless it is highly predictable that the leave-taking will have a traumatic effect, it is usually best to do nothing—to leave the informing of the residents and faculty to the resident. Chief residents and assistant RTDs should be informed and consulted with about the anticipated impact of the news. The rationale behind doing nothing is the old administrative principle: *Don't just do something, stand there!* This principle embodies the notion that when one has competent, professional, well-intended people, stepping in is likely to be intrusive and destructive to their mature efforts to cope with the problem. Taking unusual action may inadvertently convey that the problem is more serious than it really is. Exceptions to this principle may arise when there have been an unusual number of leave-takings in a short time, when the leaving resident holds a particularly important role in the program (e.g., is perceived as a "star" or class leader), or when the resident's reason for leaving involves a problem that the RTD has been attempting to address but has been frustrated about.

In small programs, the RTD will often meet regularly with all of the residents and will see most of the faculty informally. In larger programs, the RTD should meet regularly with the chiefs and with each class's elected representatives. These meetings will be opportunities to provide information and to learn whether the news of the leave-taking is evoking a strong enough response to call for active intervention. Such intervention with the residents is usually in the form of a meeting with the entire class, including free-form discussion of the impending loss. Commonly, other issues are triggered by the news of the departing resident, issues that the RTD may be unaware of or that can be worked through in an open discussion by the class and the RTD. It is common for fantasies to fly among the residents; therefore, open meetings, with information freely shared (or clear, meaningful reasons for confidentiality being expressed), are extremely useful in detoxifying these imaginings. Our program, unlike some, does not have regular annual retreats, but we have used retreats for special situations. On one occasion we had almost 50% turnover in a class. A number of conflicts emerged on different sites the following year. We supported a retreat at which the class, interestingly, requested a particular clinical faculty member, a former chief resident who started out their orientation day as interns, to be the facilitator. Another class had a member diagnosed with terminal cancer. A retreat with one of our consultation-liaison faculty who specializes in thanatology was arranged.

If the faculty is disturbed by news of a departing resident, they usually require no specific intervention, as they are much less reticent about calling up, asking what is going on, expressing their worst fears, and accepting the explanations offered.

DISMISSAL OF A RESIDENT

The dismissal of a resident from the program is an extension of the situation of voluntary departure of a resident and is complicated by the residents' feelings about one of their own being fired. Their feelings will be mixed. There is always an element of "There but for the grace of God go I," but most residents know who the weaker members of the class are and have no wish to have incompetent psychiatrists counted among their colleagues. This side of the ambivalence is often expressed as relief or anger that the faculty waited too long to act! A common compromise formation may involve questioning the process, though not necessarily the outcome. Was the dismissed resident dealt with fairly? Given fair warning? Offered fair opportunity to remediate deficiencies? And were the resident's rights respected in the process?

The faculty can be at odds over a dismissal as well. Many faculty members regard themselves as experts on teaching and evaluating residents. They are often unaware of the evaluations on other services or, if they are aware, may have their own opinions about the prejudices or blind spots of their colleagues. Thus, they may be all over the map, from "I told you so; what took you so long?" to "This was a good resident who has been treated completely unfairly."

This is one of those situations in which the process must not only be fair but also be seen to be fair. A clear procedure for handling deficient residents is crucial. An element of this procedure must be the recognition that at some point, as a problem resident is dealt with, the RTD and, one by one, the faculty members shift from an education-based "let's help out this resident" view to an employer-based "let's put pressure on this resident to improve or else" stance. The procedure begins with a clear, well-written due process document. In our program, we asked our forensic psychiatrist to write the first draft. This was then circulated to all faculty and residents for comment, was rewritten, and was then submitted to the RTC for approval. That approval was contingent on review by the university attorney, who recommended substantial revision. The RTC then re-reviewed and reapproved the procedure. Every incoming resident receives a copy of this due process document, and all faculty members and residents who are involved in a potential administrative action are offered copies to refresh their memories (Appendix 11–B).

A good due process policy is only the beginning. Every program must have a committee that implements the due process, reviews all residents' evaluations, and recommends action to the RTD. The composition and procedures of the evaluation committee must be thought through carefully.

Faculty members who are perceived to take evaluation seriously and hold high standards yet are humane, discreet, and of high integrity should be appointed. Every affiliated institution should have some representation, lest a hospital or agency feel that its observations and opinions may not be taken as seriously as are those of others. The department chair should probably not be on the committee because almost every due process will have the chair as the final level of appeal, and his or her impartiality needs to be protected. One can debate whether there should be resident representatives on the committee. Many faculty members argue that evaluation is a pure faculty function. On the other hand, without some participation by residents, the evaluation committee becomes a "black box" in the eyes of the residents and therefore becomes the object of projections. I have found it most effective to have the chief resident sit on and be a full participant in this committee. Input from a resident's perspective is often very useful, especially because the residents often know of a peer's deficiency even more clearly than the faculty. Furthermore, the chief will be in a position to say, "I was there and the resident was given a fair review/hearing."

Once the decision to dismiss a resident has been made, the RTD is in a bind. Open information would be the most effective method of alleviating residents' anxiety and enlisting faculty support, yet ethical and legal considerations require restraint and protection of the dismissed resident's privacy. There is often the potential for legal challenges that may not be apparent for months. I was once cited by the Equal Employment Opportunity Commission for being prejudiced against older East Indians a year after a resident's dismissal! Other dismissed residents have sued me in state and federal district courts. On another occasion, a resident who had been voted by the education committee to be dismissed mounted—with the encouragement, collaboration, and support of a faculty member on that committee—a major legal challenge that accused me of harassment and that led to a variety of steps being taken by our university minority affairs office and legal office to deal with the situation. As one can imagine, rumors flew; I and the rest of the committee were unhappy; but none of us were at liberty to defend ourselves against the insinuations and accusations of the resident and her supporting faculty member. In the end we were comfortable that we had done our best, whereas turning things over to other branches of the university allowed us to proceed with the business of educating the other 59 residents in the program.

Although the residents will often pressure the RTD for details, they are usually understanding of the need for judicious protection of this sort of information. This is one of those situations where one must simply take the heat if the dismissed resident chooses to slander the RTD and the department. In the long run, the residents will appreciate perspicacity, even if they get taken in by the whisperings at first. Simply saying "How much would you want me to say about you, were you in a similar position?" usually gets the point across. In the situation described in the preceding paragraph, the residents, while conflicted, were far more impressed by the professionalism demonstrated by the education committee members' silence than by the open accusations of the resident and her faculty supporter. Careful and detailed communication and heeding the advice of one's department chair and hospital or university attorney are paramount. I am aware of training directors who have lost their jobs over just such situations when the chair or university administrators were insufficiently educated about the circumstances.

There are times when *an RTD's job is to take the heat*, and this is one of them. The heat can be shared, however. The chair and the associate dean for graduate medical education should collaborate in reviewing the due process and should be kept fully informed, especially if there is any hint that legal action might result from the dismissal.

RESIDENTS WHO HAVE CHRONIC ILLNESSES OR DISABILITIES (WITH SPECIAL NOTE OF HIV ISSUES)

Perhaps it is naiveté, or it may be a product of my role as a psychiatric consultant to an acquired immunodeficiency syndrome (AIDS) clinic, but human immunodeficiency virus (HIV) seems to be much less of an issue among residents than it once was. There is no longer the terror and prejudice about HIV-positive individuals that existed 10 years ago. At that time, residents and faculty had enormous countertransference issues with patients. At this point, I rarely find faculty or residents stirred up by having to care for AIDS patients. If they are, one handles it no differently from the entire range of countertransference problems that arise daily in residency: there must be adequate didactics, appropriate supervision, and available psychotherapy.

A situation in which everyone gets distressed is when a resident or faculty member has a clinical encounter in which he or she may have been exposed to HIV (usually a needle stick). Panic runs wild among the residents, and the faculty often feel guilty. The RTD is aided in this situation by the fact that virtually every hospital now has standard procedures for responding to such situations. The more one approaches the event in a professional manner—emphasizing the known risks; the known preventive measures (acknowledging that no prevention is foolproof); and the well-established procedures for follow-up, testing, and counseling—the more settled everyone will become. A meeting with the residents emphasizing the "known risk" aspect of the event may be useful. I try to encourage the residents, as part of their professional growth, to take pride in the aspects of their chosen profession that are special by virtue of the risks and responsibilities undertaken in the cause of caretaking.

The final—and potentially the most controversial—issue that can arise is whether to consider a candidate for the program who is HIV positive, and how to react if it becomes known that a resident carries the infection. The RTD should be aware of existing legal ramifications. Specifically, the Americans With Disabilities Act of 1990 (P.L. 101-336) probably precludes any attempts to exclude HIV-positive residents from the program. But that is unlikely to mollify feelings. Residents are likely to be primarily supportive yet also resentful of any special needs an infected resident may have (e.g., easy fatigability that may influence the ability to take call). Faculty members may also be supportive but even more resentful than the residents. Part of the pleasure of teaching residents is the fantasy of reproducing oneself and seeing residents identify with you. Any resident who is clearly "different" challenges this gratification. The faculty may present the issue in terms of rationalizations about the resident's ability to do the work, to be a full team member, to practice enough to warrant the time and effort invested. On the other hand, some faculty members may see such a resident as an asset, bringing a unique and creative perspective to the field and to the other residents.

I see the issue of the HIV-positive resident as a special case like any resident with a disability. In our program we have considered applicants who had multiple sclerosis, muscular dystrophy, chronic back problems, myocardial infarction, chronic heavy metal poisoning, sequelae of polio, psychiatric disorders, debilitating rheumatoid arthritis, and Friedreich's ataxia. But this consideration can only occur after the faculty has engaged in an ongoing dialogue about the program's values. *The faculty must consider who they are, their vision of the field, and the balance between humanistic values and standards of excellence* in working with residents. Only then can applicants with disabilities be considered solely on their ability to become an effective psychiatrist and to perform the functions of a resident. Once the faculty has made these decisions, these values will be implicitly conveyed to the residents as part of their socialization into the program. The values of the program need not even be articulated by the RTD, for they will permeate the system. But *the RTD must see the need for and initiate the faculty dialogue*. The dialogue is often not explicit but implicit in discussions that occur in a variety of situations: in the recruitment committee, the evaluation committee, and the RTC and in individual discussions with faculty members about a whole host of issues. In these forums, as the program's values are being established, the RTD is in a strong position to influence the direction, but there must be a feeling of consensus. The Americans With Disabilities Act lends a legal dimension to this discussion, because this law cannot be broken in the application process. But the legal prescription should not preempt the departmental values dialogue.

In our program, after such a dialogue, we accepted the applicant with Friedreich's ataxia, but only after she had demonstrated how she would use her motorized cart to handle an aggressive patient. She performed well but ran into some resistance from a subgroup of her classmates who did not want to share one particular rotation with her. The chiefs handled this situation with a class meeting. This psychiatrist is now chief of a unit that specializes in psychosocial rehabilitation of the severely regressed, chronically mentally ill. She has been uniformly beloved by her patients, who sense her deep empathy for those with a chronic disability. My hunch is that her very presence is an inspiration for many of her patients. We have had brighter residents and others more skilled in certain areas of psychiatry, but I doubt there is any resident of whom we feel prouder. An HIV-positive resident would be no different.

As our program has become increasingly competitive in recent years, with essentially no worries about filling slots in the Match, chronic illness in applicants has become an issue that we have revisited multiple times. Not all programs are in our position—where we *could* insist that all applicants that we place on our Match list be uncomplicated by various family, life, psychiatric, or physical issues. Despite the fact that ours is in such a position, the RTC has raised the bar (e.g., the applicant with rheumatoid arthritis conveyed a certain entitlement about accommodations for her disability and was not ranked) but has happily matched with applicants with histories of bipolar disorder, multiple sclerosis, substance abuse, and other chronic conditions.

PATIENT SUICIDE

There are probably some psychiatrists who, in their entire careers, have no patient commit suicide, but if there is any universal tragedy that psychiatrists must endure, this is it. Every psychiatrist must make peace with the likelihood that it probably will happen. One of my own teachers once said, "If a psychiatrist never has a suicide, he is not treating very sick patients." I quote this often to residents who have endured their first patient suicide.

In some ways, a patient's suicide must be understood as the way a psychiatrist's patients are most likely to die. Deaths of patients is an issue all physicians must face. To the extent that residents can appreciate this fact, a patient's suicide is another part of the experience of practicing their profession. The willfulness of the act, in the face of the resident's efforts to help the patient find meaning in life, is what makes it difficult for residents to find peace with the event.

The resident whose patient commits suicide is likely to feel guilt beyond that associated with the failure of treatment efforts. This guilt involves whatever unresolved countertransference issues existed in the treatment relationship. A resident may feel overly guilty about the suicide of a patient at whom the resident was angry or whom the resident especially liked. It is the level of emotional investment, positive or negative, that makes this so difficult an issue. It may be evident to everyone, faculty and fellow residents alike, that the dead patient was an extraordinarily high-risk, chronically suicidal patient, but that is often cold comfort to the resident.

The rest of the resident group will almost always be supportive and will also experience a sense of relief that it was not their patient. The faculty, most of whom will have been there before, will be uniformly supportive, sometimes overly solicitous. Excessive solicitude gives the resident the message that the event is of greater magnitude than is realistic.

It is important that three things occur to help the resident and the entire group process a suicide (Table 11–2). First, there should be a psychological autopsy, which involves reviewing the case and treatment and paying attention to the feelings of everyone involved in the case. I encourage every site to have a standard procedure in place for dealing with suicides. An outside consultant who acts as facilitator to summarize the case and bring closure at the end of the discussion is optimal (see Appendix 11–C). Second, the resident needs an expert confidant. This will usually be the supervisor on the case, the resident's therapist, or some other trusted faculty member. It can be, but need not be, the RTD. The resident will also need a peer confidant, who will usually emerge from among the resident's friends, family, or peers. The RTD should be alert to the vulnerability of residents who are socially isolated. Asking the chief resident to check in on such a resident can be helpful. Finally, the entire resident group, and the resident, need to know that the RTD *knows* what has happened and is *attuned* to the issues. A note, a brief remark in the hall, or an invitation to drop by and visit about the suicide may be all that is necessary. Rarely, a formal meeting with the RTD may be appropriate.

TABLE 11–2.   What to do when a resident's patient commits suicide

1. Have a site-based, standard procedure for a psychological autopsy.
2. Be sure the resident has an available confidant.
3. Let the resident and the entire group know that you know what has occurred.

RESIDENTS WITH LEGAL, ETHICAL, OR MALPRACTICE DIFFICULTIES

It used to be very uncommon for legal complications to arise during residency. That is no longer true, partly due to the general increase in litigation in society, partly due to the field's greater attention to ethical and forensic issues, and partly due to the increased severity and acuity of patients seen during training. It is now fairly common for residents to be named in malpractice suits arising from emergency room encounters. This is quite a shock for a young resident the first time it occurs. The RTD must balance three separate functions in these situations: the supportive/educational role, the legal role, and the administrative role.

If a resident has transgressed a doctor-patient boundary, made a serious medical error, or otherwise compromised clinical care, the RTD's first legal and administrative responsibility is to prevent further harm to patients. If the severity of the error is not such that immediate administrative action is required, then the RTD can assume a more supportive, educational stance. Optimally, this is done through the site where the problem occurred; otherwise, formal counseling, provision of additional supervision, getting the resident into psychotherapy, and gearing up the standard administrative procedures at their usual pace become necessary. It must be clear to the resident that this is not simply a routine matter of learning and developing clinical skills. At the same time, if the problem is regarded as remediable, adequate support should be provided. The RTD must make a complicated judgment as to the origins and remediability of the transgression. Does it reflect naiveté? Personality problems? A temporary aberration? Major cognitive deficits? Serious knowledge deficiencies? This judgment will determine how much one assumes a supportive versus a potentially punitive administrative stance.

RTDs are constantly making decisions of this type. If a conflict between a resident and a faculty member results in an angry memo, should the memo go into the resident's file or should it be held awaiting other evidence of problems? An RTD must know the faculty as well as the residents in making this decision. Beginning a paper trail has repercussions for the resident and can be difficult to stop once started. It is important that a personality conflict with a particular attending physician not escalate into multiple memos that the evaluation committee must then react to. On the other hand, failure to start a paper trail can make needed administrative action impossible, despite widespread conviction among the faculty that a resident is incompetent or pathological. Therefore, it is important to make an early judgment as to the significance of a serious clinical error. In some instances a supportive, mentoring role is indicated. In others, one must request documentation in writing from faculty, place one's own memos of record in the file, and lower one's threshold for further administrative action.

Some clinical errors are so egregious that they must be acted on immediately; for example, sexual contact with a patient or wanton negligence. The due process policy must be written so that the RTD has the ability to immediately suspend a resident's clinical activities pending further documentation, information, and action by the evaluation committee. More difficult is the situation in which one concludes that a resident's problem is not likely to be remediated but does not yet justify administrative action. In such a case the RTD must move carefully but firmly and persistently in documenting the deficits so that the evaluation committee will be able to act without fear of lawsuit or other repercussions from the resident in question. Residents' rights must be sincerely respected by making their files available to them and allowing the insertion into the record of any material residents may wish to add on their own behalf. Faculty must be alerted to potential problems, but it must be done in such a way that fairness is observed and the program is not left open to charges of conspiracy or bias. Documentation must be assiduous. To accomplish this, the RTD must have worked extensively with the faculty about their feelings as evaluators. The most common problem I have observed is when faculty members see a problem, especially in the early years of residency, but are reluctant to document it, rationalizing to themselves that the resident is "still new," "will learn more," or "will grow out of it." No one is served well by reluctance to identify failing clinical accomplishments early. When documentation of an existing problem is not begun until sometime in PGY-3, the program is likely to be placed in the position of having a senior resident about whom everyone is embarrassed but whom everyone is afraid to fire. The resident's complaint that "No one told me" seems confirmed by the written record and opens the possibility of a lawsuit.

The RTD must lead persistently in this area. Whether dealing with an egregious violation, a remediable error, or an evolving movement toward administrative action, the RTD must face the dilemma of how much to share and with whom. I almost always share full information with the chief resident and the associate training directors, not only for their information but also for their input and advice. If I foresee any potential for legal or administrative entanglements, I *always* inform the department chair of what is going on. These are people whose discretion I trust. The dilemma comes with regard to protecting the resident's rights and privacy and avoiding the appearance of a conspiracy. I never share anything with additional residents until some official action occurs, and even then it may be necessary to withhold information (as with a dismissal). The faculty at the site where the transgression occurred invariably are fully informed and consulted about what action to take, but I rarely inform other faculty members except to ask the supervisors on the next rotation to let me know if there are any problems. I take considerable heat from some faculty members for this stance, although others appreciate it. The case for full disclosure to future supervisors of a resident who has made a serious and dangerous error is compelling. At the same time, the need for fully independent observations is also important. Either choice will put the RTD in a difficult position and require taking some flak.

A more pleasant task awaits the RTD when a resident is sued but is not deemed by the program to be clinically weak. In such a case, the RTD's entire energy can be directed toward supporting a young colleague-to-be in coping with every physician's worst nightmare. The most important thing is to have resources and support available to the resident. In addition to counseling and supervision, every hospital and medical school has an attorney, and every program must have a forensic psychiatry expert, if not immediately on faculty then by consultation with other programs. I find that sending the resident to speak with these people is enormously reassuring to him or her. The resident immediately realizes that he or she is not in this alone and that he or she has expert support, and it rapidly becomes apparent that many other residents have traversed this path. I often tell residents that although it may not be pleasant, being sued while still a resident offers them the maximum support possible and is much better than encountering their first suit all alone. It can be a tremendous learning experience, one that they share with their peers, as they learn extensively about the interactions of the medical and legal systems. The hospital attorney turns out to be much better than I at convincing the residents that they are not being personally or professionally attacked by a suit. There is a lot to learn about how and why people get named in suits, as well as who gets eliminated from a suit. Some residents have even developed an unexpected interest in forensic psychiatry as a result of being sued.

MIDYEAR CHANGES IN FACULTY OR SITES

One of the most shocking discoveries I encountered as a new RTD was realizing that the most conservative group I had to deal with were the residents. I had expected the residents to be natural allies in changes—especially regarding forward-looking, progressive changes in the program. In fact, residents almost invariably react to any proposed programmatic change negatively, even suspiciously. Faculty members tend to react egocentrically: "How will it affect me and my service?" Residents also become tied to the schedule as originally published. Any alteration to it, even one that residents want, is often viewed with anxiety. My best understanding of this process is that it reflects the residents' feelings of helplessness and lack of control over their lives. No matter how understandable, sensible, constructive, and positive, a midyear change of sites or faculty stirs considerable distress. Furthermore, the residents often feel they have been promised a certain program. They view changes to that program as violations of a contract or as a betrayal. Theirs is a short-term perspective, solely related to immediate training expectations. The faculty's perspective is long-term, knowing the program must evolve and change.

Training directors need to be well plugged into the departmental grapevine so that they know in advance what is happening or likely to happen. This is not always easy. I recommend to new RTDs that before accepting their positions, they negotiate to be part of whatever formal or informal "kitchen cabinet" the chair uses to help run the department. Holding regular meetings with the appropriate service chiefs is also crucial. Attendance at staff meetings of all important affiliates is useful. By keeping informed this way, any service-driven structural or faculty changes will be well known to the RTD early. This gives the RTD an opportunity to inform the service of the expected impact of contemplated changes. Over time, affiliated sites and services thus become encouraged to factor the educational impact and likely reaction of the residents into their decision making. I have been able, for example, to convince sites to delay changes until the beginning of the next academic year, when they can be included in the new schedule. There is nothing more embarrassing than having a resident ask about a faculty member leaving or the restructuring of a service when the RTD has no idea what is going on or that anything was afoot.

Once the RTD learns that a change is likely, the timing of the announcement is crucial. During the talking and planning phase, when there is great uncertainty about whether a change will occur or what form it may take, there is no point in unnecessarily stirring up the residents' "change anxiety," especially if that period includes recruitment interviewing. Applicants will hear about the still-uncertain changes or will simply sense the residents' anxiety. However, as the decision-making process goes forward, it is wise to inform the chief residents and assistant RTDs to get as much feedback as possible about the projected impact of any changes. It is also important that the chiefs inform the RTD as soon as rumors begin flying among the residents. It is important to formally inform the residents as soon as they start hearing rumors or at the time the definite decision to make a change is made. Typically, this will be several weeks or months before the actual change will occur, and time is afforded to process the change and respond to anxieties.

In addition, there is often a lag between the decision to make some change and the determination of what form those changes will take. Residents should be placed on the committee(s) or be consulted by the decision maker (as should the RTD) during this time period. The helplessness of the residents is part truth and part myth. Knowing of the RTD's involvement, the chief resident's involvement, and their peers' involvement helps to demythologize residents' feelings of being out of control. The announcement should be made either to the entire group of residents or to the class involved. A series of meetings might be necessary to ensure the ongoing flow of information, especially the reasons for the midyear change and the shape of things to come, and to provide opportunities to assuage the residents' anxieties.

In the end, however, even with the maximum preparation, the RTD will have to come up with a new schedule (or endorse restructuring an old rotation) and may have to endure the residents' rage, paranoia, and accusations. The RTD needs to take the heat—it comes with the job. Furthermore, if the RTD sees an unavoidable negative change coming up, caused by forces beyond his or her control, there is an old administrative saying, "It is easier to ask forgiveness than to ask permission." RTDs need to do what they can to make the best of things for the residents, make their own decisions, tell the residents straight out what the decisions are—and then take the heat. The residents will feel more secure with an RTD who acts and owns up than with one who seems as helpless and out of control as they feel.

In the case of a faculty member leaving, especially a beloved teacher, the residents' reaction is parallel to that of the faculty when a resident transfers electively: "What's wrong with the program?" Being in a transitional stage of not quite full-fledged working people, yet hardly students anymore, residents are not yet aware of the complexities involved in career decisions. The RTD should do his or her best to inform them. Most will accept the explanations, but some will not. In our program we have one or two older residents in every class, often physicians retraining from other specialties. They are often more convincing about the career issues than I am. In the event that the faculty member's leave-taking does reflect a problem in the program, there is no point in hiding it except to protect the privacy of the faculty member involved. The RTD should always indicate awareness of the problem and his or her plans to address it.

CHANGES IN OR ABSENCE OF THE CHAIR OR RESIDENCY TRAINING DIRECTOR

Albert Einstein College of Medicine sponsors the annual Tarrytown Leadership Conference, which is attended by most chief residents from U.S. psychiatry programs. At the conference a sophisticated introduction to group process, management, and leadership is begun by assigning groups a task but not designating a leader. Subsequently, the same task is assigned after a leader has been selected. The chiefs vividly learn the importance of an identified leader and that a bad leader is invariably far more effective than no leader at all. Most people intuitively understand this basic phenomenon of small social group behavior. In my opinion, training in this area, which was universal in the 1970s, is still central for all psychiatrists. Few experiences are more threatening than news of the leader's demise, no matter how intense the antipathy toward the leader may have been. This is what the impending or actual absence of the chair or RTD means to both residents and faculty.

The reaction is intense and unpredictable. Among the residents there may be anxiety that borders on terror, anger that verges into rage, fear that turns into paranoia, relief that becomes euphoria, or disinterest that is probably a form of denial. The faculty will be having similar reactions, although their greater experience with institutional transitions may make them more modulated, and their focus will be more on the future role of their particular service. The residents are more likely to experience their world falling apart, whether it is or not. Rumors and fantasies run wild. I have seen residents pick up and transfer to far inferior programs because they simply could not tolerate the uncertainty of lacking or changing a leader.

Oddly enough, this may be one of the easiest "special" problems to solve. If the anxiety is born of the absence of a leader, then the clear visibility and active leadership of the RTD best assuages those feelings. In so doing, the RTD becomes a lightning rod for all feelings, but this will likely reduce acting out and keep everyone focused on his or her training. Then the RTD can take the heat. Because residents are rightly regarded as novices at institutional life, some RTDs have a tendency to withhold or otherwise manage information they receive about such a transition. To my way of thinking, this infantilizes the residents and encourages regression in such times. I prefer to educate them about the nature of institutional transitions, informing them fully of all that is going on—the good, the bad, and the ugly. This treats them like junior colleagues and invites them to behave accordingly. A few years ago our department made the transition from having a psychoanalyst to having a basic scientist as chair. I did my best to follow my own advice (described above), including sharing my own anxiety about pressures I might come under to change the program in various ways. I also kept the residents apprised of my developing assessment of the new chair as I met with him. I believe that in the end, I was much more anxious about the transition than the residents were.

A special complication arises when one is either the outgoing or the incoming RTD. These are positions that every RTD will assume at some point in his or her tenure. If one is the outgoing RTD, there can be a perceived hypocrisy in continuing to act as leader while awaiting one's successor. However, a stance such as "We go about our business as usual while awaiting my successor, at which time I will happily hand over the reins to a colleague I respect," can go a long way toward assisting the next RTD, even if one is leaving unwillingly. Helping the residents with their grief, whatever form it takes—idealizing or vilifying the outgoing RTD—is the primary task. If an RTD is leaving to take a position elsewhere, he or she should call a meeting of all residents as quickly as possible to break the news. The residents most affected by this transition will be those in PGY-2. They will consider themselves as belonging to the old RTD but will spend most of their training time under the new one. Their professional identity is nearly formed yet is not sufficiently secure to see them through the change. Those in PGY-4 already see themselves as finished and thinking about their life after residency. Those in PGY-3 very much belong to the old RTD, but they usually feel secure enough in their identities to regulate their reactions. The PGY-1 residents are likely to feel as if they have been betrayed and recruited under false pretenses, yet their need for a clear leader will be strong enough that they will readily look for the best in the new RTD.

Incoming RTDs in such a transition get their first lesson in taking the heat. Connections must be made with the residents; they need to know who the RTD is and that the RTD will be their leader yet will not upset their applecart by making wholesale, rapid changes. New RTDs must be visible; speak openly and positively of their predecessor; be cautious in making any changes, addressing first those that the residents have wanted but that the former RTD was unable to make; and accept the residents' projections, good and bad. No matter how well incoming RTDs handle the change, there will come a time—best delayed by 6 months or so—when they do something that makes it clear to everyone that a new hand is on the tiller. Uproar will ensue. The RTD should not try to make sense of it. Things will settle down, at which point a new and mutually comfortable homeostasis will take hold. In my own case, the bonding occurred about 4 months after I arrived, when I was able to eliminate a neurology site that had long been a sore point for the residents. The uproar occurred about 10 months after I arrived, when I handled poor attendance at didactics in a very different and more demanding fashion than my predecessor had.

MERGINGS, CLOSINGS, AND DOWNSIZINGS

All of us who work within institutions have thought about and made our peace with the fact that when push comes to shove, the institution will invariably do what is best for it, regardless of the impact on individuals. We have accepted this insecurity, calculated our own likelihood of becoming a casualty, developed ways of functioning that we believe minimize our risk, and created whatever safety net we deem necessary. Residents have not done this. Some are aware of and are deeply worried about this aspect of being part of an institution—a few to the point that we regard them as paranoid. Others (most of them) are oblivious to this fact of life and are viewed by the paranoid residents as naive. When a training program merges with another, downsizes, or closes, it almost never does so in a positive educational spirit. Invariably, the program feels forced to take drastic action due to outside influences beyond its control. Residents are brutally confronted with their ultimate unimportance to the life of an institution. The faculty, facing their worst, dreaded nightmare, generally do not feel or act very much better than the residents. Their livelihoods and careers are on the line. Fortunately, the time of wholesale threats and actual closings, downsizings, mergers, and the like, such as occurred in the 1990s, appears to have passed.

The administrative problem raised by this restructuring is that the entire training program usually has to be redesigned. Once the shock of the announcement has worn off, this task, which logically falls to the RTD, can be used to help channel the reactions as constructively as possible. Most people will be either paralyzed by their feelings or fleeing for safer pastures. Others will be fighting a rear-guard and almost always futile action to reverse the decision. Some will be channeling their energies into maneuvering themselves into what they perceive to be safe situations. By swiftly setting up a process for redesigning the program based on the new realities of available services and residents, action can be shaped constructively.

A detailed procedure for this transition can be found in Yager et al.'s (1998) paper on downsizing. Similarly, Tasman and Riba (1993) wrote of their experience with a merger. A series of papers on a particularly painful and nasty closure from the points of view of involved residents and the training directors of the closing program and a nearby one are also helpful (Blotcky 1999; Bostic et al. 1999; Mohl 1999). The key elements involve including everyone in a process of adapting to the new environment. All concerned parties need to be involved in small, workable groups. The support of the department chair and service chiefs for the process is crucial, yet everyone must understand that, in the end, the chair has final decision-making responsibility. The RTD needs to be involved in all work groups and to lead a steering committee that sifts and evaluates ideas emerging from each group. Feedback to each group about what ideas are emerging from other task forces is also important. A fair and perceived-to-be-fair process can generate a good deal of excitement as people realize they are involved in designing a whole new clinical curriculum that is liberated from the constraints of previous ways of doing things. Above all, the RTD must be very visible to all, leading and facilitating the process. If the problem was that of a potentially leaderless group, this problem involves the group that is threatened with annihilation by decisions of the leader. Social cohesion must be rebuilt. The chair (the potential destroyer) is ill placed to do it. The RTD is ideally suited and must attend every meeting possible. The threat to the process is paralysis and passive-aggressive behavior by both residents and faculty. The group must meet, and meet, and meet some more. The RTD should be the rock around which the faculty and resident group redefine their cohesion and ideals by turning a decision that involved no concerns for education into an opportunity to improve the program. It is not a joke to suggest that the groups need to become so sick of seeing and being nagged by the RTD that they make some decisions in spite of themselves!

In the end, some very difficult decisions will have to be made. Some services will lose residents, some residents will go to institutions they never wanted to go to, and some institutions with which both faculty and residents have identified will lose their identities. As the dust settles, the RTD must take the heat. That's what we get paid the big bucks for!

Some closings of programs have tended to be abrupt, with short notice and with no consideration given to contractual or educational obligations to either residents or faculty, and have usually been instigated by outside administrators. The worst of these events appear to be in the past, but a minor form of them—namely, sudden decreases in funding for resident stipends—remains an ever-present threat. The residents and the RTD are in the same boat. At a time when it seems that the world has become arbitrary and malignant and is destroying their lives, it is important that the RTD maintain some model of integrity and stability, even though he or she is probably also looking for a job with some degree of panic. Using the RTD network through the American Association of Directors of Psychiatric Residency Training and the American Psychiatric Association clearinghouse, the residents can all be placed in a suitable and congenial program. Their world has been destroyed, but they themselves survive and can prosper, supported by their RTD's last official acts in that role.

CONCLUSION

What ties together the disparate problems described in this chapter are their potential or real traumatic qualities. They have the ability to tear a program apart, literally or emotionally. I go back to the introduction. If, taking into consideration the many roles of the RTD and the authentic basis of one's authority, an RTD establishes a system and set of procedures that are not only fair but perceived to be fair, these problems can become opportunities for strengthening and building a program. I must confess that when I first began as an RTD and one of these special problems arose, I tended to approach it with dread and a sense of crisis. Experience has transformed my response into a zest for grappling with difficult issues. Wrestling with these special problems can be one of the most exciting, meaningful, and important aspects of the RTD experience.

REFERENCES

Americans With Disabilities Act of 1990, Pub. L. No. 101-336

Blotcky MJ: The Titanic: a view from the bridge. Acad Psychiatry 23:160–162, 1999

Bostic JQ, Knezek BK, Smith H, et al: Gone with the wind: surviving the closing of a psychiatric residency. Acad Psychiatry 23:157–160, 1999

Family and Medical Leave Act of 1993, Pub. L. No. 103-3

Mohl PC: Inheriting the wind. Acad Psychiatry 23:162–164, 1999

Tasman A, Riba M: Strategic issues for the successful merger of residency training programs. Hosp Community Psychiatry 44:981–985, 1993

Yager J, Burk V, Mohl PC: Downsizing psychiatric residency programs: a pilot study. Acad Psychiatry 22:127–134, 1998

SUGGESTED READINGS

Jensen PS: The transition to residency seminar. J Psychiatr Educ 7(4):261–267, 1983

Lomax JW: A proposed curriculum on suicide care for psychiatry residency. Suicide Life Threat Behav 16:56–64, 1986

Phelan ST: Pregnancy during residency, II: obstetric complications. Obstet Gynecol 72:431–436, 1988

Pilkington P, Etkin M: Encountering suicide: the experience of psychiatric residents. Acad Psychiatry 27:93–99, 2003

Stewart DE, Robinson GE: Combining motherhood with psychiatric training and practice. Can J Psychiatry 30:28–34, 1985

Wagner KD, Pollard R, Wagner RF Jr: Malpractice litigation against child and adolescent psychiatry residency programs, 1981–1991. J Am Acad Child Adolesc Psychiatry 32:462–465, 1993

Young-Shumate L, Kramer T, Beresin E: Pregnancy during graduate medical training. Acad Med 68:792–799, 1993

APPENDIX 11–A

GUIDELINES FOR RESIDENT PARENTAL LEAVES

1. Four weeks of unpaid parental leave are available to each resident during the duration of the residency without educational payback obligations.
2. Parental leave must be initiated within 6 months of the arrival of a new child.
3. In addition to parental leave time, unused vacation time from the current academic year may be utilized as paid parental leave, and unused sick leave from the current academic year may be utilized as paid parental leave. Each resident is entitled to a total of 12 weeks of parental leave per 12-month period under the Family Medical Leave Act (FMLA).
4. Any leave time not covered by sick leave, vacation, or the 4 weeks of parental leave must be made up at the end of the residency, in order to assure proper educational achievement and credentialing.
5. With the permission of the Residency Training Director, leave time may be extended to a total of 26 weeks per parental leave, with the extended portion to be made up at the end of the residency. Any time in excess of 26 weeks seriously engenders the risk of request of the resident's resignation and must be discussed individually with the Residency Training Director, who holds the authority to make all decisions regarding extended leaves. Any time to be made up will be done on a site at the discretion of the Residency Training Director and conforming to the requirements for board eligibility.
6. Although salary to cover the time made up at the end of residency cannot be absolutely guaranteed, every attempt to work out scheduling on an individual basis will be made.
7. Although this is the department policy and is compatible with Parkland's policy, other hospitals' policies may preclude payment derived from vacation or sick leave.
8. To facilitate scheduling, residents are encouraged to notify the Residency Training Director of an anticipated parental leave as early as pos-

---

Reprinted with permission of the University of Texas Southwestern Medical Center Department of Psychiatry.

sible. Failure to give adequate notice may compromise the availability of leave. *Six months' notice* must be given before the arrival of a new child, and any changes in length of leave must be negotiated on a case-by-case basis with the Residency Training Director. Changes cannot be guaranteed but are more likely to be possible with more advanced notice.

9. All final decisions regarding leaves will be made at the discretion of the Residency Training Director.

GUIDELINES FOR RESIDENT PERSONAL LEAVES

1. No guaranteed personal leave is available during the residency.
2. All decisions regarding personal leave will be made at the discretion of the Residency Training Director.
3. Emergency leaves of less than 3 days' duration may be facilitated through the site attending physician after coverage arrangements are made by the resident.

GUIDELINES FOR RESIDENT SICK LEAVES

1. Two weeks of paid sick leave are available each academic year.
2. Although this is the department policy and is compatible with Parkland policy, other hospitals' policies may preclude payment for sick leave.
3. An additional 4 weeks of unpaid sick leave are available during the duration of the residency without educational pay back obligations.
4. Any sick leave time exceeding the above 6 weeks must be made up at the end of the residency to ensure educational achievement and credentialing. A total of 12 weeks sick leave per 12-month period is available to each resident under the FMLA. Any time to be made up will be done on a site at the discretion of the Residency Training Director and conforming to the requirements for board eligibility.
5. Sick leave may be used for the care of immediate family members who become ill.
6. Documentation may be required at the discretion of the Residency Training Director.

APPENDIX 11–B

DUE PROCESS PROCEDURES FOR PSYCHIATRY RESIDENTS

RESIDENT ASSESSMENT

1. Each resident will be assigned a faculty supervisor on each rotation or clinical experience. The level and method of this supervision will be consistent with the ACGME Special Requirements for Residency Education in Psychiatry.
2. Each resident will be given written evaluation by supervisors at the end of each rotation, or twice a year in the case of psychotherapy supervisors, or yearlong rotations.
3. The program director, and/or his/her designee, will meet with each resident at least twice yearly concerning evaluations of his/her performance and, with the resident's input, shall make recommendations for resolving deficiencies and improvement of the resident's general skills and knowledge. In the event deficiencies are identified, the program director may meet with the resident in addition to the two scheduled meetings. The program director shall document each such meeting.
4. The Progress and Evaluation Committee (the "Committee") is comprised of selected faculty of the adult, child, geriatric, and forensic psychiatry divisions, the training directors and chief residents, and is chaired by the program director. The Committee shall meet annually, or at the request of the program director, to discuss the progress of each resident. The Committee shall identify any areas in which the resident may improve his/her skills or knowledge, and any deficiencies in the resident's performance, or impediments to the resident's progress toward professional competence, and make recommendations for improvement. These recommendations shall be communicated to the resident in his/her meeting with the program director, and the resident may also meet with the Committee if disciplinary action is included in the Committee's recommendation as described more fully below.
5. The program director shall advance residents to positions of higher responsibility on the basis of the combined evaluations of the resident's readiness for advancement.
6. Each resident shall be given the opportunity to give a written evaluation of supervisors, clinical rotations, and courses at the end of each rotation.

DISCIPLINARY ACTION

1. The Committee, either at its regular meeting or a specially scheduled meeting, may additionally recommend that disciplinary action be taken. Recommendations for discipline may include: formal letter of warning; suspension from clinical duties, with or without pay; probation; or, in the most extreme situations, nonrenewal or termination.
2. Notice of disciplinary action shall be prepared by the program director and provided to the resident. Such notice shall include: the reasons for the disciplinary action, the length of time the disciplinary action will be in effect, and the corrective action the resident is required to make (unless the recommendation is termination).
3. After the program director has met with the resident regarding the recommended disciplinary action, the resident may appeal the recommendation of the Committee by giving written notice to the program director within 10 working days from the date of his/her initial meeting with the program director.
4. In cases of appeal, the program director shall convene a majority of the Committee as soon as reasonably practicable to meet with the resident requesting the appeal. Resident members of the Committee may attend and have voting privileges. The resident requesting the appeal is encouraged to bring any additional information to the Committee's attention, including other opinions that the resident believes were not sufficiently appreciated in the previous deliberations.
5. At any time during the appeal of a disciplinary action, the resident may choose to be represented by an attorney to ensure that his/her rights are appropriately protected, but must notify the program director no less than 3 working days before the date of any hearing at which an attorney shall appear on a resident's behalf.
6. After the meeting of the Committee regarding an appeal of a disciplinary action, the Committee shall provide a written response to the resident within 5 working days.
7. In all cases except for termination, the Committee's determination upon appeal shall be final. All recommendations for termination or nonrenewal, however, are subject to review by the department chair.

SUSPENSION OF PATIENT CARE RESPONSIBILITIES

1. A supervisor or director of a clinical service who believes that patient welfare may be jeopardized because of a resident's performance may

request the program director to temporarily suspend the resident's clinical activities.

2. If such a suspension is determined to be warranted by the program director, the program director shall inform the resident in writing of the nature of the observations that caused temporary suspension of clinical privileges and shall convene a meeting of the Committee as soon as is reasonably practicable. In such an event, the resident is encouraged to invite any members of the faculty, staff, or residents to provide information to the Committee for consideration.

3. The recommendation of the Committee, including the recommendation for any disciplinary action, shall be provided to the program director within 5 working days from the date of its meeting, which shall be promptly communicated with the resident. The resident may appeal this recommendation as described above.

APPENDIX 11–C

MORBIDITY AND MORTALITY CONFERENCES

Suicides and attempted homicides by clinic patients are reviewed regularly. The purpose of the conference is resident support, continuous quality improvement, and education. The focus is placed on the precipitating event, some of the ways family and environment may have encouraged suicidal crises (interaction of patient's psychopathology with family dynamics), and professional intervention. Supporting the family and documenting events are also discussed.

CHAPTER 12

SPECIAL EVENTS IN THE RESIDENCY PROGRAM

Ze'ev Levin, M.D.

Carol A. Bernstein, M.D.

Residency is a time of tremendous personal and professional growth and change. Certain events that routinely occur in training can be considered milestones. From entry into a program, marked by orientation, through departure, marked by graduation, the training experience itself helps to shape and mold the resident's identity as a psychiatrist. Other events, such as academic meetings, help promote professional development and intro-duce residents to colleagues and potential mentors from across the country. Departmental retreats allow for time away from the program to assess its strengths and weaknesses and to formulate ways of improving it. Planned social events for the residents, with and without faculty, foster morale and cohesion in the program. This chapter addresses these issues. Although they are less strictly educational, these topics have a marked bearing on the general climate of the training program. This chapter also addresses the appointment of a new department chair or training director and the impact that such an occurrence has on training. We have also included a section on terrorism and disasters and the impact of September 11, 2001, on our program.

ORIENTATION

Orientations are typically overwhelming for incoming residents. Although most residents are excited, a great deal of anxiety surrounds the beginning of internship, a year that is renowned for its intensity and challenges. A large amount of information is handed out, many forms need to be completed, and not much attention is paid to the individual resident. Most hospitals plan a general orientation for all incoming housestaff, which may be impersonal and not relevant to specific program issues. For this reason, we recommend a separate departmental orientation for all beginning and transferring psychiatry residents. This orientation offers an opportunity to introduce the resident to the department and to provide the resident with an understanding of the department's values, style, and personality from the outset.

Preparation is needed to ensure that the day goes smoothly, that all necessary information is covered, and that the residents will leave feeling more comfortable with the department and more familiar with what is expected. Planning can begin as soon as the Match results are in. Meetings involving the director, coordinator, and chief residents should be held to plan the day. We have found it useful to prepare an orientation book, which might include the following elements:

1. Contact information for residents and faculty, including pager and telephone numbers (office and home) and e-mail addresses
2. Rotation schedules, call schedules, and all switch dates
3. Departmental Web site information, including library access
4. Housestaff benefits and an explanation of salary lines
5. Residency didactic curriculum
6. Recommended reading list
7. Information on how to apply for state licensure and United States Medical Licensing Examination (USMLE) Step 3 registration
8. Promotion requirements for each clinical year and residency training program goals and objectives, including core competencies
9. A copy of the "Essentials for Residency Training in Psychiatry" by the Residency Review Committee for Psychiatry of the Accreditation Council for Graduate Medical Education (ACGME; 2004); other ACGME information, including resident work hour regulations; and institutional and departmental due process policies and procedures
10. A copy of *The Principles of Medical Ethics: With Annotations Especially Applicable to Psychiatry* (American Psychiatric Association 2001)

The residents should receive a copy of the orientation-day schedule. They should not be overwhelmed with packets of information before the meeting. Only essential forms should be included in the information that is sent out.

When should the departmental orientation take place? We recommend setting aside a morning or afternoon preferably after the hospital orientation is over.

Where should the orientation be held? Having the interns meet in the residency training office at the primary institution seems the easiest way to have them feel welcome.

A breakfast before the program, or lunch afterward, with key clinical faculty and the other residents provides a way for new residents to meet their faculty in a less formal setting.

WHAT SHOULD THE ORIENTATION PROGRAM INCLUDE?

- Introductions (30 minutes): The department chair, training director, and chief resident(s) should introduce themselves to the new residents and welcome them to the program.
- Site orientation (no more than 2 hours): In a multisite program, up to 15 minutes can be spent by each service chief from each clinical site to describe his or her site's services. This orientation should also include meeting with the service chiefs and/or chief residents from medicine, neurology, pediatrics, and any other nonpsychiatric services to which the residents rotate.
- Schedules and vacations (15 minutes): Time should be set aside to talk with the residents about their call schedules, vacations, and sick time, highlighting switch dates and whom to contact if changes need to be made to the schedule.
- Salaries and benefit information (15 minutes): Time should be spent going over salaries throughout the 4 years of training and issues such as direct deposit and on-site payrolls. Time should also be set aside to discuss issues such as medical benefits, sick leave, maternity and paternity leave, and therapy benefits.

It is helpful to provide all this information in a packet and to distribute it to each resident on orientation day.

In programs that have a high proportion of international medical graduates, special orientation events designed to help them become familiar with the American culture are extremely useful. A special summer curriculum can also provide entering postgraduates and transferring residents from other cultures with the opportunity to discuss what psychiatry is like in their home country, to raise questions about their new environment, and to orient them to cultural differences. Residents may also be helped to find examples of their native culture and to meet with faculty members and other residents from their own background.

RETREATS

Program evaluation should always be an ongoing process. Some programs set aside time for an annual retreat for residents or residents and faculty specifically for this purpose. These retreats provide residents with the opportunity to evaluate the program and make constructive suggestions for change in an atmosphere that is removed from the hospital or medical center. Depending on the program structure, it is preferable to offer faculty coverage for residents' responsibilities for these events. In larger or more service-dependent programs, a retreat can be held on a weekend to maximize residents' participation if coverage is problematic.

The most useful retreat formats provide opportunities for residents to meet alone as a group, with special times set aside for additional meetings with the training director(s) and key faculty members. The residency group in consultation with the training director may wish to consider whether such a retreat should serve a more social function for residents (thus involving significant others) or should be more program oriented.

The selection of retreat topics and mechanisms for feedback will vary depending on whether the retreat is for residents alone or residents and faculty together. The primary advantage of having a residents-only retreat is that residents will probably be less inhibited about discussing anxieties and concerns because faculty and supervisors are not present. The primary disadvantage is that residents will not have an opportunity to interact with faculty members in a setting that is unencumbered by other clinical and educational responsibilities. The training director should communicate with residents and faculty to determine what would be optimal for the program. Either way, it is important to solicit suggestions for retreat content from all participants as well as from the department chair and to make sure there is a mechanism to provide appropriate feedback.

The training director may wish to arrange a retreat to review, for example, different aspects of the clinical experience, didactic experience, or research focus of the program. Cohesion among residents is an example of a more process-oriented focus. Some programs arrange retreats to discuss more general issues that relate to the medical field, such as the involvement of the pharmaceutical industry in medicine and how it relates to residency education.

CHIEF RESIDENCY

Choosing a chief resident is a complicated process. After almost 3 years of working together, close bonds have developed between residents, and tensions may arise during the selection process. It is helpful for the training director to meet with the class from whom the chiefs will be chosen and to spell out the criteria for selection and the process itself.

Criteria: Selection of a chief resident provides an opportunity to recognize a resident who has excelled in all aspects of his or her work: clinical, administrative, leadership, and academic. Interpersonal skills are essential for this job, and the resident who is able to work well with colleagues and peers from all disciplines is best suited for the position.

Process: We have found that all unit chiefs and service chiefs should be involved in this process. Input from residents is also important. Some programs have residents from each year vote for their choices. We feel that this approach has the potential for making the choice a popularity contest, so we solicit input from the chief residents of the year ahead to represent the opinions of the residents. There is clearly no one right way, but it is important to ensure that the residents feel that they are heard in the choice for these coveted positions.

Not being chosen as chief can leave residents feeling overlooked or undervalued. The training director should make time to meet with all those who wish to discuss why they were not selected, and if there were faculty concerns about their capacity for the job, this is a useful time for positive, constructive feedback.

Being chosen as chief resident brings its own set of challenges. Although to be chosen from among one's peers can be a source of pride, it may also stir up feelings of guilt. Residents who have been selected as chief residents may feel undeserving of the honor or concerned that one of their peers should have been chosen instead. They may feel uncomfortable exerting their authority, and making difficult and sometimes unpopular decisions may leave them feeling isolated from their peers. Not yet identified as faculty and no longer fully identified with their fellow residents, the chief may feel quite alone.

Our chief residents have all found that the annual chief residents' meeting in Tarrytown, New York, has helped them learn to deal with many of these issues. Assuming a position of authority in a middle management position and tolerating the negative feelings that others may have toward them by virtue of their leadership role are examples of the issues addressed there in a supportive environment with an experienced faculty. The conference is also an opportunity for the chiefs to meet with other chief residents from across the country, to hear about other programs and the problems they face and have solved, and to network.

We have also found that a weekly meeting with the training director and the chiefs allows time to discuss these issues. Supervision for the chiefs from the training director cannot be more important. Our experience has led us to believe that the issue the chiefs struggle with the most is what many of us find difficult in a leadership role: tolerating the negative affect and negative transference of peers and colleagues. Supervision allows the chiefs to express their feelings, and shared anecdotes from the training director offer concrete ways to manage them.

Becoming a chief resident is a means of consolidating generic psychiatric skills while simultaneously functioning more independently and gaining experience in leadership and clinical administration. It is important that the chief resident have real responsibilities and accountability and also that he or she receive support. The experience of being chief resident can be a very powerful learning opportunity and can go a long way toward identifying future leaders.

NEW CHAIR OR TRAINING DIRECTOR

The appointment of a new department chair is anticipated with much excitement. There is the hope that with new leadership will come interesting challenges and great possibility for the department to expand and grow. It may also stir up feelings of unease. Faculty members are often concerned about the new chair's plans for changes in leadership roles within the department, and they may fear the unknown direction in which the department may be steered. The training office is usually most concerned about the attitude of the new chair toward education. Will he or she advocate for teaching and expect faculty involvement in supervision? Will the new chair be actively involved in the recruitment of prospective residents? Will he or she take time out to meet with residents and become involved in mentoring programs? How will the new chair become actively involved in exciting residents about research? Will he or she encourage the learning and teaching of psychodynamics?

A good relationship between the training director and the new chair is essential in determining the impact that the new chair has on the residency. The training director would be well served to arrange for frequent meetings with the chair to discuss any and all issues within the residency. Arranging meetings between the new chair and residents is an important way of having the residents feel connected to the new leadership. Asking the chair to teach in the didactic curriculum or to lead professor's rounds or case conferences is another way to actively involve the chair in the educational endeavor. It almost goes without saying, but constant collaboration between the chair and the director goes a long way toward enhancing the educational mission of the department.

Of much greater concern to the residents—because it has a much more direct impact on them—is the appointment of a new training director. If the director is chosen from outside the system, residents' involvement in the selection process is essential. If the director is chosen from within, soliciting opinions from the residents before the announcement is made is equally important. The new training director should be sure to meet with the residents and teaching faculty frequently and regularly. Listening to their concerns goes a long way toward fostering collegiality and respect.

The new director is best served by forming a good relationship with the department chair. The two should try to meet regularly and often. Knowing that the chair supports the training director's decisions is essential to the successful implementation of any unpopular policies and allows the new director to feel supported in his or her new role.

SOCIAL EVENTS

Social events during the course of the year go a long way toward diminishing potential strain, boosting morale, and dispelling the occasional misperceptions people have of one another. An early summer welcoming party is a nice complement to the formality of the orientation. A regular get-together of faculty and residents, with or without some academic task, can be useful in facilitating social rapport. An annual midwinter party at which the residents plan some type of humorous "roasting" or mockery of faculty is also an invaluable means of communication and morale building. These events allow residents to express to the faculty complex messages about their experience.

As in any working environment, these periodic social events enable residents and faculty to interact in more relaxed settings. Some institutions use the holiday season as an opportunity to bring the department together. Residents also enjoy coming to the training director's home for potluck dinners, picnics, or brunches. Sometimes other faculty members will also be encouraged to host similar events. Potluck suppers permit residents to participate actively and spare the training director from "too much work."

Journal clubs or other educational events planned at the homes of faculty members have been extremely well received in our program. For instance, our associated analytic institute arranges a monthly dinner at the home of an analyst at which a topic pertinent to psychodynamic psychiatry is discussed. This program has generated tremendous excitement and has contributed to an increase in applications by our residents to analytic training. Such dinners may do the same for research careers and other subspecialties. An off-site happy hour for residents only is another monthly event that can bring residents together to socialize, complain, and bond without faculty present.

In many areas, the local American Psychiatric Association (APA) district branch may have an active residents' committee. This is an ideal venue for residents from neighboring programs to get together; in some cities it has led to sponsorship of events such as a movie night that also provide an occasion for medical students, faculty members, and residents to interact. APA committees are also natural avenues for mentorship between residents and psychiatrists working in the community, whether they are academically affiliated or not.

Funding for these events poses its own set of issues. In this era of shrinking resources, it has become increasingly difficult for programs to find any extra funding. In our experience, some pharmaceutical companies are willing to donate support for these educational activities, but having these companies involved is complicated. Indeed, involvement of pharmaceutical companies in any educational arena is controversial; it is worthwhile to hold discussions with residents and faculty before initiating such activities. Web sites such as No Free Lunch (http://www.nofreelunch.org) can provide useful information on how the pharmaceutical industry employs marketing strategies to influence prescribing practices. If pharmaceutical company funds are obtained to support educational activities, it is important to review some of these ethical issues beforehand.

SPECIAL AWARDS

Rewarding residents through public recognition is another way for departments to communicate values and recognize superior achievement and effort. Awards named for retired or deceased faculty members are also a way of memorializing and honoring a faculty member and the values that he or she represented. Such local awards may acknowledge research productivity and accomplishment, general clinical ability, the resident as teacher, or any other skill or achievement the department wishes to recognize. It is important that the process of selecting recipients for these awards be straightforward and clear to minimize fears of favoritism and bias that so often accompany efforts to single out superior achievement.

GRADUATION

Graduation from residency is a sentinel event. For many residents it is the beginning of the first unstructured time in their lives. For all residents it is the culmination of at least 8 years of intense immersion in medicine and an event that signifies the beginning of their professional lives in psychiatry.

There are differing ideas about what is required for a resident to graduate from a program. Each department has its own list of promotion criteria, and with it, requirements for completion of training. Many programs require residents to write an evidence-based academic paper before they can graduate. Although this may foster intellectual and academic interest, it can also lead to a forced interest in a subject for the purpose of fulfilling a requirement, as opposed to a genuine interest in it. We have found that some kind of academic requirement highlights the importance placed by the department on scholarly learning and inquiry.

To celebrate this auspicious event, most programs have some type of graduation ceremony. We have chosen to honor all graduates from all our psychiatry programs at a ceremony attended by all faculty members and residents, to which family and friends are also invited. Each program director speaks briefly about each graduate—past, present, and future plans—and all receive certificates and greetings from the chair. This ceremony is followed by a wine and cheese reception. Our residents have also enjoyed having a graduation dinner. This can include time set aside for the residents to perform a "roasting" of the faculty. If possible, it is helpful if graduates can attend these events for free. Again, the pharmaceutical industry may be able to offer support, but involvement should be reviewed with residents and faculty ahead of time. It is particularly important to encourage a good turnout from the faculty. Having residents personally invite faculty members to whom they feel close and connected may encourage attendance by the faculty.

DISASTERS AND TERRORISM

In these troubled times, disasters and terrorism may have a direct impact on training programs and the resident cohort. Our experience as a training program in New York City on September 11, 2001, forced us to focus on this issue.

In direct response to the events of September 11, we attempted to create an atmosphere of containment, support, and organization for our residents to allow them to function as physicians while still finding time for their own personal recovery and healing. Hospital emergency rooms were the organizational center for all of the mental health outreach efforts, and we used these settings as the sites in which to assist our residents. We met with each residency class and emphasized the importance of their focusing on continuing to provide excellent care for their patients. At the same time, in response to many residents' need to participate in outreach in the community in general, we involved residents in efforts organized by the city, by the National Alliance for the Mentally Ill, and by Disaster Psychiatry Outreach for rescue workers, disaster victims, and their families. Schedules of these efforts were posted in our emergency rooms, and residents were given the opportunity to sign up for different shifts. Faculty members were assigned to the emergency rooms to help residents process what was happening. These opportunities were designed to combat feelings of helplessness and isolation. In this way, residents were able to use the emergency room as a family that provided community, consistency, structure, and support.

Residency process groups, which had been established at the beginning of training for each class, were used extensively during that time as a way for residents to deal with their own conflicts about being asked to remain psychiatrists and empathic listeners when filled with fear and a sense of helplessness themselves.

A special conference was set up for the residents to review the literature on disasters, and experts were invited to address issues such as debriefing and symptoms of posttraumatic stress and acute stress disorders. The training office maintained close communication with the residents through e-mail, alerting them to the progress of the department and the multihospital network in coordinating ongoing care for patients and their families.

An organized and uniform approach to outreach efforts, maintaining close communication between the administration and the residents in one common place (at the emergency room and through e-mail), and making a process group available to residents were some of the ways we discovered to be of use to help our residents deal with such unpredicted crises in the extended community.

ACADEMIC MEETINGS AND FELLOWSHIPS

An important aspect of residency training is the opportunity for residents to participate in and attend academic meetings. The APA and allied organizations representing various psychiatric subspecialties have annual meetings, and many of these organizations sponsor fellowships that enable residents to have their expenses paid to attend meetings. Some departments have resources to support attendance by residents if presentations are being made. Training directors routinely receive announcements about conferences and symposia, and it is useful to have a routine mechanism for disseminating this information to the resident group. Chief residents can be assigned the task of distributing information on meetings and fellowships to the residents through e-mail notices or by posting flyers on residents' notice boards. Weekly resident meetings are frequently the most effective way to do this. In hospitals where there are housestaff unions, there may be a means for residents to be reimbursed for conference fees through union benefits; it is a good idea to find out if these programs exist at one's institution. Obviously, it is important to develop a policy outlining how much release time for conferences will be permitted and who will provide coverage. In some places, institutional benefits determine how much conference time is permitted. Other programs have no official policy. The training director should consider whether such a policy should be developed. In general, residents who win honorary fellowships and who present research or papers at academic meetings should be accommodated whenever possible. Such opportunities can then be viewed as rewards for the presenters and as incentives to others.

When a resident has been awarded a fellowship, it not only provides the resident an excellent opportunity to participate in national academic activities but is also a source of pride for the entire residency program. Training directors or chairs must write letters of nomination, which should be in the dean's letter format and contain extensive information about the nominee. The author should be clear that he or she is familiar with the work, interests, and talents of the resident. Although this takes some time and effort, it is the best way to help one's resident come alive to members of any selection committee. It is also important to tailor the nominating letter to address the criteria outlined by the particular fellowship selection committee.

Some fellowships are more competitive than others. One issue to consider is how to disseminate information and make choices about fellowship opportunities. Although it is more democratic to notify the entire resident group and see who might be interested in a particular fellowship, the training director might also want to select residents who have a chance of winning. Whereas some programs turn the decision-making process over to residents, others have a faculty committee and may or may not request volunteers or nominations. Each process has advantages and disadvantages, and there is no absolute rule about what works best. For example, peers may know the most about an individual resident's clinical skills, but they may not be familiar with the resident's background and may choose a nominee based on popularity. On the other hand, faculty members may not know enough about the full dimensions of a resident's work. It is always best to maintain a system that allows for input from both sides and to set up a mechanism that is both fair and pragmatic. All fellowships and awards are special honors and opportunities, and they are meant for residents with interests and talents specific for the award.

Presented in Table 12–1 is a list of these fellowships, including objectives, contact information, Web site address, and application deadlines.

CONCLUSION

Residency training provides many opportunities to bolster the morale of residents and to enhance the educational environment through a series of special events. These events also provide unique opportunities for residents and faculty to interact together in more informal settings and to develop mentorship through social as well as educational arenas.

REFERENCES

Accreditation Council for Graduate Medical Education: Graduate Medical Education Directory 2004–2005. Chicago, IL, American Medical Association, 2004

American Psychiatric Association: The Principles of Medical Ethics: With Annotations Especially Applicable to Psychiatry. Washington, DC, American Psychiatric Association, 2001

TABLE 12–1. Fellowships and awards

Fellowship	Objective	Contact information	Deadline
American Academy of Child and Adolescent Psychiatry (AACAP)/Pfizer Travel Grants	To help defray the cost of attending the AACAP annual meeting.	Department of Research and Training American Academy of Child and Adolescent Psychiatry 3615 Wisconsin Avenue, NW Washington, DC 20016-3007 http://www.aacap.org/awards/pfizerTravel.htm	August
American College of Psychiatrists/Laughlin Fellowship Program	For a PGY-3, PGY-4, or child psychiatry fellow who is likely to make a significant future contribution to psychiatry.	Laughlin Fellowship Committee American College of Psychiatrists 732 Addison Street, Suite B Berkeley, CA 94710 510-704-8020 alice@acpsych.org	September
American Academy of Addiction Psychiatry (AAAP)/Janssen Research Award	Two awards are available annually and are presented at the annual meeting and symposium of the academy. One of the awards is reserved for research involving racial and ethnic minorities.	American Academy of Addiction Psychiatry 1010 Vermont Avenue, Suite 710 Washington, DC 20005 http://www.aaap.org/membership/resident.html	September

TABLE 12–1. Fellowships and awards *(continued)*

Fellowship	Objective	Contact information	Deadline
AAAP Travel Stipends	Offer the opportunity for residents who are interested in learning about the etiology, diagnosis, and treatment of substance use disorders to attend the AAAP annual meeting. Applicants are assessed on interest, abilities, and potential for contributions to the field.	American Academy of Addiction Psychiatry 1010 Vermont Avenue, Suite 710 Washington, DC 20005 http://www.aaap.org/membership/resident.html	September
Group for the Advancement of Psychiatry (GAP) Fellowship	Offers an opportunity to work with one of the GAP committees and to attend two meetings of the GAP.	Frances M. Roton Group for the Advancement of Psychiatry PO Box 570218 Dallas, TX 75357-0218 972-613-0985 http://www.groupadpsych.org	September
American College of Psychiatrists (ACP)/ Psychiatry Resident In-Training Examination (PRITE) Fellowship	To participate as a full-fledged member of the PRITE editorial board and participate in the board meetings as well as two ACP annual meetings; also to provide 40 candidate items (questions) each year.	PRITE Fellowship Selection Committee ACP Central Office 732 Addison Street, Suite B Berkeley, CA 94710 510-704-8020 alice@acpsych.org http://www.acpsych.org/prite/fellowship.html	October

TABLE 12–1. Fellowships and awards *(continued)*

Fellowship	Objective	Contact information	Deadline
ACP/Child PRITE Fellowship	To participate as a full-fledged member of the PRITE editorial board and participate in the board meetings as well as two ACP annual meetings; also to provide 40 candidate items (questions) each year.	PRITE Fellowship Selection Committee ACP Central Office 732 Addison Street, Suite B Berkeley, CA 94710 510-704-8020 alice@acpsych.org http://www.acpsych.org/prite/fellowship.html	October
American Psychiatric Institute for Research and Education (APIRE)/Lilly Psychiatric Research Fellowship	A 1-year fellowship for two postgraduate psychiatry trainees to specifically focus on research and personal scholarship.	APIRE/Lilly Psychiatric Research Fellowship American Psychiatric Institute for Research and Education 1000 Wilson Boulevard, Suite 1825 Arlington, VA 22209-3901 800-852-1390 http://www.psych.org/research/apire/training_fund/fellow/lilly.cfm	October

TABLE 12–1. Fellowships and awards *(continued)*

Fellowship	Objective	Contact information	Deadline
APIRE/Wyeth Pharmaceuticals M.D./ Ph.D. Psychiatric Research Fellowship	To provide 1 year of funding designed to support two postgraduate psychiatry trainees with research experience to focus on research and personal scholarship.	APIRE/Wyeth Pharmaceuticals Research Fellowship American Psychiatric Institute for Research and Education 1000 Wilson Boulevard, Suite 1825 Arlington, VA 22209-3901 800-852-1390 http://www.psych.org/research/apire/ training_fund/fellow/wyeth.cfm	October
American Association for Geriatric Psychiatry (AAGP)/Stepping Stones Program for Psychiatry Residents and Fellows	To showcase the benefits of fellowship training in geriatric psychiatry and to assist fellows in career planning.	American Association for Geriatric Psychiatry Attn: Stepping Stones Selection Committee 7910 Woodmont Avenue, Suite 1050 Bethesda, MD 20814 301-654-7850, ext. 112 http://www.aagpgpa.org/prof/stones.asp	November

TABLE 12–1. Fellowships and awards *(continued)*

Fellowship	Objective	Contact information	Deadline
American Association of Directors of Psychiatric Residency Training (AADPRT)/Pfizer Neuroscience International Medical Graduate Mentorship Program	Fosters career development of international medical graduate residents in psychiatry. Each year, seven outstanding residents are chosen to work with distinguished academic mentors to clarify and advance their career goals.	AADPRT Executive Office University of Connecticut Health Center Department of Psychiatry 263 Farmington Avenue, LG066 Farmington, CT 06030-1935 860-679-8112 aadprt@psychiatry.uchc.edu http://www.aadprt.org/public/2004/IMG/index.html	December
AADPRT/Peter Henderson, M.D., Memorial Paper Award	This award is given annually to the resident submitting the best paper in the general area of child and adolescent psychiatry. Papers submitted must be in the field of child and adolescent psychiatry and must not have been previously published.	AADPRT Executive Office University of Connecticut Health Center Department of Psychiatry 263 Farmington Avenue, LG066 Farmington, CT 06030-1935 860-679-8112 aadprt@psychiatry.uchc.edu http://www.aadprt.org/public/2004/henderson/index.html	December

TABLE 12–1. Fellowships and awards *(continued)*

Fellowship	Objective	Contact information	Deadline
AADPRT/Ginsberg Fellowship	The AADPRT/George Ginsberg Fellowship was established to promote the professional growth of residents who have demonstrated interest in education as a career path. Seven outstanding residents (representing each of the seven regions) are honored at the AADPRT annual meeting.	AADPRT Executive Office University of Connecticut Health Center Department of Psychiatry 263 Farmington Avenue, LG066 Farmington, CT 06030–1935 860-679-8112 aadprt@psychiatry.uchc.edu http://www.aadprt.org/public/2004/ginsberg/index.html	December
AAGP/Fellowship in Geriatric Psychiatry	To increase interest among psychiatric residents in geriatric psychiatry and to provide them with a direct vehicle for participation in the AAGP. Also to identify future clinical/academic leaders in the field of geriatric psychiatry. Five 2-year fellowships are awarded to PGY-3 residents.	American Association for Geriatric Psychiatry AAGP Fellowship Selection Committee 7910 Woodmont Avenue, Suite 1050 Bethesda, MD 20814 301-654-7850, ext. 112 http://www.aagpgpa.org/prof/fellows.asp	December

TABLE 12–1. Fellowships and awards *(continued)*

Fellowship	Objective	Contact information	Deadline
APA Minority Fellowships Program	To provide recipients with enriching training experiences through participation in the APA fall and annual meetings; to provide recipients with resources to support activities that enhance culturally relevant aspects of their training program; to stimulate their interest in pursuing training in areas of psychiatry where minority groups are underrepresented, such as research, child psychiatry, and addiction psychiatry.	APA Minority Fellowships Program American Psychiatric Association 1000 Wilson Boulevard, Suite 1825, MS #1 2038 Arlington, VA 22209-3901 703-907-8653 mking@psych.org http://www.psych.org/edu/other_res/ apa_fellowship/cmhs_index.cfm	January

TABLE 12–1. Fellowships and awards *(continued)*

Fellowship	Objective	Contact information	Deadline
American Psychoanalytic Association Fellowship	Seeks outstanding psychiatrists (full-time general or child and adolescent psychiatry residents, PGY-2 or higher), psychologists, clinical social workers, and academics at various levels of training who are curious about how the mind works, consider psychoanalytic thinking important for the future of their professional disciplines, and are likely to become or already are leaders in their fields.	American Psychoanalytic Association 309 East 49th Street New York, NY 10017 212-752-0450, ext. 12 http://www.apsa.org/fellows	January
APA Committee of Residents and Fellows	For residents and fellows (one from each of the APA's seven geographical areas), who must be in training throughout their tenure on the committee and must be APA members; appointed by the APA president.	Nancy Delanoche APA Office of Education 1000 Wilson Boulevard, Suite 1825 Arlington, VA 22209-3901 703-907-8635 ndelanoche@psych.org http://www.psych.org/edu/resoper2.cfm	January

TABLE 12–1. Fellowships and awards *(continued)*

Fellowship	Objective	Contact information	Deadline
APA/Aventis Pharmaceuticals Travel Fellowship for Women Residents	To identify and nurture future women leaders in psychiatry.	APA/Aventis Women Residents' Travel Fellowship Program 1000 Wilson Boulevard, Suite 1825 Arlington, VA 22209-3901 703-907-8636 aventisfellowship@psych.org http://www.psych.org/mem_groups/women/AventisInfopage.cfm	January
APIRE/Janssen Research Scholars on Severe Mental Illness	To identify promising PGY-1, PGY-2, and PGY-3 psychiatry residents with the potential to become leaders in clinical and health services research into severe mental illness.	Ernesto A. Guerra, Project Manager American Psychiatric Institute for Research and Education/Janssen Resident Research Scholars 1000 Wilson Boulevard, Suite 1825 Arlington, VA 22209-3901 800-852-1390 eguerra@psych.org http://www.psych.org/edu/res_fellows/res_training/janssen.cfm	January
Indo-American Psychiatric Association	To recognize a PGY-3 resident of Indian origin (United States medical graduate or international medical graduate) with outstanding clinical and leadership skills.	Nalini V. Juthani, M.D. Bronx-Lebanon Hospital Center 1276 Fulton Avenue #4 South Bronx, NY 10456 781-901-8652; fax: 718-901-8656	January

TABLE 12–1. Fellowships and awards *(continued)*

Fellowship	Objective	Contact information	Deadline
Association of Academic Psychiatry (AAP)/Bristol-Myers Squibb Fellowship	For a PGY-3, PGY-4, or PGY-5 resident or fellow with a demonstrated interest in an academic career and ability as a teacher before and during residency. (Only AAP institution members may nominate fellows.)	AAP Executive Office Attn: Carole Berney 725 Concord Avenue, Suite 4200 Cambridge, MA 02138 617-661-3544; fax: 617-661-4800 cberney@caregroup.harvard.edu http://www.academicpsychiatry.org	February
Association of Women Psychiatrists (AWP)/Wyeth-Ayerst Fellowship	This fellowship is designed in keeping with AWP goals of developing leadership in women psychiatrists as well as contributing to the overall mission of improving the personal and professional future roles of women.	Association of Women Psychiatrists Wyeth-Ayerst Fellowship PO Box 570218 Dallas, TX 75357-0218 972-613-0985 womenpsych@aol.com	February
American Association for Emergency Psychiatry (AAEP)/Janssen Resident Award	To recognize residents demonstrating excellence in emergency psychiatry.	AAEP/Janssen Resident Award Selection Committee 15731 NE 105th Court Redmond, WA 98052-2640 425-556-5430 http://www.emergencypsychiatry.org	February

TABLE 12–1. Fellowships and awards *(continued)*

Fellowship	Objective	Contact information	Deadline
AACAP/Presidential Scholar Award	This award, sponsored by Bristol-Myers Squibb, recognizes specialized competence among child and adolescent psychiatry residents in research, public policy, and innovative service systems.	Jeffrey Newcorn, M.D., Chair Department of Research, Training, and Education American Academy of Child and Adolescent Psychiatry 3615 Wisconsin Avenue, NW Washington, DC 20016-3007 http://www.aacap.org/awards/pres.htm	March
APA/GlaxoSmithKline Fellowship Program	To select outstanding residents with a potential for leadership and to assign them to components of the APA where they may contribute the residents' point of view to the development of policy.	Marla Mitnick Office of Minority/National Affairs 1000 Wilson Boulevard, Suite 1825 Arlington, VA 22209-3901 703-907-8667 mmitnick@psych.org http://www.psych.org/edu/resoper2.cfm#glaxo	March
American Academy of Psychiatry and the Law/Rappeport Fellowship	Offers an opportunity for outstanding residents with interest in psychiatry and the law to develop their knowledge and skills.	Rappeport Fellowship Committee American Academy of Psychiatry and the Law One Regency Drive, PO Box 30 Bloomfield, CT 06002-0030 800-331-1389	April

TABLE 12–1. Fellowships and awards *(continued)*

Fellowship	Objective	Contact information	Deadline
APA/Bristol-Myers Squibb Fellowship Program	To provide experiences that will contribute to the professional development of residents who will play leadership roles within the public sector in future years; to heighten the awareness of psychiatry residents of the many activities and career opportunities in the public sector.	Beatrice Edner Office of Quality Improvement and Psychiatric Services 1000 Wilson Boulevard, Suite 1825 Arlington, VA 22209-3901 703-907-8598 bedner@psych.org http://www.psych.org/edu/resoper2.cfm	April
Jeanne Spurlock, M.D., Congressional Fellowship	Administered by the APA and the American Psychiatric Foundation, in collaboration with the AACAP, this fellowship provides general psychiatry and child psychiatry residents an opportunity to work in a congressional office or committee, on federal health policy, particularly related to child and minority issues.	Marilyn King APA Department of Minority/National Affairs 1000 Wilson Boulevard, Suite 1825 Arlington, VA 22209-3901 703-907-8653 mking@psych.org http://www.psychfoundation.org/awardsandfellowships/spurlock.cfm	May

TABLE 12–1. Fellowships and awards *(continued)*

Fellowship	Objective	Contact information	Deadline
AACAP/Robinson-Cunningham Award	This award recognizes a paper on some aspect of child and adolescent psychiatry. The paper must have been started during residency and completed within 3 years of graduation; preference is given to independent work.	Department of Research and Training American Academy of Child and Adolescent Psychiatry 3615 Wisconsin Avenue, NW Washington, DC 20016-3007 http://www.aacap.org/awards/rc.htm	June
Daniel X. Freedman, M.D., Fellowship Program	Provides an educational opportunity in the area of federal health policy through work experience in a congressional office.	Barbara Matos American Psychiatric Foundation 1000 Wilson Boulevard, Suite 1825 Arlington, VA 22209-3901 703-907-8517 bmatos@psych.org http://www.psych.org/edu/resoper2.cfm#freedman	June

CHAPTER 13

RECRUITMENT OF RESIDENTS

Sidney H. Weissman, M.D.

Nyapati Rao, M.D.

Recruitment of trainees into psychiatry initially consists of developing strategies to interest diverse populations of physicians and medical students.

Usually recruitment initially focuses on a given year's senior class of United States medical students. It also includes other groups of physicians. The total number of trainees from the non–United States seniors interested in psychiatry has varied markedly over two decades. This pool includes

- International medical graduates (IMGs). This group is further subdivided into United States citizens who have obtained their medical education outside the United States, naturalized United States citizens, and citizens of other countries in the United States on various visas.
- Transfers to psychiatric residencies. This group consists of physicians who transfer into psychiatric residencies while still in residency training in other medical fields. This group includes both United States medical graduates (USMGs) and IMGs.
- Practicing physicians. These are physicians in practice in varied specialties who plan on changing medical careers.
- Graduates of osteopathic medical schools.

Each group of potential trainees has special needs and interests. The recruitment of each group into a given residency calls for unique strategies for each category of potential trainees. Not all residencies attempt to attract members of each group. However, as the number of USMGs entering psychiatry residency in the July after they graduate from medical school has fluctuated, the reliance on other groups of potential trainees has increased. Today the majority of residency programs have some trainees from the non–United States senior student group. Each residency training director will need to know which groups of potential trainees are most likely to be interested in training in his or her program. After this, the training director must then develop recruitment strategies that relate to the identified groups. For effective recruitment of the non–United States senior group, it is possible and probably essential for programs to develop recruitment strategies to reach each of the groups that have been identified. The issue in developing recruitment strategies is not simply to develop a marketing or communication program but also to develop critical elements in the actual training program that focus on the needs of each group and to then communicate effectively with potential trainees. An initial successful marketing of a program without the capacity to deliver to trainees what was promised will, in the long term, adversely affect the program's survival.

In recent years, various models of physician workforce needs for the United States have been offered. In the late 1990s and at the start of the current decade, it was argued that a period of major physician surplus was beginning. By 2004, however, some were claiming that there will be a significant shortage of physicians, particularly of specialists. How many psychiatrists the country will need partly depends on the clinical responsibilities of the psychiatrist. Will future psychiatrists perform a broad array of services, or will they limit their practice to certain diagnostic groups and perform limited services, such as only medication management? In light of the President's New Freedom Commission on Mental Health (2003) report, we can anticipate at least public statements by government officials of a potential shortage of psychiatrists. However, these statements need not translate into additional dollars for training. Funding for psychiatric residency training will depend on the long-term future of how the federal government will fund graduate medical education through Medicare and how effectively psychiatry can support its case for enhanced funding of psychiatric education.

The final word is not yet in on the nation's future workforce requirements. Rather than a final definitive policy on the nation's medical workforce, there will be shifting policy statements. These will deal with the changing political and economic realities of medical practice, the nation's political agenda, and federal budgets. In this light, training directors in the next decade must be prepared to respond to shifts in funding when they occur in terms of the resources available to their programs and the unique needs of the community in which they are located. There will not be a one-size-fits-all recruitment strategy. Taking all variables into account, however, we expect that the number of psychiatric residency trainees at the beginning of the next decade may be similar to the numbers today. Considering a growth in population, this would represent a decrease in per capita numbers.

RECRUITMENT STRATEGIES

Certain issues in recruitment are the same for whatever group of potential trainees is being targeted. These are discussed briefly below.

1. *Structure*. The training director needs to clearly understand the strengths and weaknesses of his or her program. Together with the faculty and residents, the training director should conduct an in-depth review of the structure of the program. They should clarify and distinguish between educational and service requirements and make sure that there is an appropriate balance. Presumably the program has met the requirements of the Residency Review Committee (RRC) for Psychiatry, but because these guidelines are broad, what is acceptable to the RRC will not necessarily attract trainees. For example, how often are residents on call in the program compared with other programs in the region? What are the mix and length of rotations in different participating institutions in the program? What opportunities exist for research? What different electives are offered? All will meet RRC requirements, but the mix will determine how the program is perceived or how the training director wishes it to be perceived. There is no one right mix, but it is important to know how the residency is constructed and how this construction relates to the potential trainees who are being recruited.
2. *Morale*. Morale is determined by both the faculty and staff and the residents. It is essential for the training director to keep a close watch on the program's morale and act decisively with the department chair if morale is perceived to have declined. Alteration in morale in either group demands immediate attention. In many programs struggling with the complex issues created by managed care, faculty members find their time intruded on when they must alter their practices and research activities to enable their department to survive. This burden influences

their performance and morale. It is not the training director's task to simply put the best face on a bad situation. The department must not experience itself as being in a constant crisis. It must organize and reward its faculty so that as the department responds to diverse pressures, the faculty members—although they may not like all the changes that are occurring—feel that they are able to maintain their core identities as academic psychiatrists. Loss of the connection to the faculty's core identity will lead to alienation and a deterioration of morale among staff and faculty and the creation of a destructive environment for recruiting. Although it is impossible to have positive resident morale in the absence of positive faculty morale, positive faculty morale does not, in itself, ensure positive resident morale. Departments can be constructed to support faculty activities at the expense of residents' educational experience. Some departments attempt to base their economic survival or maintain their service responsibilities on the backs of residents' service. Some say that this approach is especially common in hospitals that predominantly train IMGs. If this is done it will quickly be learned by applicants. In a resident recruitment market in which trainees can potentially pick their program, programs that are perceived as using residents for service without a clear focus on education will have difficulty filling their positions. If those programs do fill their positions, it will be with trainees who were not accepted elsewhere. Besides examining the department's mission and resources and faculty involvement in sustaining morale, the training director should look at the diverse activities that involve the residents in the program in isolation from each other. Periodically all rotation, call schedules, call rooms, and classes must be reviewed to ensure that residents' needs are addressed. Finally, if morale is poor among residents, this will be immediately communicated to applicants when they interview at the program.

3. *Marketing.* It is with some reluctance that we address this issue. If an institution has a fine program, why must it market? Perhaps one problem is confusion between advertising, which is a form of marketing, and the general concept of marketing. Marketing of a residency program means making sure the potential groups of trainees that the program wishes to attract know about the existence of the program and its strengths. Each training director needs to determine the sources from which his or her program's trainees have been recruited, for approximately a 10-year period. The programs then need to assess whether they wish to alter their source of trainees or maintain their current position. Either way, depending on their location and resources, they must develop or maintain a strategy to ensure that potential trainees know what

the program is about. Sometimes this may mean reaching out to students from medical schools in other cities. Sometimes programs based in medical schools must develop special programs to reach their own students. It is not a given that the students in a particular medical school are aware of the strengths and values of the residency in their own school or its affiliate hospitals. Some programs have developed relationships with premier medical schools in foreign countries.

Special marketing issues exist for a residency that is not the residency of a medical school department of psychiatry. Even if the residency's hospital is affiliated with a medical school, it does not follow that the medical school's students will be encouraged to enter a residency at an affiliate. The affiliated hospital will need to establish its own relationship with the medical school's students. It will also be necessary for the freestanding program or affiliate hospital program to establish effective communication with other medical schools. When asked by students about residencies, medical school core faculty members will frequently suggest medical school programs but not others.

MARKET UNIQUENESS

The unique capabilities of a program are what makes that program special. All programs meet RRC requirements, but the training director must identify and communicate to potential residents and to medical school faculty members at other schools the special elements of his or her program that distinguish it from competitors. In a city with a number of programs, the training director must be able to communicate to applicants how his or her program differs from its peers. It is not necessary to claim that it is better than the others, but it is important to explain how it differs.

PROGRAM WEB SITE

Other than talking to a residency staff member or a current or former resident, the first direct connection by a potential applicant with a program is frequently through the written material describing the program. Today almost all departments of psychiatry and their training programs have Web sites. Some give detailed accounts of learning objectives, clinical rotations, and seminars, whereas others include friendly photos and general information. There is, of course, no strict formula governing what should be included on a Web site, but the training director must consider what he or she wants to communicate. If the department and program have a strong emphasis on teaching psychotherapy, this should be stated on the Web site.

If the program has special research electives or a research track, these should be clearly communicated on the Web site. The entire faculty should become involved in contributing what they feel are the strengths of the program, and the training director should make sure that these strengths are stated on the program's Web site. A good Web site will not ensure recruitment, but a poor presentation may result in a potential applicant deciding to apply elsewhere. The presentation of information on the Web site must be clear, and the information must match what applicants receive when they visit the program. The Web site must also be easy for applicants to find. The Web sites of psychiatry departments and residency programs are frequently buried inside hospital or medical school sites. The training director should test the site himself or herself and should ensure that it is current. It is important that potential applicants visiting the Web site be able to see that it is current and that it was updated immediately before the recruitment year.

ELECTRONIC RESIDENCY APPLICATION SERVICE

The Electronic Residency Application Service (ERAS), a program of the Association of American Medical Colleges (AAMC), was established to standardize the application process to residencies for graduating United States medical students and IMGs. Under this system, the student completes a series of standard forms. These forms, the dean's letter, letters of recommendation, United States Medical Licensing Examination (USMLE) scores, Educational Commission for Foreign Medical Graduates (ECFMG) information, and other data are sent by the dean's office of the student's medical school. In the case of IMGs, the ECFMG serves as their dean's office. The training director must become familiar with the workings of ERAS, because it will be the means of communication between applicants and the program. The graduate medical education office and the AAMC can provide more detailed information on the use of ERAS.

APPLICANT INTERVIEW AND PROGRAM PREVIEW

The interview of the applicant by the residency faculty offers the faculty the opportunity to assess the applicant's abilities. Interviews also offer the applicant an opportunity to preview the residency. It is this latter function that we discuss here. The qualified applicant wants to learn about the residency, including curriculum issues, the faculty, the program's residents, and its location, as well as the possibility for doing research. When applicants visit the program they must be given an opportunity to learn about each dimension of the program. The personal style and preference of the training director will determine how the interview day will be structured. An important aspect of the visit that is frequently ignored is the time the applicant spends with current residents in the program. Just as not all faculty members are effective applicant interviewers, not all residents can effectively interact with applicants. Selection of residents to meet with applicants is best done by the training director, who knows the strengths and weaknesses of each resident, not the chief resident or a secretary. If the program has a resident who has graduated from the applicant's medical school, it is useful to have that resident also meet with the applicant.

FACULTY INTERVIEW

Prior to the first faculty interview of applicants, the training director must meet with the faculty to review the purpose of the applicant interview process in terms of the needs of the applicants and the program. The training director then works with the faculty to develop criteria for assessing each of the applicants. The applicant assessment includes a report of the interview and all application material. A rating form and a means of ensuring that rating forms are returned to the training director are essential. The rating forms and any other relevant data are then reviewed with the faculty. Finally, faculty members are walked through a model interview day for an applicant.

The next stage of the faculty interview process requires a degree of diplomacy on the part of the training director. Not all faculty members are equally effective interviewers or evaluators of candidates. Furthermore, some may feel that they have special abilities as interviewers or may believe that they should use the interview to put stress on applicants to learn more about them. Others may feel that any aspect of the applicant's life is open for their review. Because of the nature of the field, knowledge of the potential resident's psychological functioning is indeed important; however, the training director must work with the faculty to ensure that interviews elicit only appropriate information in a supportive and legal fashion. Although stress-inducing interviews were once in vogue, they have no place in the assessment situation. Besides being inappropriate (and frequently breaking the law), such interviews will cause applicants to go elsewhere.

Periodically during the interview season from November to February, it is critical to meet with the faculty to begin rating applicants and to evaluate the effectiveness of the assessment process. At times, applicants will ask after the interview where they stand in your assessment. If you wish, you may tell a resident applicant that you will offer him or her a position; however, you may not request that the applicant commit to enrolling in your program. You should also keep in touch with any applicant whom you feel would do well in your program. Make sure that when applicants leave after their interviews, they know how to contact you and at least your chief resident. If one exists, a resident from the applicant's medical school is even better.

DUAL-CAREER COUPLES

Although a dual-career couple is any couple in which each partner has specific career needs, the term generally refers to couples in which both partners are graduating from medical school and are seeking residencies. Many of these couples will seek programs located in major metropolitan areas because of the broader career opportunities that are available for the nonpsychiatrist partner. Programs in large cities need to make few special arrangements for these applicants, but programs in smaller cities may need to offer assistance in a number of areas to successfully recruit these individuals. The degree of assistance will of course vary in each situation.

THE MATCH

The National Resident Matching Program (NRMP) serves as the route for connecting nearly all United States senior students and varying numbers of all other applicants with their residencies. Individual residencies do not sign contracts with the NRMP; rather, hospitals sign contracts to offer their first-year residency positions through a notification and selection system administered by the NRMP. When a hospital joins the Match, so do all of its residencies.

Senior United States students usually join the Match. When they join the Match, they may withdraw only under special circumstances. All other applicants to residencies may also utilize the Match. IMGs, for example, may enroll in the Match. However, unlike United States seniors, IMGs may withdraw at will from the Match. This is because, unlike with United States seniors, for whom the Match can enforce their continued enrollment through their medical school's dean, the Match has no such enforcement authority with regard to IMGs. Therefore, a program can offer a position to an IMG outside the Match and, if the applicant accepts, reduce the number of positions requested in the Match. Each program needs to assess its situation in deciding how to handle such matters. It is critical for training directors to monitor NRMP dates and policies so that if necessary they can alter any of their current procedures for compliance with the Match.

THE MATCH LIST

After all applicant interviews have been completed, it becomes necessary to rank the applicants and to prepare a Match list to send to the NRMP. The list is generally prepared during an extended faculty meeting in which all of the earlier ratings of applicants are reviewed. The training director is generally responsible for organizing these data and for developing a rating score for each applicant. Each program will of course have its own criteria. There is no "correct" set of criteria with which to score applicants. A score is developed for each candidate, and a cutoff score is established such that applicants with scores below this level will not be included on the Match List. The Match List should include only those applicants whom you believe could work in your program. If your list includes IMGs, it is important to determine that they have remained in the Match. As of Fall 2004, IMGs may obtain positions outside of the Match. One can perform an initial check through the NRMP. However, not every IMG who accepts a position may have informed the NRMP. For this reason, it is wise to e-mail or phone IMGs to be certain that they are still in the Match.

The rank-order list compiled in the faculty meeting is then sent to the NRMP. Some training directors prefer to "edit" the list. If the highest-ranked applicants on your list are not likely to enter your program, then even if you fill all of your positions, it may appear to some that your program is not as desirable as others in your hospital (because you had to go "down" on your Match list) and therefore that you have weaker residents. To avoid this perception, some training directors arbitrarily place superior applicants whom they do not believe will enter their program lower on their lists. Top spots are filled with applicants whom they believe are likely to come to their program. If they guess right, it will appear to the outside world that they indeed did well on the Match. We do not recommend this kind of manipulation; in the long run, it does not help applicants or programs, but instead subverts the integrity of the Match process.

PSYCHIATRY TRANSFER RESIDENTS

Although this discussion focuses on the recruitment of trainees directly into the psychiatry residency from medical school or from nonpsychiatric residencies or practice, the same general principles apply when addressing residents who are transferring from another program. Reasons for residents changing programs are diverse. The one essential element to be addressed when a resident wishes to transfer from another program is communicating directly with the training director of the other program. Although this communication is an RRC requirement, applicants may give reasons for the transfer that they do not want conveyed to their former training director. Although the situation may be difficult, this information is essential in evaluating the transferee. Of course, the information must be obtained in a tactful way that does not subject the potential transferee to undue pressure.

SPECIAL RECRUITMENT ISSUES

United States Senior Medical Students

Although they are generally the largest single group of potential trainees, United States senior medical students are the most difficult to recruit because they have the most options. All residencies will offer positions to qualified United States seniors. Following the general principles outlined will be essential for recruiting this pool of applicants.

For a medical school–based residency program, graduates of the parent medical school should constitute the first potential applicant pool. For programs that are not based in a medical school, links can be established by way of residents or faculty members, and other schools can be cultivated. Finally, it is important to remember that of all applicant groups, United States seniors are the most concerned about other residents in the program. They see these residents as their lifelong peers and friends. The training director should keep this in mind when talking about the career paths that are followed by graduates of the program.

An additional option that is available mainly to United States medical students is to complete an elective rotation in a hospital where they are considering applying for a residency. It is important that the training director work with the department's director of medical student education to ensure the success of these rotations. The training director must also make sure that while the students are on rotation in the hospital they learn about the residency. This is a good time for these students to attend classes with the residents.

United States Medical Graduates Who Are Not Currently Seniors

Whether graduates are currently in other residencies or are in practice, recruiting from this pool requires that the residency have flexibility in how residents can be scheduled into the program. For example, if an internist wishes to enter a program, how easily can the residency schedule a 2-month neurology rotation? The department secretary needs to be able to tell these potential applicants that the program is flexible.

RECRUITMENT AND SELECTION OF INTERNATIONAL MEDICAL GRADUATES

OBTAINING AND INTERPRETING ACADEMIC RECORDS, REFERENCE LETTERS, AND OTHER DATA FOR INTERNATIONAL MEDICAL GRADUATES

In this section we describe the strategies that we use to effectively evaluate IMGs. Many if not most of these strategies should also be employed in evaluating all applicants.

IMGs are by far the most difficult group to evaluate; therefore, we explore the IMG recruitment process in greater depth. IMGs are a diverse group culturally and linguistically. They come from very diverse medical education systems and at widely differing stages of their lives. United States training directors are frequently unfamiliar with ways of obtaining information about the applicants' medical school and their performance. There are certain basic data that the training director will find useful in assessing IMG applicants.

Because IMGs' reference letters may be bland and uninformative and the medical schools and their transcripts may appear unfamiliar, the training director may be tempted to rely heavily on qualifying exam scores in screening applicants to interview (Rao et al. 1991). However, other methods will yield important additional information (Rao et al. 1994):

1. IMG applicants should be asked to submit a focused autobiographical statement about themselves and their interest in psychiatry. Such statements can give a three-dimensional picture of the applicant. The statement will also provide a very quick assessment of the applicant's writing skills. The training director may talk to the applicant during the interview about the personal statement, which will fulfill a number of functions. It can verify that the statement is the applicant's own writing; it will provide openings for a deeper discussion of the applicant's life issues and path to psychiatry; and it will serve as a dynamic example of the applicant's communication skills.
2. Further information about language skill may be obtained by asking the applicant to discuss a favorite piece of English literature and to show any examples of creative writing (poems, essays, etc.).
3. The applicant may be asked to view a videotaped psychiatric interview and discuss it with the interviewer(s). This can provide a rich source of information about the applicant's language and communication

skills within the clinical and simulated supervisory setting, as well as offering a sample of the applicant's interpersonal observation skills.

4. In addition to the specific focus produced by the preceding techniques, the entire interview, including lunch with a current resident, provides material for assessing the applicant's interpersonal and communication skills.

5. Educating oneself about foreign medical education systems and specific schools requires input from many sources, because there is no single reliable, comprehensive source. The medical school can be looked up in the World Health Organization's (2000) *World Directory of Medical Schools.* We also suggest consulting the *International Medical Education Directory* (Foundation for Advancement of International Medical Education 2003; searchable through the ECFMG Web site, http://www.ecfmg.org). This publication provides up-to-date, comprehensive information about individual foreign medical schools that are approved by the regulatory agency in each country. We further suggest that training directors subscribe to *The ECFMG Reporter,* a free electronic newsletter periodically published by the ECFMG. This publication helps readers monitor complex visa and examination-related changes that pertain to IMGs. It may also be possible to ask colleagues and residents from other countries about the medical education system there and about particular schools. Training directors might also find some useful chapters in *International Medical Graduates in U.S. Hospitals* by Khan and Smith (1995).

6. For the many IMG applicants who have worked in health-related fields in the United States before applying to residency positions, it may be possible to obtain permission to question their supervisors about their performance. We do not favor only IMGs with American hospital experience. However, we have found that having an American hospital experience will make the IMG's orientation to the residency experience less problematic.

7. Training directors should become familiar with the issues and procedures involved in obtaining J-1 and H-1 visas. The section "Visa and Immigration Issues" below contains a more detailed discussion of visa issues.

8. A selection committee can be created composed of members who have all demonstrated good interviewing skills and sensitivity to IMGs' cultural issues and the phase-specific issues of immigration. Such a committee can be very helpful in educating its members to the cultural contrasts IMG applicants encounter in the United States with respect to formality/informality, confrontation/politeness, and individual-competitive versus group-cooperative norms.

9. It would be beneficial for each candidate to be seen by at least one interviewer who is familiar with the candidate's culture. This is very important in enabling the selection committee to interpret the interview data.

10. The average IMG applicant for a residency in psychiatry has been out of medical school longer than his or her USMG counterpart. The training director should assess the applicant's experience during these extra years with respect to gaining practical knowledge of medicine, biomedical research, and life in the United States. The director should also inquire about migrations from the applicant's home country to the United States.

11. The training director should assess the applicant's motivation for entering psychiatry, including the individual's knowledge of what the field is like in the United States, and his or her motivation for undertaking a second residency, if this is the case.

12. The applicant should be asked about any experiences with psychiatry or psychiatric patients. Many IMGs do not have as well-rounded an exposure to psychiatry in their undergraduate years as do USMGs. This is due to a lack of emphasis on psychiatry in foreign medical schools' curricula as a result of workforce and educational priorities determined by their societal needs. Thus an IMG may be applying for postgraduate training in multiple specialties. The training director will be challenged to choose the potentially good psychiatric resident from this group and avoid those who are just seeking an entry into the United States graduate medical education system.

13. The training director should assess the applicant's humanistic interests and degree of acculturation, and the status of any possible value conflicts relevant to the practice of psychiatry in the United States. For example, in the United States subcultures are characterized by a strong emphasis on individuality, whereas in many traditional societies loyalty to the group takes precedence over one's own individual needs and aspirations. Similarly, value judgments regarding religion, spirituality, sexuality, gender roles, and cross-generational ties in a family may cause conflicts for the IMG and must be explored in the interview.

14. Questioning candidates about immigration-related experiences and their feelings about the process they have gone through can be a very productive approach to obtaining a fleshed-out picture of the IMG applicant.

The preceding list outlines certain strategies that will help training directors choose the most qualified IMG for their program. It must be noted that the U.S. Equal Employment Opportunity Commission (EEOC) requires that no job applicant be asked questions about his or her national origin or marital status. Any questions asked or procedures used to assess an IMG must also be used to assess a USMG. Our recommendations follow the EEOC guidelines (see the EEOC Web site, http://www.eeoc.gov).[1]

Sometimes we are asked the question of whether there is a weighting or ranking of characteristics that will predict future performance. We have no research to suggest any differential weighting of these data, but we can offer an order based on our experience: A well-written autobiographical essay that fully describes the individual, passing the qualifying exam creditably in as few attempts as possible, previous training in psychiatry, medical school honors, American hospital or research experience, and freedom from significant psychopathology are usually associated with successful performance as a resident.

VISA AND IMMIGRATION ISSUES

The Accreditation Council for Graduate Medical Education permits foreign-born IMGs with provisional ECFMG certification to enter United States residency programs if they are naturalized citizens or if they hold a permanent resident (immigrant) visa, or either one of the temporary visas J-1 or H-1B (exchange visitor), or a federal work permit. Those possessing J-1 exchange visitor visas can enter only residency programs in medical school hospitals or hospitals affiliated with medical schools. The J-1 visa permits the candidate to reside in the United States to acquire medical training for a maximum of 7 years or until completion, whichever is shorter.

In addition, J-1 visa holders must obtain permission from their government to undertake training in a specialty that is in short supply in their na-

---

[1]Because of the requirements of the EEOC and to ensure fairness for all residency applicants, we asked a number of attorneys familiar with EEOC requirements to review our initial recommendations. Questions or procedures they felt might be perceived as violating EEOC guidelines were deleted from our final proposal. All EEOC fairness requirements apply to all applicants, USMGs or IMGs. No one can be asked questions about national origin or marital status. Any questions asked of an IMG must be asked of a USMG. One area of disagreement arose among our consulting attorneys. One felt that policies could be established for psychiatry residency applicants even if the in-depth review of performance was not followed in other departments for their residency applicants. Another attorney felt that the same general procedures must be standard throughout the institution. We urge that any protocols be reviewed by the institution's EEOC counselor before they are implemented.

tive country. They are also required to commit themselves to return to their native country after completion of training in the United States to practice their specialty for at least 2 years. Exemptions for this return rule are possible, but the procedures are extremely lengthy and costly and the outcome uncertain.

The H-1B visa was originally intended only for research activities, but it has recently been broadened to include clinical training. The H-1B visa permits candidates to undergo medical training without placing any restrictions on their length of stay in the United States. However, candidates must have passed the Federation Licensing Examination (FLEX) or Part 3 of the USMLE and must hire their own attorney to process the paperwork and follow through with a labor certification process with the U.S. Naturalization and Immigration Service. The training institution hiring a candidate must participate in the certification process. The H-1B visa can eventually be converted to permanent resident status without the need to exit the United States for a period of time, as the J-1 requires (Perlitsh 1997).

The changed security climate since September 11, 2001, requires that training directors closely monitor government immigration and visa policy. Policies in existence today are likely to be altered in upcoming years. It is also essential to learn how long it takes applicants in the local community to obtain the requisite visas. The length of time to obtain visas varies throughout the country.

QUALIFYING EXAMINATIONS

To undertake graduate medical education in the United States, an IMG must be certified by the ECFMG. ECFMG certification requires passing the qualifying examinations and documenting completion of educational requirements to practice medicine in the country where the applicant attended medical school. Most states in the United States require ECFMG certification for licensure.

The ECFMG exam includes a medical science exam and an English language proficiency test. Past medical science exams included the Visa Qualifying Exam (VQE), which was last administered in September 1983; the Foreign Medical Graduate Examination in the Medical Sciences (FMGEMS), last administered in July 1993; the National Board of Medical Examiners (NBME) exam, last administered in April 1992; and the FLEX, last administered in 1993. Currently, the USMLE is given to both USMGs and IMGs. Effective July 1998, to obtain a new ECFMG certificate all IMGs must successfully complete an additional examination. This is a Clinical Skills assessment that uses standardized patients and is administered by the ECFMG currently only in Philadelphia, Pennsylvania. (It should be noted that starting in 2005, a version of this exam will be required of all USMGs. The Clinical Skills exam for U.S. students is administered by the USMLE. For medical schools in which passing the USMLE written exams, including the Clinical Skills exam, is a requirement for graduation, the training director will also need to determine that each USMG has in fact passed all required exams. Failure to pass may mean the student does not graduate from medical school, even if he or she has been accepted to a program through the Match, and thus would not be able to start a residency.) Applicants may present with complicated permutations of these exams. For example, an applicant can be eligible for ECFMG certification by having passed a part of the FMGEMS and a part of the NBME exam or a part of the USMLE. As of 1993, the USMLE replaces all other qualifying exams, but IMGs who have passed the previous examinations and have acquired the provisional ECFMG certificate will still be eligible to enter residency training.

The ECFMG encourages training directors to verify an applicant's performance with the commission. The training director must also be aware that the ECFMG process of collecting documentation from the IMG's medical school will begin only after the IMG has passed the qualifying examination. This process can be subject to considerable delays from the applicant's medical school. If time is at a premium, it may be a useful practice to interview only candidates who have acquired the provisional ECFMG certificate and have a valid visa.

CONCLUSION

As noted in the introduction to this chapter, the future number of psychiatric residents in training in the United States will depend on the political resolution of the question of how many physicians the country needs and in what specialties. After a decade of projections claiming a national surplus of physicians, current data predict a major shortage of specialists, including psychiatrists—and, in particular, child psychiatrists. As this volume is being prepared, we have no answer to this question. We believe that the next decade will bring changes in the number of psychiatric trainees, as well as in the content and process of psychiatric education. For these reasons, it will become increasingly important for all of psychiatry to present the field as an exciting career opportunity to all United States and international medical students.

REFERENCES

Foundation for Advancement of International Medical Education: International Medical Education Directory. Philadelphia, PA, Foundation for Advancement of International Medical Education, 2003

Khan FA, Smith LG (eds): International Medical Graduates in U.S. Hospitals: A Guide for Program Directors and Applicants. Philadelphia, PA, American College of Physicians, 1995

Perlitsh SM: Negotiating the Immigration Maze (February 2005 edition). Available at: http://www.perlitsh.com/maze.htm. Accessed June 2005.

President's New Freedom Commission on Mental Health: Achieving the Promise: Transforming Mental Health Care in America. Final Report (DHHS Publ No SMA-03-3832). Rockville, MD, President's New Freedom Commission on Mental Health, 2003. Available at: http://www.mentalhealthcommission.gov/reports/reports.htm. Accessed July 11, 2004.

Rao NR, Meinzer AE, Primavera LH, et al: Psychiatric residency selection criteria for American and foreign medical graduates: a comparative study. Acad Psychiatry 15:69–79, 1991

Rao NR, Meinzer AE, Berman SS: Perspectives on screening and interviewing international medical graduates for psychiatric residency training programs. Acad Psychiatry 18:178–188, 1994

World Health Organization: World Directory of Medical Schools, 7th Edition. Geneva, World Health Organization, 2000

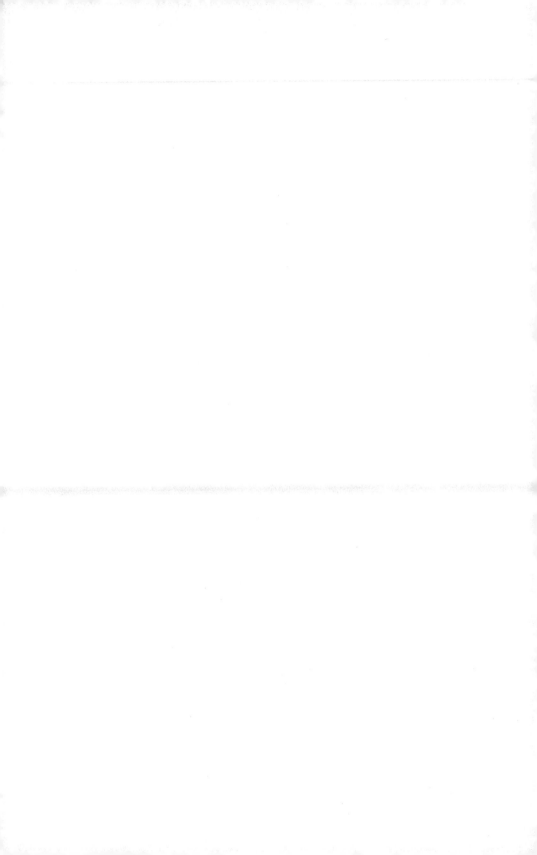

CHAPTER 14

MAJOR ISSUES IN PSYCHIATRIC EDUCATION

Joel Yager, M.D.

This chapter addresses some of the broad challenges confronting psychiatric educators in the foreseeable future and attempts to provide perspective on potentially adaptive responses to opportunities and barriers that lie ahead. Most of my comments focus on training psychiatric residents, but many apply to medical student education as well, and for good measure I further consider medical student education in later sections.

The turbulences affecting medicine as a whole and psychiatry in particular are heavily impacting psychiatric education. Some long-standing doctrines of psychiatric education are likely to stand the test of time and endure, while others will not. In examining strengths, weaknesses, opportunities, and threats (the classic "SWOT" analysis), we need to avoid kidding ourselves, to brutally examine underlying pedagogical assumptions, and to deconstruct our automatic catchphrases to challenge and get beyond them if necessary. In Postman's words (Postman and Weingartner 1969), we need to think with our best "crap detectors" and raise provocative questions to uncover mindless beliefs and empty rituals that fuel pedagogical inefficiencies we can ill afford. Along the way, we'll encounter numerous questions begging for educational research.

To start a strategic analysis, it pays to reexamine who we are and what we're trying to accomplish. These basic management questions are often posed as "What is our business?" "What are our products?" "What are we trying to market?" and "Who are our customers?" (Drucker 1993). We're pretty safe in assuming that our primary customers are always our patients and their families and that our business is enabling general physicians, psychiatrists, and other providers we educate and train to help patients and families make health choices, cope and contend with their illness, minimize their impairment and suffering, and maximize their well-being. To figure out how to effectively accomplish these goals for future practice, let's consider the following:

- What will psychiatric services look like in the future?
- How will scientific advances shape practice?
- What will psychiatrists and nonpsychiatric physicians need to know?
- How should psychiatric residents and medical students be educated?
- Who will pay for it all?
- How will we maintain professional satisfaction?

WHAT WILL PSYCHIATRIC SERVICES LOOK LIKE IN THE FUTURE?

While cottage-industry, individual private practice fee-for-service psychiatry will continue to exist in some fashion and in some markets, major forces fashioning managed care systems will increasingly define inpatient care and, for many, outpatient services as well. Most people will continue to receive their psychiatric medication and other treatment for psychiatric disorders from primary care physicians and other nonpsychiatrist providers. As in the past, it is likely that health care in America will basically correspond to the four levels that exist today: top care (out of pocket); "good enough" care (hopefully for many); "not enough" care, for perhaps most; and, unfortunately, "little or no" care, for far too many.

Even as official managed care companies may seem less relevant to a considerable amount of outpatient psychiatric practice, pressures to contain medical expenditure costs at a societal level as well as at the level of the individual pocketbook will result in care systems inexorably shaped by constraint pressures. Forces shaping these practice patterns can be envisioned as the *new* "Four A's" of psychiatry. Services will be favored that maximize *affordability*, keeping costs down; *accessibility*, offering convenience with respect to time and geography; *accountability*, offering demonstrable health benefits and good outcomes; and *affability*, offering patient satisfaction with providers and their staffs. As psychiatric educators, how focused are we on emphasizing the importance of these four A's and instilling them as core values in our trainees? *Accountability* presumably dovetails nicely with emphases on outcomes research and evidence-based practice. At least we're headed in the right directions there. But to what extent is our medical student teaching designed to most closely follow the epidemiology of clinical problems students are likely to encounter in their practices? To what extent do we foster *affability*—for example, a customer service zeitgeist—in our clinical teaching about relationship building with patients and families and in our institutions?

What about the future of the psychiatric workforce? Although previous workforce estimates using managed care models forecast an excess of psychiatrists (e.g., the 1995 Pew Commission predicted a 70+% excess [Pew Health Professions Commission 1995]), psychiatrists continue to be in reasonably high demand in most locations; subspecialists in child and adolescent psychiatry, geriatric psychiatry, and addiction psychiatry are currently in extremely high demand everywhere. The extent to which these demands will continue will depend in some degree on the demonstrable added value of psychiatric specialists in relation to other emerging "providers," a circumstance that promises Darwinian interplays of competitive and cooperative forces acting in the marketplace. What about the potential evolution of larger numbers of prescribing psychiatric nurse practitioners, or even prescribing psychologists? What long-term impacts can we anticipate from the steadily increasing "female-ization" of the psychiatric resident workforce, with women now accounting for more than 50% of trainees? Obvious effects on workforce availability and modification may result from competing family and child-rearing needs. How will training programs be modified by ever-increasing rates of intraresidency childbearing? Will there be other results of female-ization, leading to a kinder, gentler psychiatry? What about the increasing difficulty for international medical graduates to train in the United States? Can one imagine international outsourcing of psychotherapy practice via e-technology, employing English-speaking therapists in distant lands to care for our patients over broadband computer links? Is international outsourcing of psychotherapy an entrepreneurial idea waiting to happen?

HOW WILL SCIENTIFIC ADVANCES SHAPE PRACTICE?

THE NEW CURRICULUM

From the perspective of a SWOT analysis, scientific advances feeding contemporary psychiatry clearly represent major strengths. The emergence of better science to inform our evidence base, create new paradigms and theories, and improve treatments is downright exciting, all across the biopsychosocial map. How well are today's psychiatric educators doing at integrating important developments of the past few decades into the contemporary curriculum?

For example, contemporary understanding of biology, psychology, and social systems requires some familiarity with complex adaptive systems, emergence, and self-organization in biological and social systems (Johnson 2001; Kauffman 1995). The complex interplay of biology, developmental psychology, and psychopathology is perhaps best illustrated by recent research detailing quantitatively predictable effects of "long" or "short" polymorphisms of genes controlling certain serotonin receptors. These polymorphisms differentially affect how early and later adverse life events shape the subsequent appearance of depressive symptoms, depressive disorders, and suicidality in young adults. Individuals with one or two copies of the short allele of the 5-HTT promoter polymorphism exhibit more depressive symptoms, diagnosable depression, and suicidality in relation to stressful life events than do individuals homozygous for the long allele (Caspi et al. 2003). Similarly, binge-eating behaviors and binge-eating disorder among severely obese individuals have been related to melanocortin 4 receptor gene mutations (Branson et al. 2003). These and other findings are heralding an era in which psychiatry may find itself moving from the "polymorphous perverse" paradigm associated with classic psychoanalysis to a "polymorphism perverse" model, in which much more sophisticated perspectives on life events, early development, and genetic vulnerabilities interplay to generate psychiatric difficulties.

Of great intrinsic interest to many psychiatric aspirants, new paradigms that consider how specific brain processes may relate to consciousness, "mind," and personality are emerging, most anchored in scientifically derived observations such as those of Edelman (Edelman 1992; Edelman and Tononi 2000) and Damascio (1994, 1999). To what extent are we teaching these models and the neuroscience base necessary for appreciating this work?

How well are we teaching emerging perspectives in developmental neurobiology, affect regulation and attachment theory (Schore 1994, 2003), behavioral genetics (Kendler et al. 2004; Plomin and McGuffin 2003), and developmental behavioral neurobiology (Snider and Swedo 2004)? Although incompletely worked out and likely to be modified in the future, all of these "stories" deserve "airtime" and critical consideration by today's trainees. Discoveries in molecular genetics related to vulnerabilities to specific psychopathological states and their implications for clinical pharmacology are likely to become important aspects of scientific education for psychiatry (Anguelova et al. 2003; Arbelle et al. 2003; Malhotra et al. 2004). For example, vulnerability to bipolar disorder has been linked to polymorphisms of the G protein receptor kinase 3 gene (Barrett et al. 2003), and susceptibility to weight gain from clozapine (Reynolds et al. 2003) has been linked to certain serotonin transporter promoter region polymorphisms. The field of clinical pharmacogenetics is just beginning (see The Pharmacogenetics and Pharmacogenomics Knowledge Base [http://www.pharmgkb.org]). How well are psychiatric educators laying the ground for trainees to expect to fill in future factoids on these broad schemes?

Similarly, although not yet meriting widespread clinical application, progress in functional brain imaging is likely to advance to the point where we will be able to see the mind boggle. Inexpensive diagnostic tests using quantitative electroencephalography–based complex algorithms may provide bedside tools for prospectively distinguishing true medication responders, placebo responders, and nonresponders to psychiatric medication and electroconvulsive therapy (Cook et al. 2002; Leuchter et al. 2004). To what extent are trainees being introduced to these tools, their capabilities, and their limitations?

DIAGNOSTIC PSYCHOPATHOLOGY

Despite the useful features of the categorical and purely phenomenological approaches of the American Psychiatric Association's *Diagnostic and Statistical Manual of Mental Disorders*, versions III through IV-TR (American Psychiatric Association 1980, 1987, 1994, 2000), their substantial limitations are well appreciated and should be known by trainees. Accordingly, trainees should be familiar with efforts already under way to derive a DSM-V that better incorporates new information regarding biological and developmental contributions to pathogenesis, dimensional aspects of clinical phenomenology, functional impairment, and cultural factors, among other features. We may see fuzzy logic playing a greater role in diagnostic assessments (Modai et al. 2004; Yin and Chiu 2004). *Fuzzy logic*, you will recall, refers to highly mathematical methods for using (Boolean) logic in ways that have been extended to handle the concept of partial truths—truth values between "completely true" and "completely false" (Kosko 1993). Today's trainees need to be prepared for these upcoming paradigm shifts so that they don't entirely lose their bearings when the diagnostic world next changes (Helzer and Hudziak 2002; Kupfer et al. 2002).

PSYCHOLOGY, CLINICAL PSYCHOPATHOLOGY, AND PSYCHOLOGICAL THEORY

When today's psychiatric educators present broad "theories of the mind," which ones should they choose, and within what frameworks should these theories be presented and discussed (Millon 2004)? As history, Freud and his followers—other psychoanalytic theorists, Jung, Pavlov, Skinner, and other pioneers—make for good stories. But they all involve flawed and inadequate scientific theories, so that presentations of their ideas, and those of other "big thinking" theorists, demand discussions applying as much critical and skeptical thinking as we can muster, with full consideration of their serious critics such as Crews (1995) and Grünbaum (1984). But we don't want to throw out the baby with the bathwater. How well do today's psychiatric educators extract pearls from manure? Even the most "scientific" psychological assessment tools on which many of us were brought up a generation ago, such as the Rorschach and many other standardized psychological tests, are now known to have feet of clay and to be so scientifically flawed as to be clinically worthless (Paul 2004; Wood et al. 2003). In fact, all of these literatures require keen scientific deconstruction—and propaganda analyses, as described below.

Contrasting with the decreased emphasis on several of these formerly revered meta-psychological theories, certain basic themes are core to the framework of clinical practice and remain staunchly within the educational canon: stress, coping, adaptation, regression, resistance, transference, countertransference, social modeling, operant and classical conditioning, varying levels of conscious awareness, complex motivations, intersubjectivity, and developmental aspects of personality, including temperament and attachment (Mohl et al. 1990). Certain descriptive theories of human motivations and needs (Maslow 1987) and of cognitive (Flavill et al. 2001), life stage (Erikson 1980; Levinson 1978), and cultural development (Rogoff 2003) also retain some utility and can provide valuable conceptual schemas for clinicians attempting to make sense of clinical observations. Contemporary psychoanalytic researchers whose rigorous methods attempt to operationalize elusive cognitive styles and shifting ego states also merit consideration (Horowitz 1998).

In my view, several other contemporary ideas deserve attention, along with careful critical scrutiny. Based on observational studies and animal and social–psychological experiments, and serving to complement and counterpoint several psychoanalytic and family systems schools of the past century, hypotheses broadly based on evolutionary psychology and evolutionary psychiatry (i.e., theories attempting to explain how evolutionary pressures shaped genetic and cultural factors driving brain and behavior patterns in relation to adaptive success for individuals and groups) merit study (McGuire and Troisi 1998; Stevens and Price 2000; R. Wright 1995). These approaches may generate useful and increasingly testable clinical predictions based on resource availability and allocation, rank and status, mate selection and availability, power, deception, and related issues.

The curriculum can also benefit from attention to other generative literatures in clinical and social psychology. Family systems concepts retaining clinical value include those describing boundaries, structures, power relationships, family dynamic interactions, and expressed emotion, among others, and should be known by trainees (Nichols and Schwartz 2003). Interesting—if somewhat cartoonlike—models of "transactional analysis" analyzing interpersonal transactions in marriages, families, and other dyads, triads, and groups may still offer useful clinical frameworks (Berne 1961, 1996) and are occasionally taught by iconoclastic and clinically inventive psychiatrists. *Games People Play* (Berne 1996) described not only games that *patients* play, but also games played by clinicians, administrators, colleagues, and institutions. Similarly, perspectives concerning healthy and dysfunctional group and organizational dynamics (Jaques 1998; Osland et al. 2000) and group therapies (White and Freeman 2000; Yalom 1995) may be applied to institutional and administrative pathologies as well as traditional clinical settings. To what extent do psychiatric educators now attend to any of these concepts? Over the past several decades, trainees have received far less instruction in these areas than previously, and I consider that an educational loss.

Equally pertinent to our trainees, the impressive, evidence-based literature of social psychology offers an array of effective interpersonal influencing and persuading techniques, core skills required by general physicians as well as psychiatrists to heighten interpersonal attraction and rapport, foster motivational enhancement, increase the likelihood of adherence with both somatic and behavioral aspects of treatment, and contribute to symptom reduction (Kanfer and Goldstein 1991). Given that so many of these interactions inevitably occur in therapeutic encounters, often outside the awareness of both clinicians and patients and without appreciation for how subtle and effective they may be, trainees deserve to be explicitly taught about them.

PSYCHOTHERAPIES

Considerable controversy exists regarding the "what" and "how" of psychotherapy training for contemporary general psychiatrists. In part, these controversies derive from basic differences in the field regarding conceptions of what today's and tomorrow's psychiatrists actually do—or should do—in practice. Like "red states" and "blue states" in recent political elections, "red zones" and "blue zones" exist within and across academic departments and practicing psychiatric factions, delineating profound, almost cultural differences of opinion regarding what role psychotherapy training and practice should have in our profession. These long-standing historical differences were known and studied decades ago (Armor and Klerman 1968), and they are being continually challenged and updated by changing practice patterns. To what extent do current general psychiatrists actually conduct group or family psychotherapy or intensive psychoanalytically oriented psychotherapy as part of routine practice? How well do today's psychiatric educators align education and training to the real demands that practitioners will face in practice? And to what extent should the psychotherapies we teach general psychiatrists be aligned with the realities of reimbursement and practice patterns and require reasonable evidence for their effectiveness? As an aside, parallel questions concern the availability of psychiatrist psychotherapy teachers, now and in the future. To what extent do constraints and clinical productivity pressures imposed by today's academic practice plans reduce the amount of intensive psychotherapy conducted by full-time academic psychiatrists? To what extent will these forces reduce the numbers of skilled psychiatrist psychotherapy teachers and supervisors available to residents and medical students?

Regardless, the curriculum will always require that we *educate* trainees in the principles of psychotherapeutic relationships and management—the key elements of all psychotherapies (Karasu 2001)—as well as the principles of psychodynamic, interpersonal, cognitive, family, and other effective psychotherapies. Intelligent education should always embrace dissection and critical analyses of the core issues in psychotherapy research (Lambert 2004). Psychotherapy training cannot be faith based (nor, for that matter, can pharmacology training).

At the same time, current community standards in medical education require that our *training* programs mandate familiarity and hands-on experience with those psychotherapeutic approaches, packaged as "treatment manuals," that have been demonstrated to have clinical efficacy in controlled trials. We know, of course, that these manuals are at best crude guides to treatment, far from actual protocols (Parker et al. 2003). The "noise" variance in how different clinicians actually "deliver" these treatments undoubtedly often exceeds the treatments' replicability in the hands of diverse practitioners. Nowadays, such manualized approaches include interpersonal psychotherapy (IPT), cognitive-behavioral therapy (CBT), supportive therapies, short-term psychodynamic psychotherapies, and dia-lectical behavior therapy, among others. Not currently mandated by the Residency Review Committee (RRC) for Psychiatry of the Accreditation Council for Graduate Medical Education (ACGME) but equally worthy of attention are some marital and group therapies in the extended reading list. For example, in controlled trials, some CBT-oriented marital therapies have proven more effective than individual therapies for patients with uni-polar depression related to marital discord, and several CBT and IPT group approaches have been shown to be comparable in effectiveness to individual therapies in treating some disorders.

CRITICAL THINKING

We all need to respect the value—and the limitations—of so-called evidence-based medicine, a fashionable buzzword that bears careful deconstruction. Who can argue with incontrovertible evidence? Nonetheless, intelligent education requires that we understand the limitations of what is being sold as evidence based. For example, thoughtful evidence-based reviews, based on the compilation of systematic reviews requiring detailed evidence tables, can yield significantly divergent bottom-line interpretations of the data they've considered. We know that physicians develop most of their practice habits by listening to "influence leaders" or "thought leaders"—those teachers, super-visors, colleagues, and, in some instances, pharmaceutical representatives they most respect and admire (Corrigan et al. 2001). The truth is, we might be approaching "evidence informed" clinical decision making, but to believe that we can currently make most clinically complex decisions entirely on the basis of scientific evidence is a bridge too far.

How well do psychiatric educators foster trainees' critical thinking about the information they receive from these oral and written sources? How well do we teach trainees to be alert to marketing spin and propa-ganda—not only from organized industry, but also from virtually all seg-ments trying to push their opinions, including proponents of various psy-chotherapies? There's lots of snake oil in the world, and considerable effort is being expended to get into physicians' minds and wallets. Trainees are often "babes in the woods" who need some degree of psychological immu-nization to enable them to handle the onslaught (Wilkes and Hoffman 2001).

Inherent in much of what I've said is the *educational* need to foster an atmosphere of critical, skeptical thinking. As marketers and writers become increasingly sophisticated in manipulating words, statistics, and research design—and as clinicians catch on to the techniques to which they're being subjected—something of a fox-and-hounds coevolution is occurring in the development, diffusion, utilization, and ultimate effectiveness of these sales techniques. Enabling trainees to finely hone their critical discernment here goes far beyond the typical "evidence-based medicine" courses, which focus primarily on research design and the evaluation of published studies. Trainees need to see themselves as targets of aggressive influencing techniques directed toward them by marketing mavens, pharmaceutical detail representatives, industry-supported academic speakers, and zealots of any theoretical background who claim to possess the revealed word on theory and therapy (Pratkanis and Aronson 2001). Their influencing methods often incorporate body language, nonverbal and nonlexical cueing, and other "hidden persuader" techniques. The techniques emanate from fields as diverse and ancient as proselytizing by religions and cults and coercive persuasion–brainwashing to modern marketing research. Similarly, educating trainees to learn how to read between the lines of medication studies designed by industry may be built into the curriculum as serious fun, through seminars constructed primarily to thoughtfully poke holes in assigned journal articles, classic books and essays, and so forth. Although these exercises may be initially demoralizing, they ultimately empower by sharpening critical and skeptical appraisal competencies and sensitizing trainees for their entire careers.

HOW SHOULD PSYCHIATRIC RESIDENTS AND MEDICAL STUDENTS BE EDUCATED?

Louis Jolyon West, M.D., a major figure in twentieth-century American psychiatry, architect of the phenomenal growth and success of the UCLA Neuropsychiatric Institute and its Department of Psychiatry and Biobehavioral Sciences, understood what it takes to educate competent thinkers and train competent practitioners in psychiatry. "All you need," he'd say, following the tradition of his own teachers at the Payne Whitney Clinic at Cornell Medical School of the late 1940s, "are your patients, your supervisors, and a good library." This simple prescription embodies the fundamental principles of "contemporary" adult education—problem-based, case-based, and "just in time" learning. Deep wisdom from half a century ago. Since then, what have we done to muck things up?

For one, we've piled on lots of expectations for didactic teaching and coursework that take a lot of time away from "just in time" learning and from what might otherwise be discretionary time. What we teach in formal didactic seminars is rarely what trainees need to know immediately to understand and best care for their patients du jour. What we teach at those times may be valuable, but not necessarily as valuable as permitting the trainee to read up on specific concerns of the moment and to quickly review those issues with an informed supervisor. Yet we now require 70% attendance at seminars, a requirement that even most medical students won't tolerate. The 70% attendance requirement is meant to ensure that residency programs actually set aside teaching time, because some regulators thoughtfully fear that in the absence of such a requirement some programs might simply swamp trainees with work and effectively sabotage a meaningful didactic curriculum. The flip side, of course, is that requiring time-based participation does not guarantee meaningful learning. How might educators more creatively ensure that programs provide necessary learning time for trainees, without resorting to infantilizing sign-in practices? To what extent are we effectively teaching or simply ritualizing the long laundry list of curriculum topics embedded in today's RRC program requirements? Is attendance at prepared lectures by faculty or other residents the best way to learn? What better sorts of just-in-time, problem-based learning matrices should we be devising to make certain that core topics are covered? How might learning portfolios be used to document meaningful learning? And to what extent might RRC reviewers accept these alternative teaching approaches in lieu of formal topic-based lectures and seminars? To what extent are we thinking through and figuring out which topics lend themselves best to which sorts of active teaching methods?

We also know that learners do best if they are obliged to contrast and compare sometimes diverging "facts" obtained from multiple sources, so that they are stimulated to evaluate the quality of their sources. Accordingly, expecting trainees, individually or as a group, to utilize several texts and articles rather than a single source to cover a given topic will better reveal inconsistencies, gaps, and errors in the field.

READING

Do we have any idea how much trainees actually read and absorb? Or what they really find useful? Most busy practitioners learn much of what they use by reading review articles, abstract digests (Williamson et al. 1989), and, increasingly, abstracts available online via PubMed or WebMD, not complete journal articles.

What's a reasonable reading assignment for busy residents and medical students? Some insightful house officers have proposed that "xeroxing is the moral equivalent of reading," recognizing that the amount of *stuff* handed out and "assigned" always far exceeds the time available to ingest and assimilate knowledge on paper. Authors of large, substantial textbooks have quickly realized that they need to downsize their books to suit their audiences. Consequently, every major text is now accompanied by an "Essentials of...," further reduced to "Concise Guide to...," even further reduced to "Pocket Guide to...," and finally, "Psychiatry: The Postage Stamp." The "...Made Ridiculously Easy" series has been extremely popular among medical students and residents, promising easy reading requiring little or no need to think. How well do overwrought or sleep-deprived trainee brains focus on, attend to, absorb, retain, and process how many pages of what types of reading assignments, and to what end? Is assigning original research articles the best way to transmit knowledge? Or should such articles be reserved for razor-sharp critical thinking–oriented journal clubs? The deeper question is: In the finite amount of time available, and given the average throughput and carrying capacity of the average (or even above-average) trainee's brain, how can we optimize trainee learning through reading? Knowing the limits, faculty need to diligently prescreen and sift resource material before making offhand reading assignments. Of course, residents should be strongly encouraged to follow their own noses with respect to reading—to track down what they most need, when they most need it.

Along these lines, how engagingly do psychiatric scholars and educators write? How soporific is it to actually sit down and read what we're supposed to be reading, the myriad of ho-hum books and journals that come our way? While acknowledging that journal articles primarily archive new knowledge and provide print outlets for faculty obliged to publish to stave off perishing, trainees still hope that their late-night readings will not outperform medications designed for hypnotic effectiveness.

INSTRUCTIONAL INFORMATICS IN THE NEAR AND DISTANT FUTURE

Demands to increase both efficiency and effectiveness of teaching and learning (and pressures to deal with reduced educational budgets, of course) will undoubtedly push educators and learners to further utilize Web-based instruction. Web resources may enable trainees to "test out" and "certify" knowledge and "competencies" in various specific topics and fields, far more efficiently and economically than today. Online examinations linked to the American Psychiatric Association practice guidelines, for example, may acceptably demonstrate to certifying agencies that trainees have mastered desirable bodies of knowledge regarding the management of key clinical conditions. National training curricula developed by task forces in organizations such as the American Association of Directors of Psychiatric Residency Training (AADPRT), the Association of Directors of Medical Student Education in Psychiatry (ADMSEP), the Association for Academic Psychiatry (AAP), and subspecialty groups such as the American Society of Clinical Psychopharmacologists (ASCP), for specific topic areas, such as ethics, critical reading, psychopharmacology, and others, may be posted online, and trainees may be expected to complete certain modules prior to sitting down with faculty and peers in their own program's seminars. In these instances, local programs may use seminar time to clarify, supplement, provide local context, or apply to trainee's specific cases what has been learned from the national curriculum. For departments lacking faculty expertise in certain areas, such curriculum material may be a boon. As multimedia teaching material with video clips and interactive options becomes increasingly available in the future, educators will have to determine which curriculum components best lend themselves to independent Web-based learning; which absolutely require face-to-face, hands-on, or classroom interactions; what hybrids are most sensible; and what time, financial costs, and social advantages and disadvantages Web-based learning imposes.

Useful multimedia and online tools for psychotherapy training are already available for CBT. For a manualized CBT approach to the treatment of depression, for example, Jesse Wright and colleagues have recently published a CD-ROM program called "Good Days Ahead" (see http://www.mindstreet.com). At MySelfHelp.com, trainees and patients may find programs for the CBT treatment of depression (in English and Spanish), bulimia nervosa, posttraumatic stress disorder, and other conditions. Other forms of psychotherapy training will undoubtedly be offered via DVD and online as well.

Medical informatics is likely to alter psychiatric training in several other ways as well. At the simplest levels, future editions of textbooks are likely to increasingly include CD-ROMs hypertext-linked to Web sites containing illustrative video clips and other interactive teaching materials (Von Holzen 2005). Information technologies and expert systems technologies already entering some psychiatric practices offer computer-assisted diagnosis and treatment-planning algorithms and computer-facilitated expert systems interviews. Projects to develop virtual patients for psychiatric training are under development, using increasingly sophisticated Hollywood- and Silicon Valley–style avatars similar to those being continually improved for lifelike animations used in films and video games (Huang and Alessi 2001).

Just as some simple phobias may already be amenable to treatment via virtual-reality and simulation paradigms (Martijn et al. 2002), virtual-reality simulators may be developed for training purposes. Not too far off are interactive forms of interpersonal and dyadic dynamic training modeled on the methods of the Electronic Arts/Maxim company's incredibly popular series of social simulation and interpersonal interaction games (e.g., SIM City; see http://www.maxim.com or http://www.ea.com). SIMs promise to offer therapy simulators through which trainees might actually develop, polish, receive supervision in, and demonstrate psychotherapy competencies not possible in actual clinical settings. SIM psychopathology should not be too hard to evolve from current programs.

GRAND ROUNDS

Grand rounds in academic departments currently serve multiple social as well as strictly pedagogical purposes, bringing faculty and residents together (or at least those able to get away from clinical services and who believe that their time will be somewhat well spent in a passive mode), and in some instances providing lunch (and free pens). With gradual decrements in pharmaceutical funding to support calories and speakers, departments may increasingly be forced to rely on their own resources to provide these resources, even to consider "potluck" methods for both meals and wisdom. In fact, for those departments not already doing so, these sessions provide excellent opportunities for faculty and trainees to offer upscale show-and-tell sessions—for example, by asking senior faculty members who specialize in particular areas to present critical reviews of what their journals are reporting and what their fields have accomplished in the past year. Integrating journal clubs with grand rounds may serve several functions. Topics ranging from "What's new in the assessment and treatment of schizophrenia?" to "What's new in psychodynamic psychotherapy?" not only may show that faculty are keeping on their toes but also may help others in the audience. Increasing reliance on honorarium-free (or modest-fee) regional faculty trades between academic centers might accomplish a good deal of what star power and heavily subsidized grand rounds have previously achieved.

ASSESSMENT

The "competency–industrial complex" (Summers and Tracy 2001; D. Wright 1998) has achieved a sustained toehold in mainstream medical education, and we can safely predict that psychiatric educators will be required to wrestle with developing methods sufficient to satisfy the assessment beast's ever-increasing appetite for what passes for quantitative and qualitative method–rituals, if not authentic, reliable, and valid ways of demonstrating competence. Educators are still puzzling out what the basic required competencies entail and how they should be assessed. Try defining—let alone deconstructing—"systems-based competence," one of the "holy six" implemented by the ACGME for all postgraduate training. (From my perspective, *systems-based competency* may be operationally defined as knowing how to survive in the face of mind-numbing bureaucratic regulatory requirements that face patients, families, and clinicians.) How might consensus groups of psychiatric educators best come together to operationally define these core competencies for psychiatric training?

No doubt, demonstrating that trainees have actually learned and can do things in acceptable fashion has something to be said for it. Demonstrating such achievements without tying ourselves up in meaningless rituals or wasting precious time and resources in the effort is another matter. Detectors on full alert, please. Some educators would judge trainees to be acceptably "competent" if they aren't put on probation and don't get kicked out of the program. This isn't rocket science. Test trainees for the specific areas of knowledge you care about. Oral exams are always better than written exams, because trainees actually need to show that they can think and reason on their feet. Knowing how to take multiple-choice tests or to write essays using cut-and-pastes obtained via Google are less important skills. If specific skills are to be measured, trainees should document that they have in fact had the prerequisite clinical experiences by keeping records of their experiences. Faculty (or senior residents) should be able to observe and query trainees regarding these patients, read their write-ups, and ascertain that they understand what they were doing right and what they might have done wrong. For psychotherapy competencies, for example, listening to tapes and reviewing a "processfolio" of the trainee's work with a patient may be the most practical method available to us (Yager and Kay 2003).

Formal assessment poses several significant challenges: proving the reliability and validity of the assessment methods, showing that the assessments we do actually translate into competent performance in the real world, and having to do all of this without breaking the bank in terms of faculty and trainee time, administrative resources, and costs. The fact is, many of the ideas about assessment of psychiatric competencies sound great in theory but fall flat in practice when examined at all critically. While particular faculty members at some institutions may elect to devote their scholarly energies to developing new and improved methods of measurement and assessment (and in the process get all their names on published papers, and so get promoted, the primary reason for doing these activities), what's the average program to do? Here are some survival-oriented suggestions:

- Obtain copies of methods and instruments that other programs are using, and speak to other program directors about what they're actually doing. Query psychiatric programs around the country and other medical training programs at your own institution. Estimate the burden that such methods pose on administrative and faculty time, and select those that do the most with the least effort, to the degree that your sense of integrity isn't offended. With your faculty, be clear as to how much of this effort you're doing for yourselves, for the trainees, and to meet regulatory requirements. If it's primarily for the latter, there's a problem somewhere.

- If you're obliged to give formal exams of some sort, get questions from available question-banks and other sources, and don't waste time writing your own multiple-choice questions (unless what you're asking about is new or unique material).
- Observe your trainees interacting and working with patients and then discuss their actions and thoughts with them. These experiences offer irreplaceable opportunities for hands-on instruction, feedback, and the most meaningful levels of assessment.
- Ask trainees to self-assess. Help them by providing specific areas of knowledge and skills in which you'd like them to evaluate themselves.
- Bottom line: Do your best to avoid time-consuming and anxiety-provoking rituals, but make sincere efforts to know how your trainees are doing and to help them when progress isn't up to expected levels.

ADDITIONAL REFLECTIONS ON MEDICAL STUDENT EDUCATION

Among the many formidable challenges facing today's medical student educators, front and center are those of determining which key aspects of psychiatric knowledge and skills to present to students during increasingly brief periods of time (often reduced due to encroaching and competing demands of a family practice curriculum), and where and how to offer clinical training experiences.

Preclinical Teaching

The knowledge-base infrastructure medical students bring to clinical specialties such as family medicine and internal medicine is built upon premedical requirements for biology and chemistry and preclinical courses presented by medical schools' basic science departments (encompassing anatomy, histology–cell biology, immunology, infectious diseases, pathology, and so forth). By contrast, although neuroscience and neuropharmacology are included in the preclinical curriculum, behavioral sciences and psychopathology are not premedical requirements, and few medical schools host preclinical basic science departments focused on social, psychological, and behavioral matters. These realities continue to make a compelling case for strong representation of psychiatry and behavioral sciences in the preclinical curriculum. Basic concepts of psychology and psychopathology; family relationships; psychological development throughout the life span; coping responses to severe illness, injury, and other stressors; elements of physician–patient interactions; and cultural matters in health behaviors and health care are only some of the important background themes required by medical students about to encounter patients in clinical settings. Although behavioral scientists in departments other than psychiatry may contribute to this instruction, in my view departments of psychiatry ought to have a big seat at this table. Cross-matrixed curricula ought to become routine in undergraduate medical education, to ensure that key behavioral topics such as alcohol and substance use; eating behaviors and obesity; smoking; adherence to treatment; sexual behaviors; and responses by patients and families to serious threats, including bad news and terminal illnesses, are in fact covered adequately across departments and don't fall between the cracks. Wherever possible, high-quality video and interactive small-group sessions are needed to supplement lectures and reading.

A frequent problem facing preclinical psychiatric educators concerns pressures to fuse psychopathology and neuroscience courses. This can be done well for some subjects, in which certain psychiatric disorders have been illuminated by contemporary neuroscience findings. For these problems, students are usually excited by the "hard science" underpinning what we know about psychopathology and gain additional respect for clinical psychiatry as a result. However, for many important issues in psychopathology and neuroscience, the fields still go their separate ways, and attempting forced integrations on all fronts may not yet ring true.

Settings for Clinical Clerkships

To what extent should introductory clerkships be devoted to introducing the major serious psychiatric disorders—dramatic cases of schizophrenia, mania, melancholic depression, borderline personality disorder, and so forth—on the one hand, and covering other conditions likely to be encountered in nonpsychiatric practice—garden-variety ambulatory depression, anxiety and panic disorders, substance abuse, delirium, and early dementia—on the other? Although students should optimally learn as much as possible about all of these conditions, realistic trade-offs and balances must be struck.

What factors should determine local decision making? First, medical students on clerkships feel more involved, challenged, and useful when real work is expected of them as active members of a treatment team, when they sense that they're making a difference in the lives of the patients and actually helping treatment staff, not when they function as passive observers. Ordinarily, this means working side by side with residents and attendings (in some instances only with attendings) over time, as sidekicks and apprentices. Students usually do better when attached to residents than to attendings, since residents are better able to identify with trainees just a few years ahead of them, assuming that they're good residents. How can educators best use today's psychiatric inpatient services for medical student training when these settings serve primarily as psychiatric intensive care units for the sickest of the sick—chronic, treatment-intransigent cases that discourage attendings and residents alike? Second, students don't do too well when assigned to a fragmented multitude of clinical settings. Two is reasonable, three at most, if the third is very occasional.

This translates to lots of locally determined decisions based on the nature, quality, and quantity of "boots on the ground." Assignments must be made according to clinical services where good residents rotate, the strengths and weaknesses of the clinical services, and the location and availability of strong, highly cathected clinical teachers. Students paired up with residents can serve on teams in which they are expected to gather information from patients and families and be prepared to demonstrate their knowledge through case presentations in seminars, rounds, and long notes—to be "up" on their patients and their conditions, the ultimate in problem-based and case-based teaching, just as they are expected to do on internal medicine rotations. Concurrently, they benefit from "off ward" ambulatory experiences, particularly in urgent-care, emergency room, and possibly consultation-liaison services. To what extent can the pace of work in psychiatry emergency and urgent-care settings permit the luxury of assigning third-year students to conduct initial interviews under observation? How might psychiatric educators better investigate possible associations between clerkship assignments to general versus specialty units (e.g., units primarily serving only patients with chronic schizophrenia or geriatric psychiatry patients) and subsequent performance on standardized exams, feedback about the clerkships, and/or potential interest in psychiatry as a career choice?

Many clerkships lack resources to assign all students to ongoing contact with patients suffering from ambulatory depressions, anxiety disorders, substance abuse disorders, and other bread-and-butter psychiatric problems they're likely to encounter in general medical practice. Psychiatric educators may develop videotape libraries to cover common psychiatric problems not sufficiently encountered on the clerkships for use in small-group, problem-based seminars, analogous to the slide sets and film libraries of classic or rare cases often used in dermatology and radiology teaching. At the very least, we need curricula that provide the 95% of medical students who don't become psychiatrists with basic tools for screening and intervening with the "horses" (as opposed to "zebras") they're likely to face clinically. How do we ensure that *all* clinical clerks can recognize cognitive impairment and distinguish dementia from delirium? Recognize and treat mood and anxiety disorders and distinguish them from dementias and deliriums? Suspect and screen for substance abuse disorders, personality problems, psychoses, and domestic violence and other family problems? Psychiatric educators are often forced to delegate such exposure—in theory—to family practice and other primary care clerkships. But let's not kid ourselves—the extent to which students learn to assess and manage these disorders on nonpsychiatric rotations is, obviously, highly variable, often more a matter of lip service than reality. To manage such educational realities, some schools have created "cross cutting" education groups composed of all of the clerkship directors and charged with ensuring that such important topics as the "behavioral problems" of primary care, substance abuse, end-of-life care, pain, nutrition and obesity, and so forth are actually covered in the curriculum and don't fall between the cracks.

Finally, the fragmentation problem mentioned earlier is one of the primary reasons that efforts to integrate psychiatry with neurology or family practice clerkships have failed miserably in most places where they've been attempted. The impetus for such shotgun marriages has often been the desire of educational administrators to shoehorn more activities into briefer periods of time, in part to create the illusion that students who spend more weeks, nominally, in contact with each specialty actually engage in better-quality education in those fields. But students subjected to these jerry-rigged clerkship contraptions often complain about a lack of intensive patient involvement in *any* of the specialties. They often feel reduced to observer status. Students also cite lack of focus and poor integration on the part of the "teamed" departments and speak of being overwhelmed by having to simultaneously learn too many topics in too many areas. They often cope by narrowing their attention to the areas that most concern them and neglecting the others. My strong suggestion is to avoid or dismantle conjoint clerkships. However, getting some "airtime" to teach psychiatrically relevant aspects on other clerkships, such as family practice or internal medicine, where psychiatric consultation is integrated into the delivery of primary care, should be encouraged, in support of "one-stop shopping" models for primary care patients.

RECRUITING AND DEVELOPING ADEQUATE NUMBERS OF TEACHERS AND SUPERVISORS FOR MEDICAL STUDENTS

Increasing pressures on most academic faculty for "productivity" often decrease the time and enthusiasm they devote to medical student teaching. How can psychiatric educators more inventively find teaching resources for medical students? Psychiatric residents appropriately serve in a variety of instructional capacities but require tips and direction as to how to be better teachers, some of which are offered in *Psychiatric Residents as Teachers: A Practical Guide* (American Psychiatric Association Committee on Graduate Medical Education 2002). Small-group rather than one-on-one teaching for medical students is the rule rather than the exception. What aspects of psychiatric clerkships might lend themselves to teaching and learning in video labs and online training? How can educators better cultivate and incentivize volunteer faculty from the community and retired faculty members to teach medical students?

TO WHAT EXTENT SHOULD CLERKSHIPS ENCOURAGE STUDENTS TO LEARN ASPECTS OF PSYCHIATRY MOST PERTINENT TO THEIR LIKELY AREAS OF SPECIALIZATION?

Among students who have settled on non–primary care specialty choices by the time of their clinical clerkships, some see little relevance in psychiatry for their ultimate careers, particularly those headed for hospital-based fields such as pathology, radiology, and anesthesiology, and some surgical or medical subspecialties. Beyond the fact that all students should learn something about assessment of patients for the major psychiatric disorders, do all medical students really need to learn the same thing? With current resources, what's the best way to engage and assign students in ways that introduce them to aspects of psychiatry they're most likely to need to best serve their patients? Clerkships that build in psychiatric assignments around likely specialty choices via focused consultation-liaison experiences, targeted readings, short written assignments on psychiatric aspects of these specialties, or other innovations might not only engage these students but also ultimately improve the quality of care they will deliver.

RAISING THE STAKES IN ASSESSMENT

The presence of the new National Board of Medical Examiners (NBME) Step 2 CS (Clinical Skills) exam inevitably and increasingly obliges psychiatric educators to prepare students adequately to pass this hurdle. Some schools have traditionally put greater effort than others into preparing students for objective (or observed) structured clinical examinations (OSCEs). Psychiatric educators are likely to be key local players in organizing school-wide OSCE experiences as well as in developing material specific to psychiatry. Because this is a relatively new game, medical educators will need to plug into national activities through ADMSEP and regional medical school collaboratives, to benefit from materials developed elsewhere that may be accessible for pooled use, and to stay closely abreast of the specific types of OSCEs employed in the NBME examinations. Teach to an exam? God forbid. But the opportunity is here for ADMSEP to define core competencies for medical students in psychiatry and to build assessment tools—for example, using the RIME (reporter–interpreter–manager–educator) method of assessing specific abilities (Shea et al. 2004)—that may find general national acceptance and ultimately integrate with the NBME CS exams.

Parenthetically, the fact that the assessment–industrial complex, here in the form of the NBME, can so powerfully shape the content and methods of medical education bears note. This inescapable phenomenon should powerfully motivate educators to become part of the "system" in order to bring their realities, concerns, and political force to bear regarding decisions concerning national examination standards and requirements that will inevitably impact their lives and those of their students.

SUSTAINING ENTHUSIASM FOR MEDICAL STUDENT EDUCATION

Historically, medical student teaching often falls to psychiatric faculty early in their careers. As time goes on, interest in teaching medical students often wanes in favor of teaching residents and fellows. I guess I'm one of the lucky ones whose interest in medical students has, fortunately, been sustained throughout my career. First and foremost, I find teaching young and eager medical students, regardless of their ultimate career choices, to be great fun. I love to see their conceptual lightbulbs go on, to inspire those heading for nonpsychiatric careers, and to turn a few who'd never previously considered it in the direction of psychiatry. My paternal instincts are stimulated by these interactions (having two children who are now physicians hasn't hurt). Furthermore, several institutional structures at the medical schools at which I've taught reinforce the diversity of opportunities and the value of teaching medical students. If you're not too socially phobic, lectures are great opportunities to have reasonably attentive audiences—there are always at least a few rows of really interested students. My suggestion is to update lectures frequently, and to lecture on entirely new subjects every few years to avoid getting stale. My schools have also required a great deal of small-group, problem-based teaching, and here students, and their teachers, can really come alive in ways that reinforce the sense of being at a university. I've also had numerous opportunities to interact with students socially and to get to know them and their close relationships through ongoing individual and group mentoring opportunities, and as a research and scholarly mentor to many (since scholarly projects have been required of medical students both at UCLA and at UNM).

We maintain a psychiatric interest group—PIG—list of students identified by any faculty member or resident as showing some inclination toward the field. I regularly invite these students as well as students currently on the clerkship to a monthly evening "professional development seminar" we sponsor for residents and faculty at my home. The PDS, known as "dinner and a show," features faculty from our department or elsewhere in the university, or other interesting characters from the community, who engage in informal raconteuring for a few hours after ethnic food brought in from local restaurants. Students get to know our residents and faculty in this highly informal setting. Numerous medical students have developed attachments to the department through these events, and several fence-sitters have swung to careers in psychiatry.

Finally, it's been gratifying to see that our medical schools have now made preclinical medical student teaching, in addition to the usual contact on clerkships, mandatory for promotion in both the tenure and the clinician-educator tracks.

PAYING ATTENTION TO OUR SEED CORN—FOSTERING RESEARCH AND SCHOLARSHIP

As was recently underscored by a report from the Institute of Medicine, to remain vital, our profession will have to continue generating new knowledge and ideas, but recent trends suggest that inadequate numbers of today's psychiatrists are training for and being retained in careers devoted to patient-oriented research (Institute of Medicine 2003). This complex problem has multiple roots, including the recruitment of research-oriented students into medical school, the recruitment of research-oriented medical students into psychiatric careers, training and retaining residents in research, and retaining junior researchers in these roles. Numerous competing agendas are at play, including financial pressures on heavily indebted medical students; increasing percentages of female residents in psychiatry—whose childbearing clocks might compete with research training clocks and discourage some from extended periods of research training; and increasing percentages of international medical graduates in psychiatry, whose visa situations may not currently permit them to receive National Institute of Mental Health (NIMH) research training stipends or to easily remain in the United States following such training. Although substantial efforts are currently being mounted by academic leaders in collaboration with NIMH (Yager et al. 2004), each psychiatric educator and individual program ought to keep this national agenda in mind and to seek creative local ways to recruit, inspire, and foster trainees' nascent interests in furthering knowledge through research and scholarship.

FUNDING EDUCATION: WHO WILL PAY FOR IT ALL?

Who will pay? Why, your chair, of course. Maintaining adequate funding for postgraduate and medical student programs will continue to challenge the best financially savvy minds in the field while overwhelming the rest of us. Cutbacks in graduate medical education funding from the Health Care Financing Administration will continue to add to the overall financial pressures on departments. At the same time, increasing regulatory mandates regarding both graduate and undergraduate medical education, which sometimes seem to be inexorably growing and mutating, will continue to pressure academic departments faced with relentlessly squeezed financial streams. Mediating these forces, educators will be forced to clarify which of their multiple priorities are essential rather than discretionary, to juggle competing requirements, and to become politically adept at helping regulatory agencies such as the ACGME, its RRC, the Liaison Committee on Medical Education, and the NBME help local departments realistically contend with the multiple expectations and costs facing them. Imaginative solutions will be welcome everywhere.

PROFESSIONAL SATISFACTIONS OF PSYCHIATRIC EDUCATORS

How can psychiatric educators continue to deeply enjoy themselves in the process of helping trainees learn their stuff? Happily, several aspects of the educator's role dovetail closely with factors that foster professional satisfaction. We know that professional satisfaction correlates closely with keeping up with new knowledge and skills (lifelong learning); helping one's profession to grow through the creation of new knowledge (scholarship and research); helping one's profession to increase its benefits to patients, their families, and one's colleagues through political action and activity in one's professional organizations and by being part of a stimulating professional community (professional involvements); and doing what one can to improve one's work environment in small ways on a daily basis (being an all-around good person).

My own lifelong learning occurs around patients I see—when I consult or teach and encounter patients regarding whose problems I want to update, I immediately attack Google and Entrez Med/PubMed. I also learn a lot from my residents and colleagues, one of the deep benefits of academic citizenship. I try to at least read the abstracts in the various general psychiatry, specialty area, and general medical journals that flood our home, and to more seriously peruse articles of particular relevance. Because one of the deep pleasures in psychiatry concerns keeping up broadly, I read (or at least regularly skim) *Science, Science News, The New York Review of Books, The New York Times Book Review, The New Yorker* (can you tell I'm from New York?), *Atlantic Monthly, Utne Reader,* and *Wired,* because I'm impressed at how much of central importance for psychiatric understanding comes from other fields.

Finally, at the end of the day, professional satisfaction may be judged by one's ability to pass the "mirror test"—that is, to be able to look at yourself in the mirror and feel that you've been doing your best to make decent contributions in these areas (Gardner et al. 2001). Most psychiatric educators' daily activities are—and will continue to be—on track to permit them to get high marks on the mirror test, an excellent form of assessment. Perhaps that's *our* way of teaching to the exam.

REFERENCES

American Psychiatric Association: Diagnostic and Statistical Manual of Mental Disorders, Third Edition. Washington, DC, American Psychiatric Association, 1980

American Psychiatric Association: Diagnostic and Statistical Manual of Mental Disorders, Third Edition, Revised. Washington, DC, American Psychiatric Association, 1987

American Psychiatric Association: Diagnostic and Statistical Manual of Mental Disorders, Fourth Edition. Washington, DC, American Psychiatric Association, 1994

American Psychiatric Association: Diagnostic and Statistical Manual of Mental Disorders, Fourth Edition, Text Revision. Washington, DC, American Psychiatric Association, 2000

American Psychiatric Association Committee on Graduate Medical Education: Psychiatric Residents as Teachers: A Practical Guide, 2nd Revision. Washington, DC, American Psychiatric Association, 2002 (also available at: http://www.psych.org/edu/res_fellows/psychresidentguide.pdf)

Anguelova M, Benkelfat C, Turecki G: A systematic review of association studies investigating genes coding for serotonin receptors and the serotonin transporter, II: suicidal behavior. Mol Psychiatry 8:646–653, 2003

Arbelle S, Benjamin J, Golin M, et al: Relation of shyness in grade school children to the genotype for the long form of the serotonin transporter promoter region polymorphism. Am J Psychiatry 160:671–676, 2003

Armor DJ, Klerman GL: Psychiatric treatment orientations and professional ideology. J Health Soc Behav 9:243–255, 1968

Barrett TB, Hauger RL, Kennedy JL, et al: Evidence that a single nucleotide polymorphism in the promoter of the G protein receptor kinase 3 gene is associated with bipolar disorder. Mol Psychiatry 8:546–557, 2003

Berne E: Transactional Analysis in Psychotherapy. New York, Grove, 1961

Berne E: Games People Play: The Basic Handbook of Transactional Analysis. New York, Ballantine, 1996

Branson R, Potoczna N, Kral JG, et al: Binge eating as a major phenotype of melanocortin 4 receptor gene mutations. N Engl J Med 348:1096–1103, 2003

Caspi A, Sugden K, Moffitt TE, et al: Influence of life stress on depression: moderation by a polymorphism in the 5-HTT gene. Science 301:386–389, 2003

Cook IA, Leuchter AF, Morgan M, et al: Early changes in prefrontal activity characterize clinical responders to antidepressants. Neuropsychopharmacology 27:120–131, 2002

Corrigan PW, Steiner L, McCracken SG, et al: Strategies for disseminating evidence-based practices to staff who treat people with serious mental illness. Psychiatr Serv 52:1598–1606, 2001

Crews FC: The Memory Wars: Freud's Legacy in Dispute. New York, New York Review of Books, 1995

Damascio AR: Descartes' Error: Emotion, Reason and the Human Brain. New York, HarperCollins, 1994

Damascio AR: The Feeling of What Happens: Body and Emotion in the Making of Consciousness. New York, Harcourt, 1999

Drucker P: Management: Tasks, Responsibilities, Practices, Reprint Edition. New York, HarperBusiness, 1993

Edelman GM: Bright Air, Brilliant Fire: On the Matter of the Mind. New York, Basic Books, 1992

Edelman GM, Tononi G: A Universe of Consciousness: How Matter Becomes Imagination. New York, Basic Books, 2000

Erikson EH: Childhood and Society. New York, WW Norton, 1980

Flavill JH, Miller PA, Miller SA: Cognitive Development, 4th Edition. Saddleback, NJ, Prentice-Hall, 2001

Gardner H, Csikszentmihalyi M, Damon W: Good Work: When Excellence and Ethics Meet. New York, Basic Books, 2001

Grünbaum A: Foundations of Psychoanalysis: A Philosophical Critique. Berkeley, CA, University of California Press, 1984

Helzer JE, Hudziak JJ (eds): Defining Psychopathology in the 21st Century: DSM-V and Beyond (American Psychopathological Association Series). Washington, DC, American Psychiatric Publishing, 2002

Horowitz MJ: Cognitive Psychodynamics: From Conflict to Character. New York, Wiley, 1998

Huang MP, Alessi NE: Digital motion phenomenology of depression. Stud Health Technol Inform 81:30–37, 2001

Institute of Medicine: Research Training in Psychiatry Residency: Strategies for Reform. Washington, DC, National Academies Press, 2003

Jaques E: Requisite Organization: A Total System for Effective Managerial Organization and Managerial Leadership for the 21st Century: Amended, 2nd Edition. Gloucester, MA, Cason Hall, 1998

Johnson S: Emergence: The Connected Lives of Ants, Brains, Cities and Software. New York, Touchstone, 2001

Kanfer FH, Goldstein AP: Helping People Change, 4th Edition (New York, Pergamon Series). Saddle River, NJ, Allyn & Bacon, 1991

Karasu TB: The advanced practice of psychotherapy. Harv Rev Psychiatry 9:118–123, 2001

Kauffman S: At Home in the Universe: The Search for Laws of Self-Organization and Complexity. New York, Oxford University Press, 1995

Kendler KS, Kuhn J, Prescott CA: The interrelationship of neuroticism, sex, and stressful life events in the prediction of episodes of major depression. Am J Psychiatry 161:631–636, 2004

Kosko B: Fuzzy Thinking: The New Science of Fuzzy Logic. New York, Hyperion, 1993

Kupfer DJ, First MB, Regier DA (eds): A Research Agenda for DSM-V. Washington, DC, American Psychiatric Association, 2002

Lambert M (ed): Bergin and Garfield's Handbook of Psychotherapy and Behavior Change, 5th Edition. Hoboken, NJ, Wiley, 2004

Leuchter AF, Morgan M, Cook IA, et al: Pretreatment neurophysiological and clinical characteristics of placebo responders in treatment trials for major depression. Psychopharmacology (Berl) 177:15–22, 2004

Levinson DJ: The Seasons of a Man's Life. New York, Ballantine, 1978

Malhotra AK, Murphy GM Jr, Kennedy JL: Pharmacogenetics of psychotropic drug response. Am J Psychiatry 161:780–796, 2004

Martijn JS, van der Mast CA, Merel K, et al: Exploratory design and evaluation of a user interface for virtual reality exposure therapy. Stud Health Technol Inform 85:468–474, 2002

Maslow A: Motivation and Personality, 3rd Edition. New York, HarperCollins, 1987

McGuire MT, Troisi A: Darwinian Psychiatry. New York, Oxford University Press, 1998

Millon T: Masters of the Mind: Exploring the Story of Mental Illness From Ancient Times to the New Millennium. Hoboken, NJ, Wiley, 2004

Modai I, Kuperman J, Goldberg I, et al: Fuzzy logic detection of medically serious suicide attempt records in major psychiatric disorders. J Nerv Ment Dis 192:708–710, 2004

Mohl PC, Lomax J, Tasman A, et al: Psychotherapy training for the psychiatrist of the future. Am J Psychiatry 147:7–13, 1990

Nichols MP, Schwartz RC: Family Therapy. Saddle River, NJ, Allyn & Bacon, 2003

Osland JS, Kolb DA, Rubin IM: The Organizational Behavior Reader, 7th Edition. New York, Prentice-Hall, 2000

Parker G, Roy K, Eyers K: Cognitive behavior therapy for depression? Choose horses for courses. Am J Psychiatry 160:825–834, 2003

Paul AM: The Cult of Personality: How Personality Tests Are Leading Us to Miseducate Our Children, Mismanage Our Companies, and Misunderstand Ourselves. New York, Free Press, 2004

Pew Health Professions Commission: Critical Challenges: Revitalizing the Health Professions for the Twenty-First Century. San Francisco, University of California, San Francisco, Center for the Health Professions, 1995

Plomin R, McGuffin P: Psychopathology in the postgenomic era. Annu Rev Psychol 54:205–228, 2003

Postman N, Weingartner C: Teaching as a Subversive Activity. New York, Delta Books, 1969

Pratkanis A, Aronson E: The Age of Propaganda: The Everyday Use and Abuse of Persuasion, Revised Edition. New York, WH Freeman, 2001

Reynolds GP, Zhang Z, Zhang X: Polymorphism of the promoter region of the serotonin 5-HT(2C) receptor gene and clozapine-induced weight gain. Am J Psychiatry 160:677–679, 2003

Rogoff B: The Cultural Nature of Human Development. New York, Oxford University Press, 2003

Schore AN: Affect Regulation and the Origin of the Self: The Neurobiology of Emotional Development. Hillsdale, NJ, Lawrence Erlbaum, 1994

Schore AN: Affect Dysregulation and Disorders of the Self. New York, WW Norton, 2003

Shea JA, Arnold L, Mann KV: A RIME perspective on the quality and relevance of current and future medical education research. Acad Med 79:931–938, 2004

Snider LA, Swedo SE: PANDAS: current status and directions for research. Mol Psychiatry 9:900–907, 2004

Stevens A, Price J: Evolutionary Psychiatry: A New Beginning, 2nd Edition. Philadelphia, PA, Taylor & Francis, 2000

Summers BG, Tracy JS: Competency Assessment: A Practical Guide to the JCAHO Standards, 2nd Edition. Marblehead, MA, HCPro Opus Communications, 2001

Von Holzen R: The emergence of a learning society. The Futurist 39 (January–February):24–25, 2005

White JR, Freeman AS (eds): Cognitive-Behavioral Group Therapy for Specific Problems and Populations. Washington, DC, American Psychological Association, 2000

Wilkes MS, Hoffman JR: An innovative approach to educating medical students about pharmaceutical promotion. Acad Med 76:1271–1277, 2001

Williamson JW, German PS, Weiss R, et al: Health science information management and continuing education of physicians. A survey of US primary care practitioners and their opinion leaders. Ann Intern Med 110:151–160, 1989

Wood JM, Nezworski MT, Lilienfeld SO, et al: What's Wrong With the Rorschach? Science Confronts the Controversial Inkblot Test. San Francisco, CA, Jossey-Bass, 2003

Wright D: The Ultimate Guide to Competency Assessment in Health Care, 2nd Edition. Eau Claire, WI, PESI Healthcare LLC, 1998

Wright R: The Moral Animal: Why We Are the Way We Are: The New Science of Evolutionary Psychology. New York, Vintage, 1995

Yager J, Kay J: Assessing psychotherapy competence in psychiatric residents: getting real. Harv Rev Psychiatry 11:109–112, 2003

Yager J, Greden J, Abrams MT, et al: The Institute of Medicine's Report on Research Training in Psychiatry Residency: strategies for reform—background, results, and follow-up. Acad Psychiatry 28:267–284, 2004

Yalom ID: Theory and Practice of Group Psychotherapy, 4th Edition. New York, Basic Books, 1995

Yin TK, Chiu NT: A computer-aided diagnosis for distinguishing Tourette's syndrome from chronic tic disorder in children by a fuzzy system with a two-step minimization approach. IEEE Trans Biomed Eng 51:1286–1295, 2004

INDEX

*Page numbers printed in **boldface** type refer to tables or figures.*

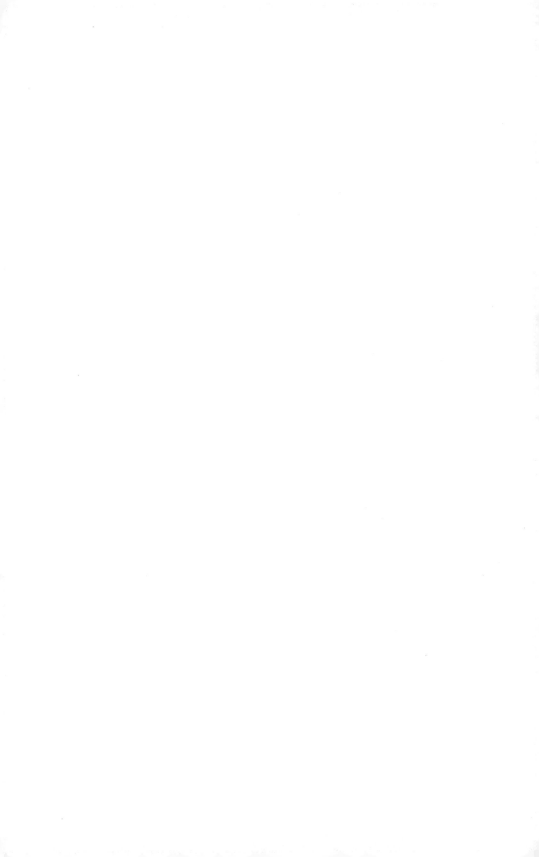